Mental Health in Historical Perspective

Series Editors
Catharine Coleborne
School of Humanities and Social Science
University of Newcastle
Callaghan, Australia

Matthew Smith
History of Psychiatry
University of Strathclyde
Glasgow, United Kingdom

Covering all historical periods and geographical contexts, the series explores how mental illness has been understood, experienced, diagnosed, treated and contested. It will publish works that engage actively with contemporary debates related to mental health and, as such, will be of interest not only to historians, but also mental health professionals, patients and policy makers. With its focus on mental health, rather than just psychiatry, the series will endeavour to provide more patient-centred histories. Although this has long been an aim of health historians, it has not been realised, and this series aims to change that.

The scope of the series is kept as broad as possible to attract good quality proposals about all aspects of the history of mental health from all periods. The series emphasises interdisciplinary approaches to the field of study, and encourages short titles, longer works, collections, and titles which stretch the boundaries of academic publishing in new ways.

More information about this series at
http://www.springer.com/series/14806

Claire Hilton

Improving Psychiatric Care for Older People

Barbara Robb's Campaign 1965–1975

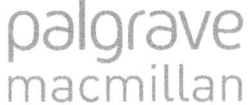

Claire Hilton
Institute of Contemporary British History and Institute of Psychiatry,
  Psychology and Neuroscience
King's College London
London, United Kingdom

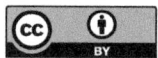

Mental Health in Historical Perspective
ISBN 978-3-319-54812-8   ISBN 978-3-319-54813-5 (eBook)
DOI 10.1007/978-3-319-54813-5

Library of Congress Control Number: 2017940474

© The Editor(s) (if applicable) and The Author(s) 2017. This book is an open access publication.
Open Access This book is licensed under the terms of the Creative Commons Attribution 4.0 International License (http://creativecommons.org/licenses/by/4.0/), which permits use, sharing, adaptation, distribution and reproduction in any medium or format, as long as you give appropriate credit to the original author(s) and the source, provide a link to the Creative Commons license and indicate if changes were made.
The images or other third party material in this book are included in the book's Creative Commons license, unless indicated otherwise in a credit line to the material. If material is not included in the book's Creative Commons license and your intended use is not permitted by statutory regulation or exceeds the permitted use, you will need to obtain permission directly from the copyright holder.
The use of general descriptive names, registered names, trademarks, service marks, etc. in this publication does not imply, even in the absence of a specific statement, that such names are exempt from the relevant protective laws and regulations and therefore free for general use.
The publisher, the authors and the editors are safe to assume that the advice and information in this book are believed to be true and accurate at the date of publication. Neither the publisher nor the authors or the editors give a warranty, express or implied, with respect to the material contained herein or for any errors or omissions that may have been made. The publisher remains neutral with regard to jurisdictional claims in published maps and institutional affiliations.

Cover illustration © David Bleeker - London / Alamy Stock Photo; all rights reserved, used with permission.

Printed on acid-free paper

This Palgrave Macmillan imprint is published by Springer Nature
The registered company is Springer International Publishing AG
The registered company address is: Gewerbestrasse 11, 6330 Cham, Switzerland

To Samuel, Jacob and Benjamin and their friends who are trying to make the world a better place.

Foreword

My beloved grandmother died frail and confused in an overcrowded long-stay ward in a decrepit Victorian National Health Service hospital. There were so many beds in the ward there was barely room to stand between them. Nurses were seemingly indifferent towards their impossible task. In 1968 I was a bewildered and angry medical student with no idea how to voice my concerns at her evident distress and the lack of personal care. My parents too were troubled by the poor conditions, my grandmother's unkempt appearance, the meals left untouched and out of her reach, the terrible ward stench. They never made a formal complaint, hardly knew where to begin, and in any case my grandmother died soon after admission. I have no doubt that this experience was one of the triggers for my choice of career in the psychiatry of old age. I did not know then that there was a battle in progress in the late 1960s and early 1970s between those who grasped how widespread was the poor care of older people in the National Health Service and were determined to improve it and those lined up against them, the forces of denial inside the service, who really believed there was not much wrong and in any case thought there was nothing to be done about any shortcomings given the resourcing and public ignorance. At the vanguard of the battlefront was one remarkable woman, Barbara Robb, who published *Sans Everything: A Case to Answer* in 1967, a searing indictment of the conditions for older people in long-stay hospital wards, initiated by her own observations of the care of one of her psychotherapy patients.

In this book, Claire Hilton has set out the campaign waged by this one inimitable woman, her organisation Aid for the Elderly in Government

Institutions (AEGIS) and the long struggles to convince the Ministry and its constituent Regional Hospital Boards that the truth was as she described it and to get them to accept that change was necessary. There could be no better qualified person to document this enlightening story than Claire Hilton. Claire is a dedicated, talented clinician, a psychiatrist working with older people, who has for some years immersed herself in the history of the development of the specialty of old age psychiatry in the twentieth century. She has illuminated the period by bringing together the characters and politics of the influential clinical professionals, policy makers, public health observers, press and government funders. In this new work, Claire has drawn on her profound understanding of the period and, through further scrupulously detailed research, has exposed a story that has wider implications, showing how policy makers can be easily misled by misinformation when the truth is unpalatable. But what she has also given us here is a cracking good read, a compelling story of one woman's battle tragically cut short by Robb's too early death in 1976.

The fact is that the scandals have continued in National Health Service hospitals, but more often today in the myriad of independent-sector nursing and care homes that now provide the majority of long-term care for those institutionalised at the end of their lives. Scandals are no longer swept under the carpet, rather under many small rugs, as psychiatrist Klaus Bergmann so memorably put it and quoted by Claire in her disturbing final analysis of what has changed for the better and how much still needs to be done. In spite of the cautionary finale, this is an uplifting story, and anyone who is interested in how to campaign on a social issue will learn some invaluable lessons from this splendid book.

Elaine Murphy,
Baroness Murphy of Aldgate

Preface

In 1967, *Sans Everything: A Case to Answer*, was a best seller, a remarkable achievement for a nonfiction book about the unappealing subject of the poor care of older people in English psychiatric hospitals. The title and scandalous content remained familiar over the years, particularly to old age psychiatrists and others who aimed to provide high-quality mental health services for older people. None of them, however, could tell me anything about its author, Barbara Robb, although at the time she wrote, she was quite a celebrity, achieving both fame and notoriety. Cabinet Minister Richard Crossman wrote in his diary that she was a 'terrible danger' to the government, and a 'bomb' who had to be defused. With such an accolade, somewhere there had to be a story.

I first read *Sans Everything* in about 2006 after my husband bought it for me as a birthday present. The contents were gruesome, and like other readers, I focused on them, paying little attention to the chapters providing direction about how to improve care. Breathing a sigh of relief, I reassured myself that things aren't nearly so bad today.

While undertaking related historical research, the names of several *Sans Everything* contributors came to light. Who were they? How did Barbara get them to write for her? Who were the people and places behind the pseudonyms? Who was 'Miss Wills' who Barbara rescued from 'Cossett Hospital'? Who was Barbara? How did she get involved with the psychiatric hospitals, and what else did she do? These and other questions aroused my curiosity.

There are many reasons Barbara Robb was forgotten. She fought to improve provision for institutionalised older people and not for personal acclaim. She was a thorn in the side of the National Health Service leadership who did not want to remember her, and both she and her husband, Brian, died prematurely. Half a century since publication of *Sans Everything*, it is time to reconsider the story behind it and its messages, much of which remains relevant to the care of unwell and frail older people today. Perhaps my sigh of relief was only partly justified.

Acknowledgements

Investigating Barbara Robb and *Sans Everything* was exhilarating, delving into archives and meeting many people who helped and offered much encouragement. Barbara's family were enthusiastic. Her cousin William Charlton and his wife, Anne, welcomed me to their home in Northumberland, and her great-niece Anna Charlton showed me round Hesleyside Hall. Barbara's niece Elizabeth Ellison-Anne lent me Barbara's photograph album depicting the years 1937–1941, and she, with friends Cynthia Bressani, John Gilliver and Colin Bowes, showed me round the family home, Burghwallis Hall, and the adjoining church. Sister Deirdre McCormack showed me round St Peter's Residence, and Constanza Isaza Martínez and Andrés Pantoja allowed me to wander round their home, the cottage where Barbara and Brian lived for many years. Charles and Robin Daniel, whose mother, Joyce, spoke out for more humane hospital provision in Cornwall, told me about her in the cottage where she lived. David Cochrane gave valuable advice at the beginning of the project, and Margaret Shepherd NDS, explained aspects of Roman Catholic practice. Other people told me about Barbara's life and times and provided archives and photographs: they are acknowledged in the endnotes. Anna Towlson, archivist at London School of Economics, was always helpful with my visits to, and queries about, Barbara's extensive archive. Many other archivists and librarians answered questions, retrieved documents and assisted with the project. Numerous historians offered constructive advice, including Tim Hurley, Michael Kandiah, Chris Knowles, Michael Passmore, Mary Salinsky, Sally Sheard, Kathleen Sherit, Mari Takayanagi and Pat Thane.

Tom Arie and David Jolley, my esteemed colleagues in old age psychiatry, read and commented on every chapter with great tact and patience. My husband, Michael, and sons, Samuel, Jacob and Benjamin, all guided me through computer hitches and accompanied me on visits to former psychiatric hospitals. Benjamin also gave advice on logical fallacies in the *Sans Everything* inquiries. Michael has been endlessly patient with the time spent on this project and has enjoyed our visits to people, places and archives from Cornwall to Northumberland.

I am indebted to the Wellcome Trust for funding this study during an eight-month sabbatical from clinical work as an old age psychiatrist. I am also grateful to Central and North West London NHS Foundation Trust for allowing me to take time off and to Lynis Lewis and North Central London Research Network for help with administrative matters.

My link to Palgrave Macmillan began with a chance meeting with historian John Stewart at a conference at the Wellcome Trust. He introduced me to Matthew Smith and Catharine Coleborne, academic editors of the series *Mental Health in Historical Perspective*. They were endlessly enthusiastic and guided me through many stages towards publication. I'm also grateful to Vicky Long who reviewed the manuscript and whose comments helped shape the book, and to Palgrave's editors, Molly Beck, Oliver Dyer and Sundar Ananthapadmanabhan, who were a pleasure to work with.

This list of helpers, encouragers and friends is not exhaustive, and I apologise to anyone missed out who thinks they should have been included. To them too I am most grateful.

Contents

1 Introduction: A Strange Eventful History   1

2 Psychiatric Hospitals and Older People: Status Quo or Making Changes?   19

3 Barbara Robb, Amy Gibbs and the 'Diary of a Nobody'   57

4 Establishing AEGIS and Writing *Sans Everything*: 'The Case' and 'Some Answers'   97

5 Reprinted Before Publication: Plotting a Route for *Sans Everything*   143

6 The Inquiries: A Lion's Den   173

7 Whitewash and After: 'Most Good Is Done by Stealth'   201

8 Then and Now: Concluding Remarks   251

Index   271

Abbreviations

AEGIS	Aid for the Elderly in Government Institutions
BBC	British Broadcasting Corporation
BGS	British Geriatrics Society
BLSA	British Library Sound Archives
BMA	British Medical Association
BMJ	*British Medical Journal*
COHSE	Confederation of Health Service Employees
CoT	Council on Tribunals
CPAG	Child Poverty Action Group
DGH	District General Hospital
DHSS	Department of Health and Social Security
ECT	Electroconvulsive therapy
GNC	General Nursing Council
GP	General Practitioner
HAC	Hampstead Artists Council
HAS	Hospital [later Health] Advisory Service
HC	House of Commons
HL	House of Lords
HMC	Hospital Management Committee
HMSO	Her Majesty's Stationery Office
IPSO	Independent Press Standards Organisation
JCC	Joint Consultants' Committee [of the BMA]
LMA	London Metropolitan Archives
LSE	London School of Economics
MHA	Mental Health Act
MoH	Ministry of Health
MP	Member of Parliament
NAMH	National Association for Mental Health [later MIND]

NHS	National Health Service
NSGHMC	New Southgate Group Hospital Management Committee
NWMRHB	North West Metropolitan Regional Hospital Board
OED	*Oxford English Dictionary*
OUP	Oxford University Press
PA	Patients Association
PEP	Post-Ely Working Party
PhD	Doctor of Philosophy
PHSO	Parliamentary and Health Service Ombudsman
QC	Queen's Counsel
RAF	Royal Air Force
RCN	Royal College of Nursing
RCPsych	Royal College of Psychiatrists
RHB	Regional Hospital Board
SWMRHB	South West Metropolitan Regional Hospital Board
SWRHB	South Western Regional Hospital Board
TNA	The National Archives
TSO	The Stationery Office
UWMRC	University of Warwick Modern Records Centre
WHB	Welsh Hospital Board
WHO	World Health Organisation
WYAS	West Yorkshire Archives Service

List of Figures

Fig. 2.1	Friern Hospital, 1957	40
Fig. 3.1	Burghwallis Hall, c.1941	59
Fig. 3.2	Barbara and her grandfather, Ernest Charlton Anne, c.1922	60
Fig. 3.3	Barbara and her brother Robert, winter 1940–1941	62
Fig. 3.4	Amy Gibbs creating a foil collage, 1961	67
Fig. 3.5	Foil collage by Amy Gibbs	68
Fig. 3.6	Service in the chapel, St Peter's, 1960s	73
Fig. 3.7	Nun feeding turkeys in the grounds, St Peter's, 1966	74
Fig. 3.8	Party on the women's ward, St Peter's, late 1960s	75
Fig. 4.1	Memorial to victims of Colney Hatch Asylum fire, New Southgate Cemetery, 1903	105
Fig. 4.2	Joyce Daniel, c.1964	117
Fig. 4.3	Russell Barton's invitation to Barbara, for dinner at Claridge's, September 1967	125
Fig. 7.1	Officials inspect a men's ward at Ely Hospital, 1969	216
Fig. 8.1	Barbara and Brian Robb, c.1972	255
Fig. 8.2	'Older women, djinns and beds' by Laura Lehman, 2016	260
Fig. 8.3	Barbara in the driving seat, 1928	261
Fig. 8.4	'Ursula' by Brian Robb, 1976	262

LIST OF TABLES

Table 4.1   The *Sans Everything* witnesses   116

Dramatis Personae

People most closely concerned with the narrative of Barbara Robb and the AEGIS campaign and those who played a part at several stages in the story:

Academics and government advisors
    Brian Abel-Smith
    Peter Townsend
Barbara Robb's family
    Ernest Charlton Anne, grandfather
    Ernestine 'Missie' Anne, aunt
    William Charlton, cousin
    Brian Robb, husband; an artist
Campaigners and supporters
    Mary Applebey, general secretary of NAMH
    Mabel Franks, an admirer from Leeds
    Audrey Harvey, Barbara's neighbour and social rights campaigner
    Helen Hodgson, founder of the Patients Association
    Lord Strabolgi
Chairmen of committees of inquiry
    First Friern Inquiry 1965
        Ann Blofeld
    Sans Everything inquiries
        Douglas Lowe, Friern
        George Polson, St Lawrence's
    Ely Inquiry
        Geoffrey Howe

Doctors
- Psychiatrists and psychogeriatricians
    - Tom Arie
    - Alex Baker, director of the Hospital Advisory Service, 1969–1974
    - Russell Barton
    - Klaus Bergmann
    - Garry Blessed
    - M David Enoch
    - Bertram Mandelbrote
    - Brice Pitt
    - Ronald 'Sam' Robinson
    - J Anthony 'Tony' Whitehead
- Other doctors
    - Malcolm Campbell, Friern Hospital, 1964–1965
    - Lionel Cosin, geriatrician
    - Geoffrey Tooth, Principal Medical Officer, Ministry of Health

Friern 'Cossett' Hospital staff, pseudonyms
- Dr Aix, consultant psychiatrist
- Miss Cloake, social worker
- Dr Giddie, ward doctor

Journalists and editors
- Anne Allen, *Sunday Mirror*
- Yvonne Cross, *Nursing Mirror*
- Anne Robinson, *Sunday Times*
- CH Rolph (Bill Hewitt), *New Statesman*
- David Roxan, *News of the World*
- Ann Shearer, *Guardian*
- Hugo Young, *Sunday Times*

RHB chairman
- Maurice Hackett, North West Metropolitan
- Isabel Graham Bryce, Oxford

Nurses in senior roles who supported AEGIS
- Keith Newstead
- WJA 'Bill' Kirkpatrick
- Doreen Norton
- Phyllis Rowe, deputy president of the RCN

Psychotherapists
    Carl Jung
    Victor White
Politicians and civil servants
    Minister of Health
        Kenneth Robinson, 1964–1968
    Secretaries of State for Social Services
        Richard Crossman, 1968–1970
        Keith Joseph, 1970–1974
        Barbara Castle, 1974–1976
    Others
        Beatrice Serota, Minister of State for Health, 1968–1970
        Arnold France, Permanent Secretary, Ministry of Health, 1964–1968
Patients, their relatives and friends
    Eric Buss, friend of Amy Gibbs
    Mrs Dickens, sister of Bob, a patient at Friern Hospital
    Amy Gibbs, 'Miss Wills', a patient at Friern Hospital
Whistle-blowers
    Sans Everything author-witnesses and their pseudonyms

Jean Biss,	Laura Heneage
Dorothy Crofts,	Elizabeth Tasburg
Joyce Daniel,	Adeline Craythorne
James Davie,	Frederick Isham
Dennis Moodie,	Michael Osbaldeston
Roger Moody	
Eileen Porter,	Emily Swinburne
Susan Skrine,	Louisa Fenton

    Ely Hospital
        Michael Pantelides

CHAPTER 1

Introduction: A Strange Eventful History

> *Last scene of all,*
> *That ends this **strange eventful history***
> *Is second childishness and mere oblivion;*
> *Sans teeth, sans eyes, sans taste, **sans everything**.*
>
> William Shakespeare, As You Like It (Act II, scene vii)

On 21 January 1965 Barbara Robb visited an elderly acquaintance, Amy Gibbs, an in-patient on a long-stay back ward at Friern psychiatric hospital, North London. There, she stepped into the murky, longstanding and hardly shifting territory of older people's institutional care. Shocked by what she saw, such as harshness from nurses and the patients' uniform haircuts, institutional clothing and lack of personal possessions and occupation, Barbara began a diary of her visits because 'I felt that I would never have another really easy moment unless I did everything I could to try to right this situation' (Allen 1967). Within months she established AEGIS, Aid for the Elderly in Government Institutions, which became one of the country's most determined pressure groups (Robinson 1970). Barbara Robb resembled earlier well-known women campaigners, such as Elizabeth Fry (1780–1845) the prison reformer, and Florence Nightingale (1820–1910) who professionalised nursing. All three women were appalled by the inhumanity they witnessed in institutions and set their minds to eliminating it. They were upper-class women of independent means with strong religious inspiration for their work. They all dedicated years to achieving improvements.

This study primarily concerns the back wards of National Health Service (NHS) psychiatric hospitals in England. These wards mainly housed people over sixty-five years of age alongside some younger people with chronic mental illness. Psychiatric hospitals were only one part of the health and welfare services used by older people, but care provided in them was particularly problematic. Patients, their families and hospital staff, all had low expectations of improvement or discharge. Staff showed little interest in older people who often received no clear psychiatric diagnosis, treatment or rehabilitation, unlike younger people in the same hospital (Martin 1962). Many staff could not 'formulate a "psychogeriatric" problem in any other terms but as the need to get it instantly off their hands' (Arie 1973, p. 541). The patients did not benefit from the expertise of geriatricians, the doctors who specialised in older people's physical healthcare. Geriatricians aimed to diagnose illness accurately and provide treatment to improve health, well-being and function, but they worked mainly in general hospitals and hardly entered psychiatric hospitals (Denham 2004, p. 357). In hospitals without geriatricians, older people were particularly at risk of poor-quality care associated with negative, ageist stereotypes, which assumed they were all afflicted with irreversible chronic illness that would result in inevitable and hopeless decline.

AEGIS's book, *Sans Everything: A Case to Answer* (Robb 1967), described scandalous inhumane and inadequate care in long-stay wards. The wards were overcrowded and understaffed. Undignified and unkind practices included teasing, hitting and swearing at patients. In many hospitals, there was no privacy for personal care, and bedtime could be as early as 5 P.M. *Sans Everything* revealed deficits and proposed remedies, including specialist psychiatric services to treat and rehabilitate mentally unwell older people to prevent admission and enable discharge, and housing schemes on surplus land around psychiatric hospitals to generate income to help pay for the services. It also recommended a hospital ombudsman, an inspectorate to monitor and ensure high standards, and better NHS complaints procedures.

Throughout AEGIS's campaign, NHS staff, patients and their relatives, the media and the wider public responded in a diversity of ways. These ranged from acknowledgement of the allegations of bad practice, such as by the press, to rejection, particularly in higher tiers of NHS administration. AEGIS struggled to convince the Ministry of Health and the Regional Hospital Boards (RHBs) about the happenings in the hospitals that they oversaw.

This study argues that Barbara Robb, AEGIS and *Sans Everything* had a far greater role than previously recognised in influencing improvements in services. *Sans Everything* was controversial, and the Ministry of Health discredited it, which obscured its centrality. However, Richard Crossman, Secretary of State for Social Services (1968–1970), and Brian Abel-Smith, Professor of Social Administration at the London School of Economics (LSE) who had a long-term interest in the NHS, regarded AEGIS as a powerful influence on NHS policy and development (Crossman 1977, p. 727; Abel-Smith 1990, p. 259). Alternative views include those in Robin Means and Randall Smith's (1985) study about welfare services for older people, which emphasised the government's role in making improvements, rather than pressure from AEGIS to ensure that it acted. Charles Webster (1998, p. 119), official historian of the NHS, regarded the Ely Hospital Inquiry as pivotal for stimulating change, rather than the events that preceded and followed it, which Barbara steered, often behind the scenes.

The primary aim of this book is to tell the story of AEGIS, *Sans Everything* and the campaign to improve older people's care. Barbara intended to do this herself, but time did not permit it.[1] Little is known of the people and events behind the allegations described in *Sans Everything*, who made them and what inspired them to do so. Published sources reveal merely summaries of the official inquiries into the allegations, the shortest being one and a half pages (Ministry of Health (MoH) 1968, pp. 82–83). These reports only glimpse at the inquiry processes, their findings and recommendations stemming from them. Barbara's tenacity to the cause was remarkable: every defeat or success increased her resolve to achieve her aims, yet little is known of her background and personality, and the support mechanisms that enabled her to do so. She organised AEGIS from her cottage home and was constantly at the helm. AEGIS's story is thus inextricably interwoven with her life. When Barbara died in 1976 at age sixty-four, AEGIS died with her. However, by then the government had initiated many of the *Sans Everything* proposals, and other campaigners, such as the Group for the Psychiatry of Old Age at the Royal College of Psychiatrists, adopted some of AEGIS's longer-term objectives (Hilton 2016b).

This book also has a secondary aim: to explore whether issues raised by AEGIS have lessons for today, because many of its themes ring true fifty years on. It aims to give insights into the reasons for repeated deficits in provision and inform current debate concerning older people's health and social care. Recent scandals have included *Care and Compassion?* (Health

Service Ombudsman 2011), the Mid Staffordshire Inquiry (2013), *Orchid View Serious Case Review* (West Sussex 2014), and the BBC Panorama documentary *Behind Closed Doors* (2014). Analysis of: how, why and by whom abuse and neglect took place in the 1960s; the recommendations made to remedy the situations; and what was (and was not) achieved, may contribute to understanding the mechanisms behind abuse in institutions and hence the steps that can be taken to prevent recurrences. Historical studies of the care of older people are particularly important as inhumanities towards them escape from public memory more rapidly than cruelties towards children. Margaret Panting, a seventy-eight-year-old woman who suffered repeated physical injury and died at the hands of relatives in 2001 is virtually unknown (Ash 2011, p. 100). In contrast, children, such as Victoria Climbié, killed by her guardians in 2000, and 'Baby Peter' who died at the hands of relatives in 2007, are embedded in public consciousness.

A study of AEGIS lies at the interface of the history of NHS policy and practice, mental health, mental hospitals, old age and gender. It reveals much about the workings of higher levels of NHS administration, such as how it managed complaints and deficits in services and its relationship with the public. It fills a gap in twentieth-century women's history, including from the slant of their position as older patients. Adequate health and welfare support in old age is particularly relevant to women because on average they live longer than men. They often live alone while suffering from frailty and age-related chronic degenerative illnesses. They may struggle to cope and require institutional care towards the end of their lives. In the 1960s, older working-class women often had particularly meagre financial resources so depended on state welfare provision and occupied a disproportionate number of psychiatric hospital beds. Other women discussed in the study besides Barbara include her supporters and author-witnesses; journalists who publicised her concerns; hospital staff; and middle-class women undertaking voluntary roles on RHBs, on Hospital Management Committees (HMCs) and with charities.

To understand the context and background of AEGIS's campaign, and to highlight this study's contemporary relevance, several further issues are discussed in this introduction: early- and mid-twentieth-century psychiatric hospital scandals; the handful of studies concerned directly with AEGIS; pressure groups; and ageism. The larger background subject of how psychiatric hospital provision developed for older people until the mid-1960s is explained in the next chapter.

Scandals of Psychiatric Hospital Care

Sans Everything was not the first or the last time poor care in psychiatric hospitals was reported and investigated. A review of existing historical studies about these episodes gives some indication of the hurdles which AEGIS might face in its endeavours. Montagu Lomax, a doctor who worked at Prestwich Asylum for a short time, wrote *The Experiences of an Asylum Doctor* (1921) about inadequate clinical practice there. It became a cause célèbre. Colleagues were hostile and accused him of sensationalism and exaggeration. The asylum regulatory authority, the Board of Control, criticised 'the methods which Dr Lomax has seen fit to adopt in preparation and publishing his book... the charges made were sheer nonsense and a gross calumny' (Harding 1990, p. 180). A committee of inquiry was unreceptive, and an anonymous contributor to an academic psychiatric journal (Anon. 1923, p. 91) praised it for a 'masterly and logical' rejection of Lomax's complaints. Despite the rejection, the committee made recommendations for improvements based on Lomax's report, as did the Royal Commission on Lunacy (1924–1926), whose conclusions underpinned the Mental Treatment Act 1930 (Harding 1990, p. 181). Harding provided insights into the way a whistle-blower can be victimised and officialdom can viciously reject constructive criticism but then use it as a basis for proposing improvements.

Relatively little historiography is available about AEGIS. Four researchers from the academic discipline of social administration and policy explored its work. Kathleen Jones and AJ Fowles (1984) included AEGIS as part of their study on the literature of long-term care and custody in the 1960s. John Martin (1984) analysed hospital inquiries from 1968 until 1984, and David Cochrane (1990) based his doctoral thesis on a case study of AEGIS and the process of health policy change in England. Some other writers have touched on *Sans Everything* but have tended to follow the Ministry of Health's interpretation, that *Sans Everything* was irresponsible scare mongering and an inappropriate smear on all psychiatric hospital nurses.[2] Although even a cursory glance at *Sans Everything* (p. xiv) shows this is incorrect, the perception has crept into secondary sources. Michael Arton (1998, p. 288), for example, stated that AEGIS gave 'the impression to the general public that mental nurses were a group of uncaring sadists', but he did not cite confirmatory evidence for his statement.

Jones and Fowles' analysis was based on a handful of published works, leading them to place little credibility on the accounts of neglect and abuse in *Sans Everything*. They accepted the official inquiry reports that most of the allegations were false. They concluded, in an uncomplimentary way, that: 'The whole affair was a very skilful exercise in public relations; and despite the flamboyance, the distortions and the inaccuracies, it worked' (p. 108). Archival sources used in the present study challenge their criticisms; the 'affair' label would be more apt for the Ministry's handling of the situation than for AEGIS's allegations.

Martin (1984) analysed the first cluster of inquiries into psychiatric hospitals, including *Sans Everything* (MoH 1968), Ely (Department of Health and Social Security (DHSS) 1969), Farleigh (DHSS 1971), Whittingham (DHSS 1972), and South Ockendon (DHSS 1974). He described them as being of the 'old order', because 'their circumstances derived from past inadequacies of provision, and from lack of new thinking'.[3] Martin concurred with the published inquiry reports into *Sans Everything* and with the Ministry's view, that almost all allegations were disproved, thus discrediting AEGIS. However, he did not discuss the incongruity of that in the context of the rapid succession of investigations into similar allegations in other hospitals that were shown to be justified.

Martin discussed patterns of malpractice. Usually there was a chain of events and a broad context of failures of care rather than a single 'bad apple'. Staff often knew what was going on but did nothing about it, partly because of the power of the work group and of staff loyalty to it (Martin 1984, p. 243). Good clinical practice was undermined when secondary aims (making things easier for the staff) were substituted for primary ones of person-centred care. This resulted in gradual deterioration of standards, and 'the ultimate exposure made by a newcomer who is not conditioned to standards which have become familiar to the long-term staff' (p. 244). Martin also noted that hospital hierarchies, especially in the nursing profession, did not encourage questioning by the all-important ward staff undertaking face-to-face work with patients, and that creativity, individuality and clinical responsibility produced better care. Failure of staff to take on as much personal responsibility as possible was 'likely to result in the quality of care sinking to that level which is most convenient for the staff to provide and which satisfies minimum standards' (p. 243). This conclusion was unnervingly close to a comment made by Andy Burnham, Secretary of State for Health, 2009–2010, to the Mid Staffordshire Inquiry (2013, p. 1378): 'the NHS is not good at giving its front-line staff a sense of empowerment. People with good ideas do not feel that they can easily put them into action.' Martin's comment about the importance of the newcomer in detecting poor standards was apparent in the role of Julie Bailey, who visited her mother in hospital and whose concerns culminated in the Mid Staffordshire Inquiry (Cure the NHS 2016).

Martin also argued that professionally isolated staff, such as in the rural psychiatric hospitals, could perceive outside influences as threatening and likely to show up their deficiencies, rather than being revitalising. On wards with inadequate staff levels and resources, complaints could be resented strongly. In such circumstances, staff stuck together, showing up 'the darker side of group loyalty', suppressing criticism and victimising the critic. Martin also noted that 'To say one is doing one's best under the circumstances is to recognise that one is *not* doing the best work. It is a defence with built-in vulnerability. It almost invites attack and it generates a guilty sensitivity to criticism' (p. 245). 'Doing one's best under the circumstances' is also heard in the NHS today, to justify inadequate clinical services associated with underresourcing.[4]

Cochrane's (1990) analysis of the important role of AEGIS in NHS policy development challenged the earlier interpretations, which were largely based on published texts. He demonstrated how it initiated the succession of scandals in psychiatric hospitals (c.1968–1974) and contributed to health service policy, including raising the priority of mental illness and mental handicap services and influencing the establishment of a hospitals' inspectorate, ombudsman and NHS complaints procedures. Cochrane documented Barbara's political career as a social reformer, but some of his conclusions, such as extrapolating her influence into the late 1980s, are hard to justify historically in view of the complex processes of social and health policy change.

Cochrane was fortunate to have Abel-Smith to supervise his thesis. He also had the advantage of being able to undertake oral history interviews with people who knew Barbara, collaborated with her or opposed her. They included Geoffrey Howe, WJA 'Bill' Kirkpatrick, Kenneth Robinson, CH Rolph (Bill Hewitt), David Roxan and Lord Strabolgi, all of whom have since died. Cochrane did not give reasons why Sir Arnold France, Permanent Secretary and Robinson's 'right hand man' at the Ministry of Health (1964–1968) (Green 2004) declined to be interviewed, and other DHSS officials and 'senior health authority officers' asked not to be named (Cochrane 1990, p. 389).

The present study differs from Cochrane's in several ways. First, it is outside the constraints of a social science discipline and aims to explore what happened historically rather than relate events to a theoretical model. Second, it is more people focussed. Who was Amy Gibbs, 'Miss Wills' in *Sans Everything*? Who were the pseudonymous contributors to the book? How did Barbara cope with the hostility and discrediting of her work? Third, now that the closure period for official archives has expired, more sources are available so it is possible to explore the *Sans Everything* allegations and inquiries in greater depth. This supports the timeliness of a further study of AEGIS's work.

Social Justice, Pressure Groups and the Emergence of AEGIS

Societal changes in the 1960s included a focus on personal autonomy and individuality with less submissiveness to authority. This affected lifestyles, expectations about standards of living and demands for humane and safe public services and environments. Despite greater affluence for many people, disturbing large-scale poverty, especially affecting children, large families and older people, was 'rediscovered' by researchers at LSE (Thane 2011). LSE academics particularly conspicuous in this work included Abel-Smith and Peter Townsend. Abel-Smith supported and gave credence to several campaigns, such as the Child Poverty Action Group (CPAG) (Townsend 2004; Sheard 2014, pp. 224, 256). Townsend (1962, 1963) published in-depth sociological studies, including about the needs of older people. He wrote about their poverty and the disadvantageous health inequalities that accompanied it. He cited a 1950s estimate that up to 75 percent of retired people had incomes low enough to qualify for means-tested National Assistance (Townsend 1963, p. 186). Poverty became an important social justice issue and a matter for 'pressure groups'.

Pressure groups, and lobbying and petitioning governments and leaders, were well-established mechanisms for conveying public unease and encouraging social change. For example, 150 years before Barbara formed AEGIS, Elizabeth Fry established a small campaign organisation, Association for the Improvement of the Females at Newgate, after her first visit to the London prison (Howard League 2016). In the 1960s many new organisations emerged, expressing concerns and aiming to generate action. They campaigned on issues such as the environment, nuclear disarmament, abortion, homosexual and women's rights and other 'conscience' issues. The broadly focussed Consumers' Association, founded in 1957, became a powerful representative of this general trend (O'Hara 2013). Crossman was wary of well-run pressure groups, like AEGIS and CPAG: 'these small splinter groups, can be extremely powerful if they provide the press with hot poisonous news. They can really damage our image.'[5]

Investigative journalism and a less deferential media emerged in the 1960s, with some newspapers 'geared to shaking and rattling', seeking justice and making 'people sit up straight'.[6] One journalist, Andrew Roth, contrasted the changes in his profession from the 1950s to the 1960s:

> Pressmen, political correspondents like myself, for example, would know a great deal more than they would report because they didn't think it was 'nice' to report about certain things.... Now that's changed very considerably, thanks to a number of institutions like *Private Eye* and the breakout of the BBC in *That was the week that was* (Davies 1985, pp. 17–18).

This gave opportunities for professionalised, media-aware campaigning organisations to publicise their concerns to help achieve solutions. The BBC, for example, showed *Cathy Come Home*, Ken Loach's film that told the bleak tale of Cathy, who lost her home, husband and eventually her child through the inflexibility of the British welfare system. The film was central to founding the housing charity Shelter (Shelter 2016).

Before the creation of the NHS in 1948, financing of hospitals and long-stay care was largely addressed through philanthropic and Poor Law mechanisms. The donor–beneficiary relationship inhibited protest about substandard practice or facilities, a deeply engrained pattern that, to some extent, recurs or has continued. In the 1960s, patients generally expressed their appreciation and uncritical acceptance of the care they received (Cartwright 1964, pp. 8, 203). Older people rarely complained then or now (Parliamentary and Health Service Ombudsman (PHSO) 2015). The authorities interpreted lack of complaints to mean that provision was satisfactory.[7] They did not take into account that many patients and their relatives feared the consequences of complaining or did not know how to complain (also PHSO 2015), and there were no guidelines informing them how to do so.

Although patients had individual contact with doctors, the paternalistic doctor–patient relationship in the 1960s discouraged patients from asking questions about their own health or commenting on aspects of the service they received. Societal changes away from conformity towards greater personal autonomy were associated with less acceptance of medical paternalism and a shift away from the assumption that the doctor and the NHS always knew best. Disquiet about experiences of NHS patients received public airing, such as in Gerda Cohen's *What's Wrong with Hospitals?* (1964), based on her own frustrating and depersonalising experience of hospital care. She wrote that patients of all ages had 'no rights, no dignity, no status', were treated 'like chipped flower-pots in for repair' and were kept in ignorance 'merely because it's no one's job in a hospital to tell the patient what is happening' (pp. 7, 9).

In contrast to pre-NHS days, after 1948, general taxation funded the NHS. Public funding meant public ownership. In the early 1960s this linked to the idea of patients as 'consumers' of health services with some control of the 'product' they used (Anon. 1961). This connected to the creation of NHS-focussed pressure groups, which concentrated on efficacy of official policy, or post-policy failure, rather than on individual needs (O'Hara 2013). Helen Hodgson, a teacher, set up the Patients Association (PA) in 1963 following reports about the drug thalidomide that caused severe physical deformities in children born to mothers who took it during pregnancy, and Maurice Pappworth's (1962) revelations in 'Human guinea pigs: a warning', about doctors' experiments on unknowing patients (Mold 2012, p. 2032). The PA aimed to be a nationwide patient-participatory organisation, focussing on a growing tide of discontent with NHS services, particularly hospitals, doctors and bureaucracy, including the paucity of information on how to make a complaint. It aimed to educate the public on their rights and responsibilities as patients and to improve care across the NHS (Macfarlane 2009). Pressure groups developed various styles, ranging from the antagonistic (such as the PA) to the National Association for the Welfare of Children in Hospital (founded 1961) (Action for Sick Children 2016), whose members were afraid of being seen as difficult, partly out of a fear that hospital staff would exact reprisals on their children (Mold 2013, p. 238).

Alex Mold's study (2013, p. 240) of the changing role of the patient and NHS consumer groups concentrated on acute hospitals, only once mentioning long-stay patients. The care of older, mentally ill and mentally handicapped people on long-stay wards was peripheral to health service pressure groups such as the PA. Concerning older people, the National Old Peoples' Welfare Committee (founded 1944; later Age Concern) mainly provided practical philanthropic support and lobbied the government about community provision for older people, and Help the Aged (founded 1961) emphasised social support and relief of poverty (Age UK 2016).[8] Neither had specific expertise or interest in mental health. The National Association for Mental Health (NAMH; founded 1946; later MIND) focussed mainly on younger people. Nevertheless, in 1963, NAMH devoted one issue of its journal to older people. An editorial, 'The elderly: "Living and partly living"' (Anon. 1963) referred to many older people 'with little sense of usefulness, little interest in anything, and little affection from anyone'. It was hardly optimistic, but did suggest that interested psychiatrists could work together with 'the many other workers in this field—within the health service and outside'.

AEGIS emerged into this climate of more pressure groups eager to make improvements in NHS and social care. AEGIS was the only one doing that specifically for around 60,000 older people in NHS long-stay psychiatric wards (Townsend 1962, p. 282).

Ageism

New social constructs in the 1960s included *ageism*, a term coined by Robert Butler (1969) in the United States, and *gerontophobia*, which was coined by Alex Comfort (1967) in England. These terms reflected excessively negative attitudes and practices, or age discrimination, that could affect provision of services for older people. Ageism is unlike many other sorts of discrimination, such as gender, sexual orientation, race and religion because most of us will live into old age. Ageism means that paradoxically we treat ourselves as 'other'. It is self-perpetuating: ageist stereotypes may be internalised in childhood and reinforced across the life span, often unconsciously, so that when someone becomes old they may adopt the stereotypes themselves (Levy 2009, p. 333).

Pat Thane (1993, 2000) took up some of the issues around ageism and stereotypes in her historical studies of old age. She noted that the 'cultural conservatism' of the 'continuing belief that it is "common sense" to expect inequality past a certain age' was used to justify ageist attitudes (Thane 2010, p. 22). She also explored the complex issue of mass retirement in the mid-twentieth century, which had an impact on ageist ideas. In her view, it was one of several changes that 'increasingly defined old people as a distinct social group defined by marginalisation and dependency' (Thane 2000, p. 406). Socially accepted marginalisation can affect expectations of people providing services and older people receiving them. It can legitimise governments overlooking older people's needs, thus affecting the resources allocated to them. Paul Bridgen (2001, pp. 507–508), in his analysis of geriatric medicine and long-term care, concluded that the early NHS was disappointing from the old age perspective: despite relative improvements in provision in acute hospitals, ideas about rehabilitating older people were slow to be integrated, and no firm strategy for long-term care provision was established, either by the NHS or by local authorities. Marginalisation of older people could also affect historians' interest in them, as Webster commented (1991, p. 165): 'Considering the importance of the elderly as users of the NHS, remarkably little retrospective analysis has been written about the health services from their perspective.' Since 1991, more historical research has been undertaken, including about psychiatric services for older people (Hilton 2015, 2016a, 2016b), considered in the next chapter.

Methodology

If Barbara had persisted with her initial idea to destroy her archive, far fewer sources about the AEGIS campaign would be available today. In a letter in 1970 to her executor, her brother 'Darling FJ', Frederick John Charlton, she said she had changed her mind because someone at the DHSS 'surprisingly enough' suggested that many files 'had a certain sociological interest'. She bequeathed her files to Abel-Smith.[9] He arranged for them to be deposited at LSE. The AEGIS archive, as far as we know, is as Barbara left it. It did not encounter pruning after retirement or weeding, common to organisational archives when a new leader takes over or the organisation changes its archives policy. It takes up eight metres of shelf space and includes thousands of letters and hundreds of cuttings from newspapers, magazines, medical journals and nursing journals about positive and negative aspects of the NHS and related subjects. It records Barbara's campaign in minute detail but contains little autobiographical material. A separate personal archive appears not to have survived. Most biographical information was drawn from private archives, *The Jung-White Letters* (Lammers and Cunningham 2007), and other people's memories and memoirs. Much was recorded by the author in semistructured oral history interviews (2015–2016). Interviews quoted in Cochrane's thesis provided valuable insights where other sources were unavailable. Unfortunately, Cochrane's original interview transcripts have not survived.[10]

Other public and private archive collections were used, to ensure inclusion of different perspectives. The National Archives (TNA) and county record offices hold extensive relevant official documentation. The London Metropolitan Archives (LMA) holds records of Friern Hospital, central to the AEGIS story. The Royal College of Nursing (RCN) unfortunately lacks archives relating to nurses' roles in, or perspectives on, *Sans Everything* and AEGIS.[11] The University of Warwick Modern Records Centre holds the unedited typescripts of Richard Crossman's diaries, which provide his personal perspectives on Barbara and her campaign.

Some terms used in this book require clarification. A challenge of writing about stigmatised people and places is that terminology changes frequently in the hope that new language will be associated with less stigma and kinder attitudes and practices. The Mental Treatment Act (1930), for example, replaced *asylum* with *mental hospital*, which became *psychiatric hospital* after the Mental Health Act (MHA) 1959. Uptake of new terms was inconsistent, and, for example, well after the MHA 1959, the terms mental hospital and psychiatric hospital were used interchangeably in official sources for no apparent reason. Around 1970, *mental subnormality* changed to *mental handicap*, and the terms *a dement* and *senile* became offensive. Colloquially, out-dated language risks being used pejoratively, but I have used terms when they convey meanings, attitudes and expectations in the historical context better than modern alternatives.

The term *the elderly* is avoided. Geriatrician Bernard Isaacs (1982) and Pat Thane (2010, p. 19) criticised its use because it reinforces a stereotype of older people, conveying an unhelpful and inaccurate impression that they are a homogeneous group, rather than being as diverse as the rest of the population. *Psychogeriatric* is used only to refer to modern proactive psychiatric services for older people, which began in a few hospitals by the end of the 1960s (Hilton 2016b). It is not used to refer to the earlier passive custodial system of care for older people in the psychiatric hospitals. Another inconsistency in official documents was the spelling of *inquiry* and *enquiry*. I have used the former throughout except where *enquiry* appears in quotations.

Writing about Barbara Robb, I have referred to her as 'Barbara' throughout. Letters in Barbara's archives reveal her often informal approach, and Ann Lammers (2007, p. 258) noted her ability to 'melt' formality; she would have been comfortable with a respectful but casual approach. More difficult to deal with historically is the blurring of identities between Barbara and AEGIS. Taking into account that AEGIS would not have existed or functioned without Barbara, it is sometimes unclear whether to refer to 'AEGIS' or 'Barbara'. The Ministry, for example, was uncertain whether to blame her or AEGIS for fanning criticism[12] and accused her of 'making as damaging a case as she can'.[13] Crossman and Rolph, in diaries and memoirs, tended to refer to her by name rather than the organisation she represented, both because of her influence and because she was unforgettable as a person (Rolph 1987, p. 183). This account uses both 'AEGIS' and 'Barbara', whichever seems most appropriate and accurate in each context.

Barbara was conscious of the huge trust people put in her by revealing sensitive information. She did not want a witch-hunt or for individual staff who revealed their concerns to be scapegoated by the authorities. Nor did she want a backlash of reprisals by angry staff against their colleagues, patients or their visitors who made criticisms, a fear that prevented many from doing so.[14] Similarly, it is not my intention to embarrass the descendants of the staff discussed whose behaviours were allegedly unsatisfactory. Most were not deliberately cruel but thought they were practising according to professional standards (Whitehead 1970, p. 13). I have therefore identified them by their pseudonym, if Barbara allocated one, or by a single initial. In contrast, for the author-witnesses in *Sans Everything*, except in quotations, I have used their real names. Fifty years on, the pseudonyms are no longer required: the course of events showed the legitimacy of the allegations, and the witnesses' courage and humanity in revealing them.

Notes

1. Robb, in 'Record of a Campaign', which describes the AEGIS campaign in 'chapters'; Letter, 'Bill' Rolph to Robb, 1 April 1968, AEGIS/B/3. (AEGIS archive, London School of Economics).
2. Kenneth Robinson, in *Man Alive*, BBC2, 16 July 1968, transcript, 18, AEGIS/2/7/A.
3. Martin included Napsbury (DHSS 1973) but the type of issues raised were different from those of the other inquiries. Napsbury is not further discussed in this study.
4. Comment made to the author in the course of her clinical work.
5. Crossman Diaries, May 1970, 168/JH/70-27 (University of Warwick Modern Records Centre).
6. Anne Robinson, investigative journalist with the *Sunday Times* (1968–1978). Reported on the AEGIS campaign and conditions in psychiatric hospitals, including South Ockendon. Interview by author, 2015.
7. Meeting, Robb and Geoffrey Tooth, 25 May 1965, AEGIS/1/1.
8. Help the Aged merged with Age Concern to become Age UK in 2009 (Age UK 2016).

9. Letter, Robb to FJ Charlton, 19 August 1970, AEGIS/1/10/B.
10. David Cochrane, discussion with author, 2015.
11. Neasa Roughan, archives assistant, RCN, email to author, 2015.
12. Memo, C Benwell, 'Condition of the elderly in mental hospitals', 10 March 1967, MH150/349 (TNA).
13. Memo, C Benwell to Miss Hedley, 20 June 1967, MH150/350 (TNA).
14. Memo, H Yellowlees to Mrs Croft, 27 July 1967, MH159/213 (TNA).

Bibliography

Abel-Smith, Brian. 1990. Interviewed by Hugh Freeman. *BJPsych Bulletin*, 14, 257–261.
Action for Sick Children. 2016. http://www.actionforsickchildren.org.uk, accessed 23 January 2016.
Age UK. 2016. 'Our history'. http://www.ageuk.org.uk, accessed February 2016.
Allen, Anne. 1967. 'One woman who refused to pass by..'. *Sunday Mirror*, 9 July.
Anon. 1923. 'The administration of public mental hospitals in England and Wales'. *British Journal of Psychiatry*, 69, 90–98.
Anon. 1961. 'Patients as consumers: wants and needs'. *Lancet*, i, 927–928.
Anon. 1963. 'The elderly: "Living and partly living"' *Mental Health*, 21, 210–211.
Arie, Tom. 1973. 'Dementia in the elderly: diagnosis and assessment'. *BMJ*, iv, 540–543.
Arton, Michael. 1998. 'The professionalisation of mental nursing in Great Britain, 1850–1950'. PhD thesis, University College London. http://discovery.ucl.ac.uk, accessed 16 September 2016.
Ash, Angie. 2011. 'A cognitive mask? Camouflaging dilemmas in street-level policy implementation to safeguard older people from abuse'. *British Journal of Social Work*, 43, 99–115.
Bridgen, Paul. 2001. 'Hospitals, geriatric medicine, and long-term care of elderly people 1946–1976'. *Social History of Medicine*, 14, 507–523.
Butler, Robert. 1969. 'Age-ism: another form of bigotry'. *Gerontologist*, 9, 243–246.
Cartwright, Ann. 1964. *Human Relations and Hospital Care*. London: Routledge and Kegan Paul.
Cochrane, David. 1990. 'The AEGIS campaign to improve standards of care in mental hospitals: a case study of the process of social policy change'. PhD thesis, University of London. http://etheses.lse.ac.uk, accessed 17 September 2016.

Cohen, Gerda. 1964. *What's Wrong with Hospitals?* Harmondsworth: Penguin Books.
Comfort, Alex. 1967. 'On gerontophobia'. *Medical Opinion and Review*, 3, 9, 30–37.
Crossman, Richard. 1977. *'The Diaries of a Cabinet Minister'. Vol. 3. Secretary of State for Social Services 1968–1970.* London: Hamilton and Cape.
Cure the NHS. 2016. http://www.curethenhs.co.uk, accessed 24 August 2016.
Davies, Malcolm. 1985. *Politics of Pressure: The Art of Lobbying.* London: BBC.
Denham, Michael. 2004. 'The history of geriatric medicine and hospital care of the elderly in England between 1929 and the 1970s'. PhD thesis, University College London. http://www.discovery.ucl.ac.uk, accessed 17 September 2016.
DHSS. 1969. *Report of the Committee of Inquiry into Allegations of Ill-Treatment of Patients and Other Irregularities at the Ely Hospital. Cardiff.* Cmnd. 3975. London: HMSO.
DHSS. 1971. *Report of the Farleigh Hospital Committee of Inquiry.* Cmnd. 4557. London: HMSO.
DHSS. 1972. *Report of the Committee of Inquiry into Whittingham Hospital.* Cmnd. 4861. London: HMSO.
DHSS. 1973. *Report of the Professional Investigation into Medical and Nursing Practices on Certain Wards at Napsbury Hospital.* London: HMSO.
DHSS. 1974. *Report of the Committee of Inquiry into South Ockendon Hospital.* HC. 124. London: HMSO.
Green, Arthur. 2004. 'France, Sir Arnold William 1911–1998'. *Oxford Dictionary of National Biography.* http://www.oxforddnb.com, accessed 15 September 2015.
Harding, Tim. 1990. '"Not worth powder and shot": a reappraisal of Montagu Lomax's contribution to mental health reform'. *British Journal of Psychiatry*, 156, 180–187.
Health Service Ombudsman. 2011. *Care and Compassion? Report of the Health Service Ombudsman on Ten Investigations into NHS Care of Older People.* London: TSO.
Hilton, Claire. 2015. 'Psychiatrists, mental health provision and "senile dementia" in England, 1940s–1979'. *History of Psychiatry*, 26, 182–199.
Hilton, Claire. 2016a. 'Psychogeriatrics in England in the 1950s: greater knowledge with little impact on provision of services'. *History of Psychiatry*, 27, 3–20.
Hilton, Claire. 2016b. 'Developing psychogeriatrics in England: a turning point in the 1960s?' *Contemporary British History*, 30, 40–72.
Howard League for Penal Reform. 2016. http://howardleague.org, accessed 1 September 2016.
Isaacs, Bernard. 1982. 'Let's abolish "the elderly"'. *BMJ*, 284, 112.

Jones, Kathleen and Fowles, AJ. 1984. *Ideas on Institutions*. London: Routledge and Kegan Paul.
Lammers, Ann. 2007. 'Jung and White and the God of terrible double aspect'. *Journal of Analytical Psychology*, 52, 253–274.
Lammers, Ann and Cunningham, Adrian. eds. 2007. *The Jung-White Letters*. London: Routledge.
Levy, Becca. 2009. 'Stereotype embodiment: a psychosocial approach to aging'. *Current Directions in Psychological Science*, 18, 332–336.
Lomax, Montagu. 1921. *The Experiences of an Asylum Doctor: With Suggestions for Asylum and Lunacy Law Reform*. London: G Allen and Unwin.
Macfarlane, Ross. 2009. 'Patients Association archive available in the Wellcome Library'. http://blog.wellcomelibrary.org, accessed 17 September 2016.
Martin, Denis. 1962. *Adventure in Psychiatry*. Oxford: Bruno Cassirer.
Martin, John (with Evans, Debbie). 1984. *Hospitals in Trouble*. Oxford: Blackwell.
Means, Robin and Smith, Randall. 1985. *The Development of Welfare Services for Elderly People*. Kent: Croom Helm.
Mid Staffordshire NHS Foundation Trust. 2013. *Mid Staffordshire NHS Foundation Trust Public Inquiry*. HC. 947 (Francis Report). London: TSO.
Ministry of Health. 1968. *Findings and Recommendations Following Enquiries into Allegations Concerning the Care of Elderly Patients in Certain Hospitals*. Cmnd. 3687. London: HMSO.
Mold, Alex. 2012. 'Patients' rights and the National Health Service in Britain, 1960s–1980s'. *American Journal of Public Health*, 102, 2030–2038.
Mold, Alex. 2013. 'Repositioning the patient: patient organizations, consumerism, and autonomy in Britain during the 1960s and 1970s'. *Bulletin of the History of Medicine*, 87, 225–249.
O'Hara, Glen. 2013. 'The complexities of "consumerism": choice, collectivism and participation within Britain's National Health Service, c.1961–c.1979'. *Social History of Medicine*, 26, 288–304.
Panorama. 2014. *Behind Closed Doors: Elderly Care Exposed*. BBC1, 30 April.
Pappworth, Maurice. 1962. 'Human guinea pigs: a warning'. *Twentieth Century*, 172, 66–75.
Parliamentary and Health Service Ombudsman. 2015. *Breaking Down the Barriers: Older People and Complaints About Health Care*. http://www.obudsman.org.uk, accessed 22 August 2016.
Robb, Barbara. 1967. *Sans Everything: A Case to Answer*. London: Nelson.
Robinson, Anne. 1970. 'Whitewash in the old folks' wards'. *Sunday Times*, 5 April.
Rolph, Cecil. 1987. *Further Particulars*. Oxford: OUP.
Sheard, Sally. 2014. *The Passionate Economist*. Bristol: Policy Press.
Shelter: the housing and homelessness charity. http://www.shelter.org.uk, accessed 29 March 2016.

Thane, Pat. 1993. 'Geriatrics' 1092–1115. In *Companion Encyclopedia of the History of Medicine*, eds. William Bynum, Roy Porter. London: Routledge.

Thane, Pat. 2000. *Old Age in English History: Past Experiences, Present Issues*. Oxford: OUP.

Thane, Pat. 2010. "Older people and equality' 7–28. In *Unequal Britain*, ed. Pat Thane. London: Continuum.

Thane, Pat. 2011. 'There has always been a "big society"'. *History at Large*, 30 April. http://www.historyworkshop.org.uk, accessed 1 August 2015.

Townsend, Peter. 1962. *The Last Refuge*. London: Routledge and Kegan Paul.

Townsend, Peter. 1963. *Family Life of Old People*. Harmondsworth: Penguin Books (First published 1957).

Townsend, Peter. 2004. 'Smith, Brian Abel- 1926–1996'. *Oxford Dictionary of National Biography*. http://www.oxforddnb.com, accessed 1 December 2015.

Webster, Charles. 1991. 'The elderly and the early National Health Service' 165–193. In *Life and Death and the Elderly*, ed. M Pelling, R Smith. London: Routledge.

Webster, Charles. 1998. *The National Health Service: A Political History*. Oxford: OUP.

West Sussex Adult Safeguarding Board. 2014. *Orchid View Serious Case Review*. http://www.westsussex.gov.uk, accessed 17 September 2016.

Whitehead, Anthony. 1970. *In the Service of Old Age: The Welfare of Psychogeriatric Patients*. Harmondsworth: Penguin Books.

Open Access This chapter is licensed under the terms of the Creative Commons Attribution 4.0 International License (http://creativecommons.org/licenses/by/4.0/), which permits use, sharing, adaptation, distribution and reproduction in any medium or format, as long as you give appropriate credit to the original author(s) and the source, provide a link to the Creative Commons license and indicate if changes were made.

The images or other third party material in this chapter are included in the book's Creative Commons license, unless indicated otherwise in a credit line to the material. If material is not included in the book's Creative Commons license and your intended use is not permitted by statutory regulation or exceeds the permitted use, you will need to obtain permission directly from the copyright holder.

CHAPTER 2

Psychiatric Hospitals and Older People: Status Quo or Making Changes?

Huge and forbidding, Friern Hospital, where the AEGIS (Aid for the Elderly in Government Institutions) campaign began in 1965, had 2,250 beds and an unwelcoming, dimly lit corridor more than one third of a mile long, which connected most of the wards. The corridor lights could go off unexpectedly as Friern's electricity supply needed upgrading:[1] 'it would not do to ask a nervous person to visit' said Barbara Robb (1967, p. 78). A male junior doctor recollected:

> You were a bit fearful walking down the corridor. It was the most peculiar experience...you would see a furtive head looking quietly out of a little nook or cranny, which was actually an entrance to a ward...so you would wonder what was going to happen to you. You had to be rather bold.

While working at Friern in 1964–1965, that doctor hardly mentioned to his colleagues in other hospitals that he was employed there: 'I think it was regarded as being rather a tainted claim to fame.... I don't think my peers were aware of it, to be honest.... It wasn't something you wanted to crow about or boast about amongst other trainees or amongst your seniors.'[2]

Friern Hospital was originally named Colney Hatch Asylum. It opened in 1851, the largest and most modern institution of its kind in Europe (Hunter and Macalpine 1974, p. 11). It was one of a network of county asylums built in the mid-nineteenth century, based on humanitarian principles and optimism by the 'mad doctors' that they would find treatments for insanity. Alongside demographic changes of an increasing population, tolerance of bizarre behaviour lessened, particularly in more urbanised and regulated environments, and demands for beds rose. Hopes of effective treatment diminished and a custodial approach became common (Rogers and Pilgrim 1996, pp. 46–50). In 1884 the Lunacy Commission (renamed Board of Control in 1913), the public authority overseeing the asylums, commented that older people at Colney Hatch occupied disproportionately more beds than would be expected from their number in the population, and that 'special provision for the aged' was essential to reverse the trend (Hunter and Macalpine 1974, p. 62). The Commissioners observed the pattern elsewhere and in 1897 reported their concern to the responsible authorities (Lewis 1946, p. 151). The government ignored the worsening situation, fearing the economic costs of providing for more older people. The medical profession lacked interest, and there was no public pressure to make changes (Hilton 2016, p. 20). By 1963, people over age sixty-five made up 12 percent of the population but occupied 39 percent of psychiatric hospital beds (47,782 of 123,744), and startlingly, women over age seventy-five (making up 5 percent of the female population) occupied 25 percent of all female beds in those hospitals (Brooke 1967, p. 4).[3]

The most progressive psychiatric hospitals functioned therapeutically despite antiquated buildings. During the 1950s and early 1960s, they were led by dynamic psychiatrist 'medical superintendents', such as Bertram Mandelbrote at Littlemore (Oxford), Denis Martin at Claybury (Essex) (Martin 1962), and Russell Barton at Severalls (Colchester) (Jolley 2003).[4] Other hospitals, such as Friern, lacked a forceful leadership.[5] The medical superintendent, together with the senior nurses and administrative staff of the hospitals—usually a matron, chief male nurse and hospital secretary—were expected to liaise with their voluntary Hospital Management Committee (HMC). The Minister of Health, through the Regional Hospital Boards (RHBs), appointed HMC members, based on their 'knowledge and experience', without defining what that meant (Ministry of Health (MoH) 1966, p. 6). HMC members were usually highly committed and well intentioned,[6] and the Ministry delegated a high level of financial and organisational responsibility to them (MoH 1966, p. iii). The National Association for Mental Health (NAMH), however, regarded HMCs as 'too often ill-qualified—by reason of their age, their backgrounds, the rigidity of their outlook, or their sheer ignorance and inexperience of the matters with which they must deal'.[7] The Patients

Association (PA) had other concerns about the effects of delegation to RHBs and HMCs because it resulted in lack of ministerial control over the hospitals, to the extent that 'guidance' or 'advice' that the Ministry sent to RHBs was usually ignored.[8]

HMCs faced numerous challenges in their hospitals, including ensuring adequate staffing and standards of care, managing overcrowding, and maintaining and modernising buildings. When the Mental Health Act (MHA) 1959 abolished the Board of Control, responsibility for inspections and maintaining standards passed to HMCs who would 'visit' their own hospitals. HMCs received little guidance about how to determine quality. A senior member of the hospital staff usually accompanied them during their visits, which discouraged patients and most staff from voicing concerns. HMC visitors focussed on the physical environment rather than what went on in it. Good interior decor led to glowing reports when psychological and social care was atrocious (Barton 1959, p. 48).

To contextualise the situation that so disturbed Barbara Robb when she visited Amy Gibbs in 1965, it is necessary to understand the interactions between older people and the hospital wards and community services, research and innovation about their needs and the government's standpoint on service provision. During the period from the early 1940s until the mid-1960s, these strands had no clear single chronology and only limited overlap, so in this chapter they are explored thematically. Research on diagnosis and treatment of mental illnesses in older people, for example, had little effect on clinical practice, and government initiatives for older people did little to implement the research findings or remedy overcrowding in back wards. The relevant developments during the same period at Friern are described at the end of the chapter.

THE PSYCHIATRIC HOSPITAL WARDS

In the mid-twentieth century, some patients with mental illnesses were discharged from hospital in an improved state, but there were, and are, always some who require on-going care. Proportions of short- and long-stay patients varied, depending on a combination of factors, which Kathleen Jones (1993, pp. 150–158) optimistically alluded to, in the 1950s and 1960s, as the social, pharmacological and legislative 'revolutions' of psychiatric care. Social developments included day hospitals, therapeutic communities and the 'open door movement' (p. 151). Pharmacological treatments, research and greater understanding about mental illness helped shape medical practice and enabled more people to be discharged. New legislation—the MHA 1959—facilitated and encouraged, but did not mandate, more liberal and community approaches. Another factor noted around the same time was the psychological damage resulting from long-stay custodial care. In 1959, Barton coined the term *institutional neurosis* to describe this. Hallmarks of institutional neurosis comprised apathy, loss of interest, submissiveness and social withdrawal. Barton identified seven causes: ward atmosphere; bossiness of staff; medication; enforced idleness; loss of personal friends, possessions and life events; loss of contact with the outside world; and loss of prospects outside the institution (Barton 1959, p. 17). He did not claim to have introduced a new neurotic illness, despite the name he gave it, but aimed to use his observations as a means to improving care (Jones and Fowles 1984, pp. 71–78).

In 1961, Erving Goffman, a sociologist in the United States, wrote about 'total institutions', including 'stripping', a dehumanising removal of all personal belongings as part of the process of complying with group living on admission to an institution. Uniform haircuts, enforced bathing or showering on entry and other demeaning practices, accompanied stripping. Officials could rationalise the practices, such as being for safety or hygiene, but they cumulatively destroyed individuality and ensured compliance in an institution segregated from the outside world. Compliance, by staff and 'inmates', was key to managing large numbers in a limited space with inadequate resources, as in prisons, concentration camps and custodial back wards (Goffman 1961, pp. 8, 119–220).

Psychiatrists and nurses in the hospitals often held unhelpful attitudes about their older patients, with low expectations about improving their health. In 1952, three well-regarded and experienced psychiatrists suggested:

> we must be practical and temper our remedies to the gravity of the situation. It is more economical... to treat—say—60 patients in two wards, than the same number in three wards. We are forced... to overcrowd in the mental hospitals, and senile patients have proved to be the patients least affected by this (Cook et al. 1952, p. 382).

These psychiatrists did not explain how they assessed older people to be the 'least affected', but older people characteristically stoically accepted the care they received and the restrictions placed on them in an institution.

The psychiatrists also did not mention how they ascertained that their patients were 'senile', raising the possibility that some were apathetic associated with undiagnosed depressive illness that could have been actively treated leading to discharge. They stated that they did not advocate a lower standard of care for older people, although it is impossible to see how their proposal to overcrowd wards could be interpreted otherwise.

Nurses on psychiatric wards mainly dealt with physical aspects of care, with a focus on neatness rather than therapy. For older patients they typically provided passive physical care and, fearful of reprimand, would overprotect their patients, such as wheeling them in a chair rather than allowing them to walk unsteadily, and other restrictions that undermined their independence (Whitehead 1970, pp. 26–29). They also removed patients' belongings, such as spectacles, to avoid them being lost or broken (Townsend 1973, pp. 132–135), concerning themselves with the loss of the objects for which they might be reprimanded, rather than on the benefits to the patient. In 1957, an enlightened textbook by Annie Altschul (a psychiatric and general trained nurse, later professor of nursing in Edinburgh) taught about encouraging older patients to lead fulfilling lives either within the hospital or aiming for discharge. Altschul's chapter on 'habit training' optimistically tackled rehabilitating demented patients who had lost skills due to being nursed in bed. She warned that nurses must 'never ... allow patients to deteriorate to the degree to which they did in the past' (Altschul 1957, pp. 131–150, 145). Her teaching was radical in the 1950s: modern geriatric nursing became a compulsory component of training only in 1979 to comply with European Union requirements (Norton 1956, 1988, p. 34).

In understaffed wards, nurses often worked under pressure to complete the practical tasks delegated to them, and time-saving regimes could result in undignified care. Nurses interviewed in Jane Brooks' oral history study recollected lack of privacy, 'open bed-panning' (without screens between beds, visible to all on the ward), and the feeling of nursing a 'body' without being aware of the 'person' (Brooks 2009). Tommy Dickinson (2015, p. 114), in his study of 'mental nurses' in mid-twentieth-century psychiatric hospitals, commented on other harmful practices, including physical force and 'production line' bathing, where several people were bathed speedily at one time in a communal bathroom. One nurse he interviewed told him that 'because it was the norm you didn't question it' (Dickinson 2015, p. 110). The issue of communal bathing is worthy of discussion because it highlights grey areas encountered when deciding whether practices were acceptable or degrading.[9] For standards of institutional care to be humane, they should be appropriate to the age, gender, physical, psychological and cultural needs of the individual. This necessitates modelling them on accepted practices outside the institution at the same time. In their own homes, older people usually bathed in private. Based on their practices before admission, older frail people, some of whom might be embarrassingly soiled due to incontinence, would have likely found the rushed process of communal production line bathing degrading. However, in some other contexts shared bathing was socially acceptable, such as for sports teams, creating a degree of subjectivity. Although some practices were categorically unjust, when techniques acceptable to staff but not to patients passed unchallenged, and were condoned by seniors, they became established as standard care.

Changing practice away from custodial methods towards rehabilitation was difficult to achieve. A cultural conservatism existed in many isolated, inward-looking psychiatric hospitals, which made introducing new practices difficult (Carse et al. 1958). A charge nurse who was previously a miner demonstrated this when he likened his hospital to 'a close knit mining community where relationships are very strong'.[10] In such communities, established traditions and practices may be resistant to criticism and slow to change. In addition, after the Second World War, mental nursing was an attractive occupation for demobilised soldiers, especially those who felt comfortable in a conforming, hierarchical organisational structure (Nolan 1995, p. 13). Thus in some hospitals, almost military hierarchies, consisting of the incontestable and fear-provoking senior nurses plus many inadequately trained staff, reinforced regimented obeying of instructions, inflexibility and task-driven rather than individually focused nursing practices. Patients who conformed to rules were easier to manage and less labour intensive than individuals with personalised programmes of treatment or rehabilitation, thus the rigid system helped maintain a custodial approach. This corroborates the views of one psychiatrist in the 1960s, who recollected some ward-level obstacles to change, when interviewed in 2016:

> So far as the charge nurses were concerned,...[wards] were run by the nurses, they belonged to the nurses, the patients belonged to the nurses, and they felt they were their property, and they wanted people who were reasonably easy to look after, because that made life a lot easier.[11]

Dickinson's analysis revealed punitive aspects of the rigid staff hierarchy: staff disobedience, complaints or questioning of practices, even if trying to introduce more therapeutic regimes, could be, and was, punished by instant dismissal (DHSS 1971, p. 21; Dickinson 2015, pp. 112, 179–199). Other penalties included banishing a nurse to a less prestigious or 'punishment' ward, often one caring for the most impaired older patients (Dickinson 2015, p. 114; Norton 1988, pp. 25–27). Former staff recalled seniors using underhand bullying tactics to 'get rid of oppositional people' or 'make the complainant see the error of his ways' (Dickinson 2015, pp. 183, 185). Most nurses accepted their role, to carry out, uncritically, whatever medical staff or their nursing superiors prescribed. A few took subversive action and maintained their careers, but the overall pattern was of passive obedience (Dickinson 2015, pp. 179–199; Brooks 2009, p. 2768). According to Barton, a regimented approach could not fully succeed as 'kindness, pleasantness, sympathy and forbearance cannot be commanded by giving orders or passing resolutions' (Barton 1967, p. x). Nurse Bill Kirkpatrick (1967, pp. 52, 55) noted that the problem was compounded when the hospital leadership did not fully understand the challenges of nursing older people and showed lack of interest towards patients and staff on the back wards, which contributed to nurses feeling unwanted. He wrote, 'anyone who feels unwanted becomes apathetic towards all those in his care, to say the least'(p. 52).

Social factors also influenced nurses' approach to criticising. They often had a long-term relationship with their hospital. Their relatives worked there and they lived, with their families, in tied accommodation. Antagonising the hospital authorities could risk losing job, home and family life, and according to Abel-Smith, some feared that their children would be beaten up by members of staff against whom they lodged complaints.[12] Junior doctors, as the nurses, had cultural norms concerning challenging their superiors. They could also be victimised if they criticised.[13] However, junior doctors often had short-term contracts, lived outside the hospital and, although they feared a detrimental reference for their next post, were in less personal jeopardy if they spoke up.

Comments made to external independent researchers were likely to have been more honest. In a study by social scientists Kathleen Jones and Roy Sidebotham (1958–1959), student nurses described their experiences in three mental hospitals. On one ward in a large hospital the nurses' role was 'chiefly that of custodian and domestic help' (Jones and Sidebotham 1962, p. 204). Nurses were 'full of genuine care and interest' for their patients but did not seem to understand the important part they could play in helping them with social activities. Patients who exhibited difficult behaviours were treated like naughty children and the ward lacked a 'fundamental attitude of respect towards patients, that they were adult human beings' (p. 204). Nurses feared the sister's wrath if they sat and talked to a patient, or attempted psychological and social therapeutic interventions, because it was considered 'slacking' (p. 203). By contrast, in another hospital in the study, the ward doors were unlocked, and nurses 'acted as friend and companion rather than as warder' and helped the patients to preserve their independence and autonomy (p. 198).

By the early 1950s, many mental hospitals implemented successful open-door policies. Jones referred to this as part of the 'social revolution' of psychiatric treatment, alongside industrial therapy, therapeutic communities, social clubs for patients and other 'normal' activities (Jones 1993, pp. 150–154). Mandelbrote (1964, pp. 268–270) evaluated an open-door policy in his hospital. He found that a therapeutic ward environment that gave patients greater autonomy meant that 'locked doors and physical barriers against escape were no longer necessary.' Incontinence, incidents requiring seclusion, and destructive and impulsive behaviours also declined, to about one fifth, one year after introducing the policy, with minimal increase in absconding, no increase in serious injuries, and reduced use of night sedation (pp. 272–273). By contrast, Friern maintained a policy of locked wards into the 1960s (MoH 1968a, p. 22).

Hospitals usually began to implement liberal policies on wards with patients perceived as most likely to benefit. This strategy was logical because success would build staff confidence and therefore help alter a large institution that was resistant to change. Thus wards for younger patients became hotbeds of innovation, with active treatment and rehabilitation (Martin 1962). Patients perceived as difficult or less likely to benefit, such as older people, were left until last for experimental approaches (Barham 1997, p. 22). This created a two-tier system within the institution. Psychiatrist Brice Pitt (1968, p. 29) wrote:

> Claybury's present reputation rests largely on these units. There are, however, snags, and instead of the whole hospital going on to develop similarly, a sizable split has appeared between these wards where the action is, which get lots of visitors and publicity, and the 'Chronic Hospital' which feels more out of things than in the bad old days when there was little treatment.

Whether the Ministry understood the pitfalls of two-tiers is unclear (Jones and Sidebotham 1962, p. 62) but it added to staff tensions in many hospitals, including Friern.[14] In 1958, Friern opened Halliwick, a separate treatment and rehabilitation hospital in the grounds. It was better staffed than the main hospital and there were no long-stay patients. Only 5 percent of admissions were older than sixty-five years of age, compared to 23 percent in the main hospital.[15] Staff in the main hospital perceived Halliwick as attracting the 'cream' of the staff, the most 'rewarding' patients and better resources.[16] Few staff crossed the metaphorical fence between them.[17] When Barbara discussed the two-tier system with Richard Crossman in 1969, she told him that she declined Friern's suggestion that she should visit Halliwick because she had received reports about it from the family of a peer's wife. Crossman responded that 'it would probably be impossible to get into Halliwick unless you are at least a peer's wife' and it staggered him 'that this could be allowed under socialism'.[18]

Secondary historical sources rarely mention complications associated with the two-tiers. Progress towards community care is celebrated, while those patients who were most disabled and mainly older remained in the hospitals as late as the 1990s and are hardly mentioned. Peter Barham wrote about the resettlement of long-stay patients to the community, mentioning one study about the most mentally disabled and hardest to discharge long-stay patients, which, curiously, excluded people with dementia (Barham 1997, p. 22). This hardly clarified the issues as they related to older people. Antipsychiatry, which emphasised personal autonomy and criticised the way society defined mental illness through social, political and legal means, also affected hospital practice in the 1960s. It particularly encouraged rehabilitation programmes and more liberal care regimes, but it too overlooked older people. A handful of antipsychiatry writers, psychiatrists among them, advocated primarily for younger mentally ill people. For example, RD Laing and Aaron Esterson (1964, pp. 31–264) described patients under forty years of age, mainly with schizophrenia, and Goffman (1961, 1963) hardly mentioned older people in his monographs on discrimination and institutionalisation despite their increasing presence in psychiatric hospitals. Any influence of antipsychiatry on services for older people was incidental to its main objectives.

Social scientists documented, and attempted to improve, care for older people. In Townsend's (1965) chapter 'Prisoners of neglect', he noted that levels of function of many older people on back wards were similar to those in local authority care homes, suggesting that they did not need specific psychiatric hospital placement. Townsend also reported boredom, uniform haircuts and disrespect for personal identity on the back wards. Some older people on these wards were very lucid, but had hearing, visual or speech impediments, and staff labelled them as mentally impaired. Many lacked aids that could enable communication and improve function. Deplorably,

> A considerable number possess capacities and skills which are held in check or even stultified. Staff sometimes do not recognise their patients' abilities, though more commonly they do not have time to cater for them (Townsend 1965, p. 229).

Many older people were trapped in psychiatric hospitals because of lack of more appropriate alternatives, including geriatric medical wards, domiciliary support and residential care homes. With older people's needs straddling health and social care, the authorities argued about which of them should take financial responsibility for providing support, rather than ensure the most appropriate use of resources (Means and Smith 1985, p. 173).

Townsend criticised the authorities for hiding the worst aspects of the psychiatric hospitals when, in his view, the defects were remediable. Although hospital conditions for older people were by no means uniform, his negative experiences lingered:

> It is not just the appearance, the coarseness to the touch, the noise or the impenetrable silence but the smell of neglect that remains imprinted on the mind: the sweet but slightly rotting smell of an assortment of bewildered human beings who exist in claustrophobic proximity like wrinkling apples spaced fractionally apart in a dark cupboard (Townsend 1965, p. 135).

Wards and Community: Getting the Balance Right

Ward environments were often inadequate, but many domestic dwellings were also impoverished, especially in urban areas. Doctors visiting patients in Birmingham in 1949 described some homes as 'dark, infested slums' (Thomson 1950, pp. 930–931). A survey in Glasgow in the late 1950s, where housing was particularly bad, indicated that 'in spite of housing difficulties, almost all the old people we met had no desire to make a change and any suggestions to this end were usually met with hostility' (Thomson 1959, p. 447). Older people perceived the hospitals as institutions with the stigma of workhouses and asylums. Their own homes, though poor and lacking in facilities, were more than buildings. They contained personal possessions and memories that contributed to the occupier's sense of identity, security, self-esteem and perceived roles in their family and community (Macmillan 1960). Long-term hospital admission deprived older people of these assets, but their wishes were often not acknowledged. Wealthier older people could choose to stay in their own homes, but poorer people usually had no choice and little was done, such as through welfare schemes, to enable them to do so (Harvey 1965). Community welfare provision was insufficient in many places. John Welshman (1996 p. 89), in his study of public health and older people, concluded that stagnation, patchiness and haphazard local authority social care was common, associated with financial constraints, and that central government encouraged, rather than insisted, that services were provided.

According to psychiatrist Cecil Kidd (1962a, p. 457) younger people were admitted to hospital because they needed treatment for their illness, whereas older people were admitted because 'either they cannot be treated *or cannot be tolerated at home*' (italics in original). Thus for some older people assumed to have no hope of recovery, who could not be supported at home by their families and for whom no alternatives existed, psychiatric hospitals were 'dumping grounds' (Strabolgi 1965; DHSS 1972, pp. 20–21). Assumptions about irreversible decline were associated with older people bypassing the hospital assessment wards and being admitted directly to long-stay psychiatric wards (Robinson 2009, pp. 9–10). This precluded thorough medical assessment, so remediable physical illness, which in older people could be masked by mental disturbance ('acute confusion' or 'delirium'), would remain undiagnosed and untreated. This relationship was known to general practitioners (GPs) in the 1950s: 'The noisy, restless, agitated old person will often die if moved to a mental hospital' (Batt 1949; Taylor 1954, p. 414).

Evidence accumulated from the 1940s about the need to support families caring for an older person to prevent them despairing and giving up, but little was done to remedy the situation (Rowntree 1947; Sheldon 1948). Families were often 'unreasonably willing' to provide care at home (Lowther and Williamson 1966, p. 1460) but a sudden deterioration in an older person's level of confusion 'nearly always precipitates a crisis in the patient's family' (Anderson 1956, p. 343), the final straw for a family lacking practical support and without emotional reserve to cope with additional stress. Townsend reiterated the need for more support for older people living alone, and for families caring for them, to prevent 'dumping' (Townsend 1962, pp. 106–108, 1965, p. 233).

GPs held the key to community medical and nursing resources and to hospital services. Stephen Taylor (later, Lord Taylor of Harlow), a physician, investigated thirty outstanding general practices, aiming to depict practice worthy of adoption elsewhere. Taylor noted diverse views about older people. Some GPs thought that, with time and patience, working with them could be rewarding. Others viewed them as 'difficult, and even unpleasant...often inarticulate, hard to get to know, and slow to respond' (Taylor 1954, p. 413). One husband and wife GP team, Cuthbert and Beatrice Watts, wrote gloomily that 'senile dementia' (*sic*) is common in the 'last decade of life', 'Nothing can be done for these unfortunate people' and older people 'can be most difficult and trying' (Watts and Watts 1952, pp. 140,145). Some GPs were aware of the need to support families, but others thought it best to advise them that providing care 'can only have an adverse effect on their own lives, without benefiting the patient's in the slightest', and because 'no additional help can be sufficient to make it bearable', admission to long-stay care was preferable (Gibson 1957, p. 111). Conveniently for GPs, this fitted with psychiatrists' views that their hospitals had an obligation to fulfil GPs' requests 'to admit the elderly dementing type of patients from the catchment area'.[19] Psychiatrists genuinely tried to help older people by admitting them when they had nowhere else to go and no one to help them with the essentials of daily life,[20] but neither GPs nor psychiatrists were keen to actively work with them (Watts and Watts 1952, p. 140). Tensions existed between GPs and the psychiatric hospitals, as David Enoch, a consultant psychiatrist at Shelton Hospital, Shrewsbury, described in the early 1960s:

> GPs used to ring us up and say: 'An old bird is on the way to you.' Sometimes we were lucky if we even had a message at all! When we went round in the week we were told that there were three people over 80 that had been 'pushed in.' The matron and the chief male nurse just had to find a bed. These patients merely appeared. I have great respect for the local authority and those trying to deal with the chronic sick – but Shelton was the 'dumping ground' for this county. I think the hospital deserves a medal.[21]

Webster noted that GPs perpetuated adverse assumptions of the irreversibility of the problems of old age (Webster 1991a, p. 181). GPs' comments suggested lack of motivation to attempt to improve community psychiatric care for older people, or lack of understanding that it might be possible. How widespread those attitudes were is unclear, but they indicate the depth of pessimism that needed to be overcome to provide psychiatric care in the community.

Research and Innovation: Challenging Medical Doctrine About Older People

In the 1940s, some psychiatrists in Britain began to challenge the medical profession's clinical negativity towards mentally unwell older people. One surveyed his older patients, concluding that their mental illnesses were not inevitable, that depressive illness could be distinguished from dementia and that interventions could help (Post 1944). Successful treatment of depressed older people using the new electroconvulsive therapy (ECT) (Mayer-Gross 1945, p. 101) and evidence that social interventions could prevent admission and enable discharge of confused older people (Lewis and Goldschmidt 1943) surprised the clinicians.

In 1950, the Bethlem and Maudsley Hospital in South London was the only mental hospital in the country to have a psychiatrist working specifically with older people—Felix Post. He aimed to diagnose their illnesses accurately and actively to treat depression, schizophrenia and other disorders. He achieved good results (Hilton 2007). Post's work was reinforced by Martin Roth's meticulous study (1955), which demonstrated conclusively that the practice of labelling all 'confused' older people as having irreversible 'senile dementia' was obsolete. He identified five psychiatric disorders in its place, of which delirium, depressive illness and 'late paraphrenia'[22] were particularly important because they were often reversible. The medical profession paid little attention to Post's and Roth's findings, which challenged time-honoured teaching and the common stereotypes of old age (Robinson 2009, p. 8; World Health Organisation 1959, p. 10). Failing to take heed of their discoveries prolonged unnecessary suffering. Psychiatrist Anthony 'Tony' Whitehead (1974), commented:

> Old people may spend their last years in dreadful misery because severe depression has been wrongly diagnosed as senile decay.... If you are anxious and depressed, and more and more people start treating you as if you were a

difficult child, and you are finally incarcerated in a ward full of other elderly people who are being treated in the same way, it is likely that in time you will give up and take on the role of not just a child, but a baby.

The new ideas about older people's mental illness emerged in tandem with geriatric medicine (Warren 1943). Geriatric medicine had a slow start, and in the 1950s, geriatricians were few and far between. In general hospitals without them, consultant physicians often resisted admitting older people because they feared that these patients' illnesses were chronic, and that they would remain in hospital and 'block beds' (Howell 1951, p. 505). Brice Pitt recollected in an oral history interview about his experience as a junior doctor in the 1950s:

> Even my very good mentor had the attitude that a good registrar did not admit an old person. A bad registrar did...
>
> The hospital...was like a castle, a good registrar would fend off the elderly, as those who got in were bound to stay, bound to be dumped by their family.[23]

The general hospital consultants held disproportionate power in local hospital hierarchies, so a GP's request for admission to their hospital could be rejected on the basis of the patient's age, before the hospital made a clinical assessment. Admission to a psychiatric hospital was often the only alternative.

Sometimes geriatricians, notably, Lionel Cosin in Oxford, attempted to treat and support older people suffering from mental illness (Anon. 1954). Cosin's innovations included a day hospital plus respite beds to help families undertaking long-term care. However, the local psychiatrists' priorities mainly concerned younger patients, and they were often unsupportive of him.[24] In Cosin's view, and that of other eminent geriatricians,[25] psychiatrists were clinically inept with older people, an attitude unlikely to promote collaboration.

Geriatricians had plenty to do in general hospitals and rarely worked in mental hospitals, and most psychiatrists had little enthusiasm to implement the principles of geriatric medicine (Denham 2004, p. 357). One nurse in 1967 gave her view of the attitude of many psychiatrists towards older people: 'Oh! They're just Anno Domini, any old thing will do.'[26] This might have allowed interested psychiatrists carte blanche to work with older people. However, such freedom was moderated by complex interactions in the psychiatric hospitals, such as weighting the salaries of some senior hospital staff by the number of beds standing,[27] which would not incentivise rehabilitation and discharge. Nevertheless, in 1958, psychiatrist Ronald 'Sam' Robinson established a proactive, assessment and rehabilitation-based psychiatric service specifically for older people, at Crichton Royal Hospital, Scotland, which gradually inspired practice south of the border (Bergmann 2009; Gulland 2014). It comprised outpatient, domiciliary, in-patient (including respite) and community services. Sam Robinson incorporated principles of geriatric medicine into his psychiatric wards, which contrasted with practices observed in the 1960s at Friern and in other hospitals. He took into account, for example, that incontinence was unintentional and was associated with toilet facilities at a distance and poor mobility and that regular toileting minimised daytime incontinence, even for people with dementia. At Crichton Royal, good-quality flooring and shoes encouraged mobility and minimised falls, occupational therapy reduced agitation and 'wandering', men and women shared the same wards and wore their own clothes, and staff found that respecting the patients' dignity and wishes gained their cooperation. Sam Robinson achieved high discharge rates compared to other hospitals (Robinson 1965), demonstrating what could be achieved, even for incurable disorders such as dementia. Unfortunately, the Ministry of Health oversaw the NHS only in England and Wales, so Sam Robinson's scheme was outside their watch. Evidence is lacking that they sought to find out more about it when results were published.

In 1961, inspired by the scheme at Crichton Royal, Barton and Whitehead, introduced similar plans at Severalls Hospital.[28] Severalls' service operated on the principle that older people should remain in their own homes as long as possible and that admission was primarily short-term for active treatment. The total number of beds used by older in-patients fell by a quarter (374 to 296) over sixteen months, despite more brief admissions for assessment and treatment (Whitehead 1965). Barton and Whitehead helped staff overcome deeply embedded unhelpful attitudes towards older people, including lack of interest, infantilising approaches to dependency (such as referring to patients in cot beds as 'babies') and harsh undignified criticism ('You filthy old thing. I shall smack you if you do that again') (Whitehead 1970, p. 28). The Ministry attributed the scheme's success to local circumstances rather than envisioning wider application and encouraging its adoption elsewhere (Brothwood 1971, p. 110). Barton and Whitehead also encouraged older people to have a say in their care, acknowledging that 'doctors and nurses do not necessarily know best' (Whitehead 1970, p. 35). This concurred with Cohen's (1964) observations, that the paternalistic style of the NHS had not yet adopted values centred on patient autonomy and individuality.

Several well-constructed epidemiological studies in the early 1960s indicated scope to improve the mental health of older people, avoid admission to hospital and alleviate the stresses on families caring for them (Kay et al. 1957, 1964a, 1964b). Recommendations included health and welfare services complementing the work of GPs, housing schemes for older people and appropriate social and recreational facilities. Registers of vulnerable older people could facilitate assessments to help detect mental and physical disorders at an early stage and provide treatment and support (Kay et al. 1964b, p. 681). This was important because GPs were often unaware of disabilities, depression and dementia. Although GPs' expectations and knowledge were crucial to awareness, other contributory factors included older people and their families not reporting ailments to their GPs, and, linked to age stereotypes, attributing symptoms to age rather than treatable illness and assuming that nothing could be done to help. Thus under-diagnosis and treatment was associated with avoidable and neglected illness that contributed to crises and emergency hospital admissions (Williamson et al. 1964). Post, Roth, Cosin, Sam Robinson, Whitehead and Barton demonstrated what could be achieved, but they were a minority. More common was the fear of the 'looming geriatric impasse' (Kingston 1963) and the assumption, based on demographic change and increasing demand, that it would be impossible to prevent overcrowding the hospitals. To achieve widespread active treatment and rehabilitation for older people required: a culture shift among GPs, doctors and other staff in psychiatric and general hospitals; higher expectations by the public of what could be achieved; and support from central government.

The Government's Standpoint

William Beveridge's (1942, p. 92) proposals for the welfare state included older people, but lacked enthusiasm, precision or a sense of priority about them. Nevertheless, Minister of Health Aneurin Bevan stated optimistically in the House of Commons in 1947: 'The workhouse is to go.' In their place, a five-year goal was set to achieve better domiciliary support to enable older people to remain longer in their own homes, and to provide small attractive community residential units each accommodating twenty to thirty people.[29] The leadership did not enforce provision, a pattern of failed implementation for older people's services recognised before the NHS (Webster 1991a, p. 166). Webster (p. 188) noted that 'the elderly bore their disappointment with dignity, and general public indignation was slow to materialise.' Some doctors and administrative authorities blamed older people for the inadequacy of hospital and community services: beds were 'blocked by cured cases' (MoH 1957, p. 27), reflecting the 'burden of those old people' (Bickford 1955). Postwar austerity complicated planning, and demographic predictions created unease about the effect of older people on the economy and how the country would provide for them (Political and Economic Planning 1948). Ominous speculations surpassed the optimistic (Thane 1990, p. 292). The Royal Commission on Population (1949, p. 113) commented: 'It is the fact that (with some exceptions) the old consume without producing which differentiates them from the active population and makes of them a factor reducing the average standard of living of the community.' Little account was taken of many retired people who continued to contribute to society, by doing voluntary work and supporting their families, friends and neighbours, rather than requiring care.

The complex needs of unwell older people and the families who supported them, required planning and coordination across several professions and at all levels of health and social services administration. This received much discussion during the 1940s, such as by the British Medical Association (BMA) and the NHS mental health specialist advisory committee (Webster 1991b, p. 103). They helped shape two government circulars, *Care of the Aged Suffering from Mental Infirmity* and *Treatment of the Elderly Chronic Sick* (MoH 1950a, 1950b). The circulars recommended joint psychiatric–geriatric assessment schemes, but were noncommittal about funding and did not inspire or entice clinicians into the field. Joint schemes hardly materialised (Hilton 2014; Webster 1991a, p. 178). The titles of the circulars also revealed prevailing attitudes and expectations: passive 'care' for mental disorders compared to active 'treatment' for physical conditions. Assumptions about the need for passive care underpinned other proposals, such as by Donald Johnson, a medically qualified Conservative MP, who described day-care facilities, in a caring and thoughtful manner, as places where older people 'can be parked for two or three days a week'.[30]

The Board of Control expressed ambivalence about modernising mental health services to coincide with proposals for the NHS. Mental health legislation, it said, would need to change first, but that would require a review on the scale of a Royal Commission (Rogers and Pilgrim 1996, p. 65). A Cabinet memorandum in 1950 indicated that Bevan was uneasy about the mental hospitals: some 'are very near to a public scandal and we are lucky that they have not so far attracted more limelight and publicity'.[31] Merrick Winn (1955) wrote in the *Daily Express* that most mental hospitals are 'a disgrace to a nation that calls itself civilised. They [nurses] are doing a magnificent job. But they often do it in conditions in which, had I not seen them, I would not have believed could exist in Britain.' With little public pressure or motivation by the Ministry to back improvements, poor standards persisted.

Postwar, health and social care provision for mental illness and for older people lagged behind other clinical services. Widespread excessively negative beliefs about chronicity, mental illness and old age and increasing demands on the NHS to provide highly technical investigations and treatment for acute physical illnesses, influenced government priorities. 'Cinderella' services became casualties of unremitting retrenchment in the 1950s and victims of broken promises, such as those made in election manifestos (Webster 1991a, p. 188). The UK was not alone in its deliberations, and the World Health Organisation (WHO 1959) issued pragmatic and far-sighted recommendations, influenced by Roth and Post, about mental health and older people. WHO's report, like others from reputable bodies (e.g., National Old People's Welfare Council 1958) created little professional, public or government interest or activity.

Speculative estimates of NHS costs dominated the government's and society's perceptions and discouraged spending (Rowntree 1947, p. 2; Mass Observation 1948). A Commons debate in 1954 estimated that it cost £20 a week to keep a patient in a teaching hospital and £5 a week in a mental hospital. Precise comparisons are difficult because of technological input and higher rates of acute physical illness in the former, but MPs did not raise the possibility that underspending in the mental hospitals might be detrimental.[32] From the government's perspective, fitting more people into mental hospitals was economical. The same year, the title of another government report, *The Economic and Financial Problems of the Provision for Old Age*, hardly indicated impartiality (Phillips 1954). It focussed mainly on social needs but acknowledged that there were more admissions of older people to mental hospitals, often for social rather than health reasons (p. 74). It commented wishfully that 'their discharge rate will also increase in the near future' (p. 9), an assertion attributed to a recent report by the Board of Control. Evidence of that trend beginning was lacking, but citing it unquestioningly supported the committee's objective of minimising expenditure (Webster 1998, pp. 32–33). By contrast, the Guillebaud Report (MoH 1956) on the cost of the NHS indicated that, in the context of relatively stable NHS costs during the previous five years, additional funding for the needs of older people was affordable. It concluded with a much needed but unheeded message, to give older people 'their due priority in the allocation of additional resources' so that they are 'not overlooked amid the pressure of other competing needs' (p. 219). Guillebaud's report was unpalatable to the Conservative government, which expected it to provide evidence of excessive expenditure to enable tighter retrenchment of the NHS (Webster 1998, pp. 32–33).

The attitude that old age was a burden (rather than an achievement to be celebrated) reduced in the late 1950s (Thane 2000, pp. 475, 479). That linked to a persistently higher birth rate, the baby-boomers, some of whom were coming close to school-leaving age and could supplement the workforce to care for older people. This helped diminish the panic of the 'menace' of an ageing population (Thane 1990), but more younger people to care for them also lifted pressure from the government to improve services. With greater prosperity towards the late 1950s, provision for older people changed little: in austerity everyone waited, and when the economy improved, older people waited until last.

At the end of the 1950s in England and Wales, about 300,000 people out of a population of 6.7 million of pensionable age (4.5 percent) lived in institutions of some sort. Approximately 60,000 lived in mental hospital back wards compared to 6,000 in modern purpose-built care homes. Former workhouses housed 30,000; 85,000 lived in geriatric wards of non–mental hospitals; and 120,000 lived in private, charitable and other communal establishments (Townsend 1962, pp. 44, 282). Unwell, frail older people were generally hidden in their homes or in institutions. They were invisible to most people and politically could be ignored. In 1961, the Ministry commented: 'One of the most urgent and complex problems is the care of mentally enfeebled old people.' It 'hoped' that more geriatric–psychiatric links would be forged (MoH 1961, p. 98). That a problem could be described as 'urgent' and the response as 'hope' suggested lack of commitment to resolve it.

Broad plans for the NHS had potential to improve older people's provision. The MHA 1959 permitted modernisation of mental health services, such as relocating them from the psychiatric hospitals into the community and to district general hospitals (DGHs). In 1961, Minister of Health Enoch Powell optimistically addressed a NAMH conference (Powell 1961). He included the well-being of older people, the need to close the psychiatric hospitals and provide more community services and referred to the *Hospital Plan* (MoH 1962), a five-year national scheme for which fresh capital sums were allocated to build DGHs. Powell's *Health and Welfare*, a ten-year plan for community care, lacked dedicated resources or leadership (MoH 1963). Government proposals failed to delineate lines of responsibility for funding, organising and integrating services within the NHS and between the NHS and social welfare authorities, as needed to provide for the most vulnerable older people (Means and Smith 1985, p. 167). Implementation was predictably slow, with lack of direction, and perhaps will, to fulfil commitments to enable older people to remain in their own homes as long as possible.

In 1963, a flurry of activity resulted from an alarming study that found that older people admitted to the wrong sort of hospital—to a psychiatric hospital when they needed physical healthcare and vice versa—had worse prognosis (Kidd 1962b). This rekindled the idea of joint psychiatric–geriatric assessment units. The Ministry drew on its broadly unimplemented guidance issued in 1950,[33] but evidence is lacking that it explored reasons for the failure of the earlier proposals. Dr Geoffrey Tooth, head of mental health at the Ministry was involved in planning for older people. Although he was not always effective (some psychiatrists nicknamed him 'the carious Tooth'[34]) his report in 1964 mentioned the need to prevent older people becoming mentally ill, such as with depression. For admission to psychiatric hospitals, he was aware of the clinical and social dangers:

> a combination of superficial assessment and expediency leads to the filling of mental hospitals with old people whose physical needs are unrecognised and many of whom do not require in-patient treatment. The uprooting of such old people usually exacerbates their mental condition and, once in a mental hospital, it is exceedingly difficult to get them out. Added to which most mental hospitals lack the facilities for the assessment and treatment of the organic conditions that so often complicate or cause mental disorder.[35]

By 1964, every RHB in England except Oxford had some wards of over seventy people (MoH 1968b, p. 11). A Ministry of Health report admitted that 'their sheer size makes it virtually impossible to provide a satisfactory standard of nursing care' (MoH 1968c, p. 52). A memorandum on older people in 1965 reiterated earlier recommendations, such as better collaboration for planning services and joint domiciliary assessment of patients by health and welfare staff to decide the most appropriate place for admission (MoH 1965, p. 4). It did not mention the specific problems in psychiatric hospitals.

Townsend (1962, p. 7) regarded information about the care of older people in official reports as 'extraordinarily scanty and inept' and it 'did not speak much for the importance attached to these services by the central government.' He asked: 'Why, after 12 or 13 years' experience of post-war legislation, are the problems of the aged so insistent and disturbing and so far from amelioration, still less solution?' (Townsend 1961). No answer was forthcoming, but Webster (1991a, p. 166) offered the explanation that, alongside 'the mentally handicapped', as more people survived into old age, they were regarded negatively as part of the dependent 'growing tide of the unfit' about which little could be done.

By the mid-1960s, particularly for older people, underresourcing, understaffing, dilapidated buildings, and stagnation or good intentions hampered by professional and political paralysis, characterised the psychiatric hospitals. Despite evidence from a few places that improvements were possible, negativity towards unwell older people, and expectations that their demand on NHS resources would increase overwhelmingly, compounded the difficulties. In the competition for NHS resources, mentally unwell older people never reached top priority.

Introducing Friern Hospital

Many of the broader concerns described earlier set the backdrop for the circumstances that shocked Barbara Robb in 1965 when she first visited Friern (Fig. 2.1). The rest of this chapter explores some of the issues at Friern directly pertinent to the AEGIS campaign and *Sans Everything*. It focusses on older people on the back wards, especially facilities, personal possessions, activities and staffing, but it draws on evidence about younger people or the entire hospital when necessary. Most information about Friern was obtained from HMC and RHB archives, but General Nursing Council (GNC) inspections, to licence the nurse-training school, provide an independent source.[36] Another valuable autonomous perspective was given by Malcolm Campbell in an oral history interview in 2015. He worked as a locum junior doctor at Friern from November 1964 until

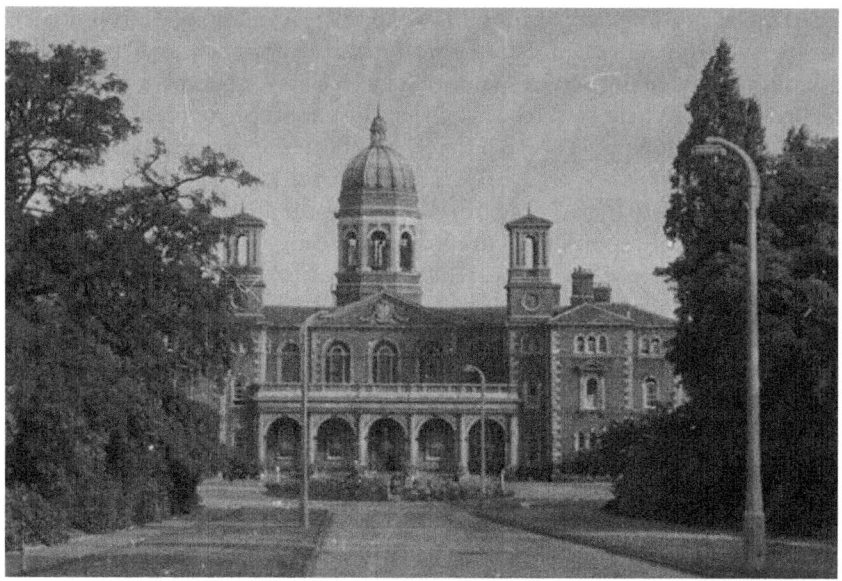

Fig 2.1 Friern Hospital, 1957. Photograph by Karl Ruge, reproduced courtesy of Friern Barnet and District Local History Society.

March 1965, between training posts in neurology, his chosen career. He worked in no other psychiatric hospitals so his recollections relate solely to Friern. His first impressions, vivid fifty years later, were of horror, 'Bedlam', or 'a dumping ground', which provided custodial care and where little medicine was practiced.[37]

The HMC faced numerous challenges. Second World War bombing destroyed five of the six villas in the grounds and damaged the main building, contributing significantly to overcrowding of patients and to Friern's dilapidated state. Friern was not alone in suffering in this way, but other hospitals affected, such as Claybury and the Bethlem, modernised their clinical work significantly more than Friern, despite structural limitations.[38] In 1959, the GNC compared its findings to those in 1951, noting some environmental improvements, such as 1,500 new beds and 'plastic curtains giving a degree of privacy in bathrooms'. It also reported difficulties, including severe overcrowding and lack of storage space for patients' belongings so that 'day clothes are made into bundles at night' rather than being stored in bedside lockers.[39] Lack of storage space meant lack of personal possessions, which could affect self-esteem, behaviour and rehabilitation (Barton 1959, p. 41). In 1963, the GNC made some positive comments, noting more lockers, pictures and plants, to make wards more home like. Many male patients had their own clothes,[40] although female patients still wore hospital clothes, which Campbell described as 'very much a pre-war poor-house style.' Another positive factor was the opening of new facilities in the grounds the same year, for social activities and for patients to have refreshments with their visitors at visiting time.[41]

In 1964–1965 the HMC acknowledged overcrowding and lack of personal possessions. Some wards had up to 90 beds. On some wards, all patients had lockers, on others, none.[42] To provide space for every patient to have a locker, 195 more beds would have to close.[43] The HMC also recorded that about eight older people sustained fractures each month, mainly due to falls, more than in comparable psychiatric hospitals. Adequate nursing supervision and good-quality flooring and footwear could have prevented falls,[44] as Sam Robinson (1965, pp. 188–190) found at Crichton Royal. Inspections revealed inadequate facilities for personal care and privacy, such as patients' toilet doors without locks.[45] Ward E3, where Amy Gibbs spent a year, had no heating in the large, communal bathroom, hardly ideal for bathing dependent older, frail people, although the ward sister 'in charge of the ward for some years...had no complaint about lack of warmth.'[46] This was alarming, considering that the HMC noted punishingly low ward temperatures at night,[47] and Campbell remembered seeing urine frozen in a bed pan. Hospital hygiene was also poor. In 1965 the hospital suffered a typhoid outbreak (Anon. 1965). Typhoid spreads only in environments where human faeces or urine come into contact with food or drinking water. Campbell recalled 'a fairly strong smell, urine, faeces, or perhaps of disinfectant [and] when I went home at night I would feel the need to have a wash and totally change my clothes because it was all pervading'.[48]

Student nurse recruitment was difficult. Much nurse training comprised direct patient care on the wards, so nursing school underrecruitment meant understaffed wards, resulting in excessively busy trained staff and lack of teaching and supervision for students. Promising students were disenchanted by the training received at Friern, some preferring to become bus conductors.[49] In 1951 the GNC noted a 'great wastage amongst female students': fifty of the sixty-eight who entered training in 1950 left within a year,[50] significantly worse than the usual one third dropping out of training in general hospitals (Lyth 1988, p. 45). In 1963, the GNC inspected one geriatric ward with forty-five patients, average age eighty-four years, staffed during the day by one qualified nursing sister, three unqualified nursing assistants and one ward orderly. Nursing tasks included personal care, serving meals, washing up, cleaning and administration, so there was little time available to interact meaningfully with patients. Some practices were unsafe, such as dispensing medication from memory without referring to written prescription cards.[51]

In 1965, the HMC commissioned expert help to ascertain reasons for nursing shortages. Two surveys were undertaken, one on the 'female side' and another on the 'male side'. Miss Craig, a researcher from the King Edward's Hospital Fund (later, King's Fund, an independent charity working to improve health and care in England) asked nurses and doctors on twenty-three female wards why they thought the hospital was short of nursing staff. She was unaccompanied by senior staff, in whose presence juniors might have been unwilling to criticise, but it is unclear whether she spoke to nurses in groups or individually, which could also have affected their answers. Overall, discontent was common and mutual. Doctors criticised nurses for low standards, and nurses complained about lack of medical attention for patients on the back wards. Nurses disliked working on understaffed wards and those with poor facilities. Understaffing meant less attention for patients, who consequently stayed longer and increased the overcrowding, which made the hospital a less desirable place to work and undermined recruitment. Senior staff criticised 'The calibre of student nurses in mental hospitals to-day' who had no sense of ambition or vocation and who 'only come into hospital to have a roof over their heads and some money in their pockets',[52] a hostile attitude that would hardly entice them in.

The HMC feared that Craig's report, and a similar one on the male side, would generate unfavourable publicity, damage their reputation and further discourage recruitment. They therefore concealed the full reports, alleging that some conclusions were based on 'misapprehension or lack of knowledge of the situation'[53] or 'false information'.[54] Deliberate distortion by independent researchers was unlikely, and the HMC did not reveal how they reached their conclusions. Condemning parts of the reports was easy compared to dealing with the problems. There is no evidence that the

HMC used the reports constructively to exert pressure on the RHB to allocate more money or as tools to stimulate thought about how to reverse the trends.

A memorandum from the Ministry (MoH 1964, pp. 1–4) on improving psychiatric services recommended more outpatient clinics, day services and community resources and emphasised rehabilitation, with patients having suitable occupation, their own clothes and greater privacy and autonomy, such as deciding when to go to bed. It placed little emphasis on hospital buildings, in accordance with plans for closing them and moving services to DGHs and into the community. It also noted the gradually widening chasm between standards in the best and the worst psychiatric hospitals. It required HMCs to inform their RHBs about recent and proposed improvements. Most psychiatric hospitals within the North West Metropolitan region responded with patient-focused plans for therapy and rehabilitation. Friern HMC, however, outlined rudimentary needs:

> Upgrading of existing lavatory and sanitary accommodation has been dealt with over the years, but new standards are constantly being set. In the 50 wards of this hospital there are no low level suites and the old fashioned type of chain-pull cistern continues to exist.... not in the bulk of the ward lavatories is there a washhand basin.... Half-doors to the lavatories have been replaced in many wards with a modern door.[55]

The HMC's grumble that 'new standards are constantly being set' gave the impression that it considered that making basic improvements was burdensome. The medical superintendent, Isaac Sutton, appeared indifferent to the inadequacies. Campbell contrasted him with Barton: 'Sutton was the absolute opposite, [wanted] the quiet life and didn't want to make any disruption or say boo to a goose really, and that was one of the big problems with Friern, why it lagged behind and didn't change.'[56] Apathy and resignation from Sutton and the HMC, and the 'vicious cycle where apathy hinders staff recruitment' were consistent with the hurdles to improvement that the memorandum envisaged in some hospitals (MoH 1964, p. 6). Barbara also detected Friern's fatalistic attitudes, when, early in her campaign, she spoke with HMC member Rose Hacker. Hacker doubted whether the recruitment cycle could be broken so Barbara informed her about hospitals where it had been. Hacker replied: 'It's all very well for them. They've all got really good senior medical staff.'[57]

PATIENTS AND COMPLAINTS AT FRIERN

Generally, patients in the 1960s accepted NHS care uncritically (Cartwright 1964, pp. 8, 203) but occasionally complaints reached the RHB and the Ministry. Examining complaints can shed light on standards of clinical practice and administrative procedures, such as how the authorities responded to the complainant and proposed to remedy the situation to avoid similar incidents in the future. At Friern, reports of good practice to balance against the complaints were not identified in archives or oral sources, although amid her criticisms, Barbara praised two helpful and empathetic ward sisters (Robb 1967, pp. 91, 102–103).

In April 1964, one complaint concerned an older man who sustained rib fractures while being looked after by nurses. His son, a senior academic at the University of London, wrote that the ward had a 'para-military atmosphere', that wearing clothes from a pool was depersonalising and that it was 'increasingly difficult [for staff] to treat people as individual human beings'. The staff were humane but the work atmosphere and environment were unacceptable. The complainant offered to talk to the HMC about his concerns rather 'than weigh in on an undiscriminating public campaign'.[58] The HMC minutes contain the written complaint but lack evidence of action to improve the situation. Perhaps pressure from a 'public campaign' might have achieved more.

Another complaint in 1964 related to alleged violence towards a patient named Bob. Staff told the family that he had fallen out of bed, but Bob's brother Fred noted that 'Bob would not tell me anything no matter how I tried to get it out of him but it looked to me that he had a wallop from somebody.' The family also complained about his belongings going missing, for which the staff blamed Bob: he was absentminded, left his belongings lying about or gave them away.[59] The family was distraught about his ongoing care: 'no social life, no change of scene, just an overcrowded ward, unsuitable company, drugged and in bed by 7.30 to 8 o'clock every night, sometimes earlier.'[60] Bob's sister, Mrs Dickens, described him as 'a frightened crushed man due to the treatment he has received in this hospital'. She also described one occasion after she took him out and returned with him to the ward, that just after she left 'I heard my brother cry out "Leave go of my arm!" and then I looked through a slit in the side of a curtain on the ward door, and my brother was then pushed and was staggering along the corridor trying to keep his balance.' She reported this but received no adequate explanation.[61]

Mrs Dickens contacted the RHB. The Board replied that Bob's illness, rather than his care, was the cause of her unhappiness, that he experienced 'delusions and is apt to make up stories about imaginary happenings', and that the consultant thought his mental illness explained his allegations about being attacked by another patient.[62] No change in his care took place in response to her letters.[63] Negative responses stopped Mrs Dickens complaining: 'I dare not complain any more about anything as I have already been called a "Paranoid case"'. After Mrs Dickens involved her MP, the hospital offered to transfer Bob to Hill End Hospital, St Albans, within the same region, but inaccessible by public transport from where she lived in Muswell Hill.[64] As Bob's only regular visitor, she refused the offer: she could not manage the thrity-mile round trip for each visit instead of the two-mile local bus ride.

Campbell recollected another complaint about a married middle-aged woman with multiple sclerosis who developed disturbed behaviour. She was put into a seclusion room that had a mattress on the floor and no heating. The family

> kicked up a tremendous stink, which, I might say was reinforced by us as doctors. We were keen for them to kick up a stink with the superintendent at the time, MPs and everyone else, about these *terrible* conditions.... We saw it as a wedge in the door for getting things changed.[65]

The hospital authorities removed the patient to another institution. In Campbell's view, the hospital responded by: 'Sweeping it under the carpet... shift the problem onto somebody else. Back to the quiet life.'

In this small sample, the hospital authorities were evasive, blamed the complainant and the patient, and provided no convincing evidence that the criticisms were investigated or attempts made to remedy deficits. In two cases, the authorities aimed to appease the family by offering to move the patient to another hospital, with the effect of removing the complainant without dealing with the underlying causes that initiated their grievances.

Comment

A handful of psychiatrists, geriatricians and social scientists, beginning in the 1940s, demonstrated that older people's mental health and well-being could improve with better diagnosis, treatment, rehabilitation and social support. Many doctors overlooked this evidence, which contradicted established teaching and confounded stereotypical low expectations of well-being in old age. Compounding this, rigid hierarchical management in many psychiatric hospitals resisted change and punished staff who criticised disrespectful treatment and care regimes. In a few hospitals with dynamic and supportive leadership, therapeutic environments for older people began to emerge, but these innovative and effective models of psychiatric treatment and care were hardly replicated. Pressure for change in psychiatric hospitals from the antipsychiatry movement hardly touched older people, for whom, in the 1960s, lobbying was largely concerned with poverty, pensions, social welfare and employment rights, rather than with health (Thane 2010, pp. 13–14, 22).

Government plans and recommendations had the potential to improve services for older people, including Bevan's five-year plan to close the workhouses and improve community support, Guillebaud's proposal to spend more on services for older people, and Powell's long-term, time-bound plans. However, recommendations for older people were permissive, lacked dedicated funding, clear lines of responsibility and sense of direction; and implementation was negligible in the broader context of competition for resources and NHS and welfare priorities. Older people and their families were frequently resigned to chronic impairment and decline with increasing age and rarely complained if services were inadequate. The Ministry used a simple economic plan of presumed cheapest provision for older people's custodial care, rather than genuinely exploring alternatives, in particular, that improving their health, preventing admission and enabling discharge might prove clinically possible, cheaper and more humane. In the twenty-first century, as in the 1960s, compared to services for younger people, older people's psychiatric provision lags behind, with inequitable allocation of revenue, despite evidence of benefit from interventions (Faculty 2011).

Friern's HMC swept complaints under the carpet and removed the need for the RHB or the Ministry to ask searching questions about the quality of services provided. An 'undiscriminating public campaign', which one complainant mentioned but did not undertake, might have had more impact than his private letter to the HMC, given the HMC's fear of negative publicity about their hospital and the broader lack of public, political and professional understanding of the psychiatric hospitals and what could be done to improve them. At Friern, little changed, but in November 1965, at the start of Barbara's campaign, the RHB informed the HMC that standards were inadequate and the hospital was under greater scrutiny than most.[66]

Notes

1. North West Metropolitan Regional Hospital Board (NWMRHB), Board meeting, 13 November 1967, 11 (London Metropolitan Archives, LMA).
2. Malcolm Campbell, interview by author, 2015.
3. Figures are for England and Wales; New Southgate Group Hospital Management Committee (NSGHMC) minutes, 23 July 1964, 5799. At Friern, women over sixty occupied 60 percent of beds on the female side, one third of them age over seventy (LMA).
4. Others included TP Rees (Warlingham Park, Surrey) and Duncan Macmillan (Nottingham).
5. Robb, note of phone call with Rose Hacker, 1966, AEGIS/1/3 (AEGIS archive, London School of Economics).
6. Anne Shearer: journalist, including at the *Guardian*. Reported on Harperbury Hospital. Learning disability campaigner and Jungian analyst. Member of Davies Committee, 1971–1973. Interview by author, 2015.
7. Robb, citing NAMH newsletter, June 1965, AEGIS/1/4.
8. Final report, meeting, Robb and Tooth, 25 May 1965, AEGIS/1/1.
9. United Nations, *Universal Declaration of Human Rights* (1948). Article 5: 'No one shall be subjected to torture or to cruel, inhuman or degrading treatment or punishment.'
10. South West Thames Regional Health Authority, 'Report of Committee of Enquiry, St Augustine's Hospital, Chartham, Canterbury' 1976, typescript, 3–4 (Royal College of Psychiatrists Archives).
11. Anon psychiatrist, interview by author, 2016.
12. Memo, Abel-Smith to Mottershead, 'Report of working group on complaints procedures', 6 August 1969, 154/3/DH/46/1 (University of Warwick Modern Records Centre, UWMRC).
13. Letter, André Masters to Russell Barton, 12 December 1970, AEGIS/1/10/B.
14. Blofeld, Ann. 1965. 'Report of the committee of inquiry on Friern Hospital' (Blofeld Report), 14. NWMRHB, Mental Health Committee, minutes and papers, 7 January 1966 (LMA).
15. An average of 17 percent across the region's psychiatric hospitals. NWMRHB, Mental Health Committee, minutes and papers, 18 March 1963, 5 (LMA).
16. Blofeld Report, 14.
17. Malcolm Campbell, interview by author, 2015.
18. Meeting, Robb and Crossman, 12 November 1969, AEGIS/6/16.

19. NSGHMC minutes, 23 July 1964, 5799 (LMA).
20. Malcolm Campbell, interview by author, 2015.
21. David Enoch, Discussion, 26–27 in JC Barker, Mabel Miller, 'The problem of the chronic psychiatric patients', Shelton Hospital, post graduate education programme, 14 December 1967, AEGIS/2/3.
22. Similar to schizophrenia.
23. Brice Pitt, psychogeriatrician, interviewed by Margot Jefferys, 1991 (BLSA).
24. Crossman Diaries, September 1968 (Visit to Littlemore and Cowley Road hospitals) 152/JH/68/86-87 (UWMRC).
25. George Adams, geriatrician, interviewed by Anthea Holmes, 1991 (BLSA).
26. Phyllis Rowe, AEGIS meeting, 16 March 1967, 12, AEGIS/B/2.
27. Carrick McDonald, 'A rehabilitation programme for chronic psychogeriatric patients', 1977, 3 (Tom Arie's archives).
28. Russell Barton, interviewed by Diana Gittins, 1995, transcript, 14, WL/GC/244/2/19 (Wellcome Library).
29. 'National Assistance Bill' *Hansard* HC Deb 24 November 1947, vol 444 cc.1603–1716.
30. 'Chronic Sick and Elderly (Services)' *Hansard* HC Deb 29 November 1957, 578, cc.1443–1525.
31. Aneurin Bevan, 'NHS Control of Expenditure (England and Wales), Memorandum by the Minister of Health' 10 March 1950, 3, CAB129/38/31 (The National Archives, TNA).
32. 'Mentally Sick (Care and Accommodation)' *Hansard* HC Deb 19 February 1954, 523 cc.2293–2379.
33. Memo, DS Todd-White to Dr Shaw, RHB (50)26, 29 April 1963, MH160/95 (TNA).
34. Information from David Jolley, 2015.
35. Memo, Geoffrey Tooth, 18 November 1964, 'Care of old people in hospitals and welfare homes', MH160/95 (TNA).
36. GNC, New Southgate: Friern Hospital, inspections 1948–1972, DT33/768 (TNA).
37. Malcolm Campbell, interview by author, 2015.
38. Letter, Felix Post to secretary of Medical Committee, 13 October 1949, GPD31/49, MCD73/49 (Bethlem and Maudsley Hospital Archives).
39. GNC, Friern Hospital, March 1959, DT33/768 (TNA).
40. GNC, Friern Hospital, 1963, DT33/768 (TNA).
41. Blofeld Report, 4.
42. NSGHMC, agenda papers, 'Survey of bed accommodation at Friern Hospital with recommendations for the reduction of overcrowding to an acceptable level', November 1964 (LMA).
43. NWMRHB, mental health committee, minutes and papers, 26 April 1965 (LMA).

44. NSGHMC, minutes, 26 March 1964, 5598 (LMA).
45. Friern joint consultative staffs committee, 11 June 1964, J1092 (LMA).
46. NSGHMC, minute book, 'Ward E3 – Bathroom Heating', 28 October 1965, 6266 (LMA); Robb, 'Record of a campaign' vol. 1, 3, Aegis/1/1; Many family houses did not have heating in the bedrooms or bathroom at this time.
47. NSGHMC, minutes, 27 February 1964, 5609 (LMA).
48. Malcolm Campbell, interview by author, 2015.
49. GNC, Friern Hospital, 20 February 1948, DT33/768 (TNA).
50. GNC, Friern Hospital, 1951, DT33/768 (TNA).
51. GNC, Friern Hospital, 1963, DT33/768 (TNA).
52. Miss Craig, 'Loss of nursing staff: Report of a small survey made in the female wards of Friern Hospital during the first week of January 1965', THC65/170, July 1965, NSGHMC, agenda papers (LMA).
53. NSGHMC, agenda papers, Doc65/11 (LMA).
54. NSGHMC, minute book, 28 October 1965, 6271 (LMA).
55. NWMRHB, mental health committee, minutes and papers, 'Plans drawn up by CH Pearsall' NSGHMC, 26 April 1965 (LMA).
56. Malcolm Campbell, interview by author, 2015.
57. Robb, notes of phone call with Rose Hacker, 1966, AEGIS/1/3.
58. Letter, RP to NSGHMC, agenda papers HMC 64/58, 21 April 1964 (LMA).
59. Letter, undated, Fred to Mrs Dickens, AEGIS/4/1.
60. Letter, Dickens to MoH, 1 September 1967; Letter, Dickens to Robb, 5 March 1968, AEGIS/4/1/A.
61. Letter, Dickens to Kenneth Robinson, July 1967, AEGIS/4/1.
62. Letter, BS Lord, NWMRHB, to Dickens, 24 September 1964, AEGIS/4/1/A.
63. Letter, Dickens to MoH, 1 September 1967; Letter, Dickens to Robb, 5 March 1968, AEGIS/4/1/A.
64. Letter, Hugh Rossi to Dickens, 27 July 1967, AEGIS/4/1.
65. Malcolm Campbell, interview by author, 2015.
66. Letter, G Weston, RHB, to CH Pearsall, NSGHMC, Doc 65/110, 12 November 1965 (LMA).

Bibliography

Altschul, Annie. 1957. *Aids to Psychiatric Nursing*. London: Baillière, Tindall and Cox.

Anderson, William Ferguson. 1956. 'Difficulties in the management of sick old people'. *Medical Press*, 236, 341–345.

Anon. 1954. 'Helping the elderly and the confused to carry on: year's success at an Oxford Day Hospital'. *Guardian*, 15 January.
Anon. 1965. 'Eleven typhoid suspects in London'. *Times*, 2 September.
Barham, Peter. 1997. *Closing the Asylum: The Mental Patient in Modern Society*. London: Penguin Books.
Barton, Russell. 1959. *Institutional Neurosis*. Bristol: John Wright and Sons.
Barton, Russell. 1967. 'Foreword' ix–xi. In Robb, 1967.
Batt, JC. 1949. 'Confusional mental states'. *Medical Press*, 222, 15–18.
Bergmann, Klaus. 2009. In *The Development of Old Age Psychiatry in Britain 1960–1989*, (Guthrie Trust Witness Seminar 2008) ed. Claire Hilton. http://www.gla.ac.uk, accessed 18 September 2016.
Beveridge, William. 1942. *Social Insurance and Allied Services*. Cmd. 6404. London: HMSO.
Bickford, J. 1955. 'The forgotten patient. (i). The problem reviewed'. *Lancet*, ii, 917–919.
British Medical Association. 1947. *The Care and Treatment of the Elderly and Infirm*. London: BMA.
Brooke, Eileen. 1967. *A Census of Patients in Psychiatric Beds 1963*. London: HMSO.
Brooks, Jane. 2009. '"The geriatric hospital felt like a backwater": aspects of older people's nursing in Britain, 1955–1980'. *Journal of Clinical Nursing*, 18, 2764–2772.
Brothwood, John. 1971. 'The organisation and development of services for the aged with special reference to the mentally ill' 99–112. In *Recent Developments in Psychogeriatrics: A Symposium*, ed. David Kay and Alexander Walk. London: RMPA.
Carse, Joshua. Panton, Nydia and Watt, Alexander. 1958. 'A district mental health service: the Worthing experiment'. *Lancet*, i, 39–41.
Cartwright, Ann. 1964. *Human Relations and Hospital Care*. London: Routledge and Kegan Paul.
Cohen, Gerda. 1964. *What's Wrong with Hospitals?* Harmondsworth: Penguin Books.
Committee on the Economic and Financial Problems of the Provision for Old Age. Cmd. 9333. (Phillips Report) 1954. London: HMSO.
Cook, Leslie. Dax, Eric Cunningham and Maclay, Walter. 1952. 'The geriatric problem in mental hospitals'. *Lancet*, i, 377–382.
Denham, Michael. 2004. 'The history of geriatric medicine and hospital care of the elderly in England between 1929 and the 1970s'. PhD thesis, University College London. http://www.discovery.ucl.ac.uk, accessed 17 September 2016.
DHSS. 1971. *Report of the Farleigh Hospital Committee of Inquiry*. Cmnd. 4557. London: HMSO.

DHSS. 1972. *Annual Report of the Hospital Advisory Service to the Secretary of State for Social Services and the Secretary of State for Wales for the Year 1971*. London: HMSO.

Dickinson, Tommy. 2015. *'Curing Queers': Mental Nurses and Their Patients, 1935–1974*. Manchester: Manchester University Press.

Faculty of the Psychiatry of Old Age, General and Community Psychiatry Faculty. 2011. *The Equality Act 2010 and Adult Mental Health Services: Achieving Non-Discriminatory Age-Appropriate Services*. Occasional Paper OP82. London: RCPsych.

Gibson, Ronald. 1957. 'The care of the elderly in general practice'. *Research Newsletter*, 4, 99–114.

Goffman, Erving. 1961. *Asylums: Essays on the Social Situation of Mental Patients and Other Inmates*. New York: Anchor Books.

Goffman, Erving. 1963. *Stigma: Notes on the Management of Spoiled Identity*. New York: Simon and Schuster.

Guillebaud Report. See Ministry of Health 1956.

Gulland, Anne. 2014. 'Ronald Arthur "Sam" Robinson'. *BMJ*, 348, g3581.

Harvey, Audrey. 1965. The unknown prisoners'. *Guardian*, 10 August.

Hilton, Claire. 2007. 'Felix Post (1913–2001) pioneer in the psychiatry of old age'. *Journal of Medical Biography*, 15, 31–36.

Hilton, Claire. 2014. 'Joint geriatric and old age psychiatric wards in the United Kingdom, 1940s – early 1990s: a historical study'. *International Journal of Geriatric Psychiatry*, 29, 1071–1078.

Hilton, Claire. 2016. 'Psychogeriatrics in England in the 1950s': greater knowledge with little impact on provision of services'. *History of Psychiatry*, 27, 3–20.

Howell, Trevor. 1951. 'The problem of the chronic sick'. *Medical Press*, 225, 505–507.

Hunter, Richard and Macalpine, Ida. 1974. *Psychiatry for the Poor: 1851 Colney Hatch Asylum – Friern Hospital 1973: A Medical and Social History*. London: Dawson of Pall Mall.

Jolley, David. 2003. 'Remembering Russell Barton'. *BJPsych Bulletin*, 27, 233–234.

Jones, Kathleen 1993. *Asylums and After*. London: Athlone Press.

Jones, Kathleen and Fowles, AJ. 1984. *Ideas on Institutions*. London: Routledge and Kegan Paul.

Jones, Kathleen and Sidebotham, Roy. 1962. *Mental Hospitals at Work*. London: Routledge and Kegan Paul.

Kay, David. Beamish, Pamela and Roth, Martin. 1957. 'Some medical and social characteristics of elderly people under state care'. *Sociological Review Monograph*, 5, 173–193.

Kay, David. Beamish, Pamela and Roth, Martin. 1964a. 'Old age mental disorders in Newcastle upon Tyne: a study of prevalence'. *British Journal of Psychiatry*, 110, 146–158.

Kay, David. Beamish, Pamela and Roth, Martin. 1964b. 'Old age mental disorders in Newcastle upon Tyne: a study of possible social and medical causes'. *British Journal of Psychiatry*, 110, 668–682.
Kidd, Cecil. 1962a. '"Rejection of the seventh age": society and the aged sick'. *Almoner*, 14, 452–457.
Kidd, Cecil. 1962b. 'Misplacement of the elderly in hospital: a study of patients admitted to geriatric and mental hospitals'. *BMJ*, ii, 1491–1495.
Kingston, Frank. 1963. 'The demands for psychiatric beds'. *Lancet*, i, 107–108.
Kirkpatrick, WJA. 1967. 'Conscience and commitment' 48–57. In Robb 1967.
Laing, RD and Esterson, Aaron. 1964. *Sanity, Madness and the Family*. London: Penguin Books.
Lewis, Aubrey. 1946. 'Ageing and senility: a major problem of psychiatry'. *British Journal of Psychiatry*, 92, 150–170.
Lewis, Aubrey and Goldschmidt, Helen. 1943. 'Social causes for admission to a mental hospital for the aged'. *Sociological Review*, 35, 86–98.
Lowther, CP and Williamson, James. 1966. 'Old people and their relatives'. *Lancet*, ii, 1459–1460.
Lyth, Isabel Menzies. 1988. 'Social systems as a defence against anxiety' 43–88. In *Containing Anxiety in Institutions: Selected Essays*. Vol. 1, ed. Isabel Menzies Lyth. London: Free Association Books.
Macmillan, Duncan. 1960. 'Preventive geriatrics'. *Lancet*, ii, 1439–1441.
Mandelbrote, Bertram. 1964. 'Mental illness in hospital and community: development and outcome' 267–290. In *Problems and Progress in Medical Care*, ed. Gordon McLachan. London: Nuffield Provincial Hospitals Trust, OUP.
Martin, Denis. 1962. *Adventure in Psychiatry*. Oxford: Bruno Cassirer.
Mass Observation. 1948. 'Old Age'. *Mass Observation Bulletin*, October–November, 21, 1–4.
Mayer-Gross, Willy. 1945. 'Electric convulsion treatment in patients over 60'. *British Journal of Psychiatry*, 91, 101–103.
Means, Robin and Smith, Randall. 1985. *The Development of Welfare Services for Elderly People*. Kent: Croom Helm.
Ministry of Health. 1950a. *Care of the Aged Suffering from Mental Infirmity*. HMC (50)25.
Ministry of Health. 1950b. *Treatment of the Elderly Chronic Sick*. HMC (50)38.
Ministry of Health. 1956. *Report of the Committee of Enquiry Into the Cost of the National Health Service*. Cmd. 9663. (Guillebaud Report). London: HMSO.
Ministry of Health. 1957. *Survey of Services Available to the Chronic Sick and Elderly 1954–1955*. Boucher Report. London: HMSO.
Ministry of Health. 1961. *Report for the Year 1960. Part II: On the State of the Public Health*. Cmnd. 1550. London: HMSO.

Ministry of Health. 1962. *A Hospital Plan for England and Wales.* Cmnd. 1604. London: HMSO.

Ministry of Health. 1963. *Health and Welfare: The Development of Community Care: Plans for the Health and Welfare Services of the Local Authorities in England and Wales.* Cmnd. 1973. London: HMSO.

Ministry of Health. 1964. *Improving the Effectiveness of Hospitals for the Mentally Ill.* HM (64)45. London: HMSO.

Ministry of Health. 1965. *Care of the Elderly in Hospitals and Residential Homes.* HM (65)77. London: HMSO.

Ministry of Health. 1966. *Handbook for Members of Hospital Management Committees.* London: HMSO.

Ministry of Health. 1968a. *Findings and Recommendations Following Enquiries Into Allegations Concerning the Care of Elderly Patients in Certain Hospitals.* Cmnd. 3687. London: HMSO.

Ministry of Health. 1968b. *The Activities of Psychiatric Hospitals: A Regional Comparison. Mental Hospitals and Units 1964.* Statistical Report Series no. 3. London: HMSO.

Ministry of Health. 1968c. *Psychiatric Nursing Today and Tomorrow: Report of the Joint Sub-committee of the Standing Mental Health and the Standing Nursing Advisory Committees.* London: HMSO.

National Old People's Welfare Council. 1958. *Notes on Mental Frailty in the Elderly.* London: National Council of Social Services.

Nolan, Peter. 1995. 'The development of mental health nursing' 1–18. In *Stress and Coping in Mental Health Nursing,* ed. Jerome Carson, Leonard Fagin and Susan Ritter. London: Chapman and Hall.

Norton, Doreen. 1956. 'The place of geriatric nursing in training'. *Nursing Times,* 6 July, 621–624.

Norton, Doreen. 1988. *The Age of Old Age.* London: Scutari Press.

Phillips Committee. See *Committee on the Economic and Financial Problems.*

Pitt, Brice. 1968. 'Attempting to solve staffing problems' 29–30. In *Improving the Effectiveness of Hospitals and Services for the Mentally Ill and Mentally Subnormal: A Collection of Papers Presented at Conferences Held at the Hospital Centre in 1966 and 1967,* ed. Anthony Whitehead and D. Cortazzi. London: King's Fund.

Political and Economic Planning. 1948. *Population Policy in Great Britain.* London: PEP.

Post, Felix. 1944. 'Some problems arising from a study of mental patients over the age of 60 years'. *British Journal of Psychiatry,* 90, 554–565.

Powell, Enoch. 1961. 'Opening speech' ('Water Tower') 5–10. In *Emerging Patterns for the Mental Health Services and the Public: Proceedings of a Conference at Church House Westminster,* 9–10 March 1961. London: NAMH.

Robb, Barbara. 1967. *Sans Everything: A Case to Answer.* London: Nelson.

Robinson, Ronald 'Sam'. 1965. 'The organisation of a diagnostic and treatment unit for the aged in a mental hospital' 186–205. In *Psychiatric Disorders in the Aged*, ed. World Psychiatric Association. Manchester: Geigy.

Robinson, Ronald 'Sam'. 2009. In *The Development of Old Age Psychiatry in Britain 1960–1989*, (Guthrie Trust Witness Seminar 2008) ed. Claire Hilton. http://www.gla.ac.uk, accessed 18 September 2016.

Rogers, Anne and Pilgrim, David. 1996. *Mental Health Policy in Britain: A Critical Introduction*. Basingstoke: Macmillan Press.

Roth, Martin. 1955. 'The natural history of mental disorders in old age'. *British Journal of Psychiatry*, 101, 281–230.

Rowntree, B. Seebohm. 1947. *Old People: Report of a Survey Committee on the Problems of Ageing and the Care of Old People*. London: Nuffield Foundation.

Royal Commission on Population 1949. Cmd. 7695. London: HMSO.

Sheldon, Joseph. 1948. *The Social Medicine of Old Age*. London: OUP.

Strabolgi. 1965. 'Dumping ground for the aged'. *Catholic Herald*, 19 November.

Taylor, Stephen. 1954. *Good General Practice*. London: OUP.

Thane, Pat. 1990. '"The debate on the declining birth-rate in Britain" the "menace" of an ageing population, 1920s–1950s'. *Continuity and Change*, 5, 283–305.

Thane, Pat. 2000. *Old Age in English History: Past Experiences, Present Issues*. Oxford: OUP.

Thane, Pat. 2010. 'Older people and equality' 7–28. In *Unequal Britain*, ed. Pat Thane. London: Continuum.

Thomson, A. 1950. 'Discussion on the problems of old age'. *Proceedings of the Royal Society of Medicine*, 43, 929–933.

Thomson, W. 1959. 'The elderly who live alone'. *Medical Press*, 242, 477–480.

Townsend, Peter. Cited in Anon. 1961. 'Old people's welfare services'. *Almoner*, 14, 379.

Townsend, Peter. 1962. *The Last Refuge*. London: Routledge and Kegan Paul.

Townsend, Peter. 1965. 'A national survey of old people in psychiatric and non-psychiatric hospitals, residential homes, and nursing homes' 223–232. In *Psychiatric Hospital Care: A Symposium*, ed. Hugh Freeman. London: Baillière, Tindall and Cassell.

Townsend, Peter. 1973. *The Social Minority*. London: Allen Lane.

Warren. Marjory. 1943. 'Care of chronic sick'. *BMJ*, ii, 822–823.

Watts, Cuthbert and Watts, Beatrice. 1952. *Psychiatry in General Practice*. London: J and A Churchill.

Webster, Charles. 1991a. 'The elderly and the early National Health Service' 165–193. In *Life and Death and the Elderly*, ed. M. Pelling and R. Smith. London: Routledge.

Webster, Charles. 1991b. 'Psychiatry and the early National Health Service: the role of the Mental Health Standing Advisory Committee' 103–116. In *150*

Years of British Psychiatry 1841–1991, ed. German Berrios and Hugh Freeman. London: Gaskell.
Webster, Charles. 1998. *The National Health Service: A Political History*. Oxford: OUP.
Welshman, John. 1996. '"Growing old in the city": public health and the elderly in Leicester 1948–74'. *Medical History*, 40, 74–89.
Whitehead, Anthony. 1965. 'A comprehensive psychogeriatric service'. *Lancet*, ii, 583–586.
Whitehead, Anthony. 1970. *In the Service of Old Age: The Welfare of Psychogeriatric Patients*. Harmondsworth: Penguin Books.
Whitehead, Tony. cited in: Anon. 1974. 'Aged "could be spared misery"'. *Guardian*, 7 October.
Williamson, James. Stokoe, I.H. Gray, S. and Fisher, M. 1964. 'Old people at home: their unreported needs' *Lancet*, i, 1117–1120.
Winn, Merrick. 1955. 'Britain's shame'. *Daily Express*, 19 September.
World Health Organisation. 1959. *Mental Health Problems of Aging and the Aged*. Geneva: WHO.

Open Access This chapter is licensed under the terms of the Creative Commons Attribution 4.0 International License (http://creativecommons.org/licenses/by/4.0/), which permits use, sharing, adaptation, distribution and reproduction in any medium or format, as long as you give appropriate credit to the original author(s) and the source, provide a link to the Creative Commons license and indicate if changes were made.

The images or other third party material in this chapter are included in the book's Creative Commons license, unless indicated otherwise in a credit line to the material. If material is not included in the book's Creative Commons license and your intended use is not permitted by statutory regulation or exceeds the permitted use, you will need to obtain permission directly from the copyright holder.

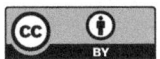

CHAPTER 3

Barbara Robb, Amy Gibbs and the 'Diary of a Nobody'

'Mrs Robb has always been a terrible danger to [the government].... I knew we had to defuse this bomb', wrote Richard Crossman in November 1969 (1977, p. 727), a fine compliment from a Cabinet Minister to a woman who emerged from the shadows to fight for improvements in the care of older people. How did she build such a fearsome reputation? What was her background? How did she acquire her skills? What made her take on the cause? What gave her the 'uncrushable belief in the need to expose what was going on'?[1] How did she cope with Hospital Management Committees (HMCs), Regional Hospital Boards (RHBs) and officialdom's tendency to reject critics and criticism and to maintain the status quo? The biographical element of this book seeks to illuminate the aspects of Barbara's background and personality that motivated her and sustained her in her campaign, and to introduce Amy Gibbs. Their life stories lead into the 'Diary of a Nobody', the visit-by-visit record that Barbara felt compelled to start writing on the first day she visited Amy in Friern Hospital, the events of which inspired the founding of AEGIS (Aid for the Elderly in Government Institutions). The Diary ensured that Barbara had an accurate description of happenings that she observed directly or was told about by patients and visitors on the ward in order to achieve her objective of making improvements.[2] It was not written for publication. She used Amy's real name, only later giving her the pseudonym 'Miss Wills'. Barbara did not explain the title.[3] Amy, an ordinary patient, could have been the Nobody, or Barbara, accorded the low status of a visitor or non-NHS professional in the hospital hierarchy, especially when criticising it. Both interpretations fit with Cohen's analysis (1964, p. 7), which she italicised for emphasis, that even where treatment of the illness was good, *'patients do not count'*.

Building on Amy's story, and linking to Townsend's (1965, p. 229) observation that many older people in psychiatric hospitals did not need long-term admission, we explore evidence about Amy's mental health and consider whether a twenty-month admission was in accordance with recognised good practice at the time. This chapter also covers the events of Barbara's campaign, based on the Diary, until November 1965 when she 'went public'. It includes the outcome of Lord Strabolgi sending a copy of the Diary to Kenneth Robinson (Member of Parliament for St Pancras North, where Amy lived; Minister of Health 1964–1968), Barbara's meeting with Dr Tooth at the Ministry, and Strabolgi's speech in the House of Lords, prompted by lack of constructive response from the Ministry.

Barbara: An Anne of Burghwallis

In the absence of a personal archive, clues to researching Barbara's background initially came from the dust jacket of *Sans Everything*. It states that she was convent-educated, trained as a psychotherapist during the Second World War and was married to artist Brian Robb, although scanty biographical material about him fails to mention Barbara. Three other clues in the AEGIS archive were the lynchpins to uncovering her life story: a police statement on which she was obliged to give her maiden name, Anne[4]; a biographical note for a conference programme that stated her place of birth as Thorner, Yorkshire[5]; and a cutting from the *Sunday Times* in 1972 which stated that she had been married for thirty-five years.[6]

Barbara Robb (née Anne) was born on 15 April 1912,[7] the second child of Major George Charlton Anne (1886–1960) and Amy Violet Anne (née Montagu 1885–1935). The Annes were an affluent Yorkshire recusant Roman Catholic family. They intermarried with other Catholic families, fairly openly adhered to the Catholic faith and harboured Catholic priests (Kingsley 2016). A plaque at the entrance of St Helen's chapel in the family home, Burghwallis Hall (Fig. 3.1), near Doncaster, records the ancestral martyrs who died 'for the faith': George Anne, Elizabeth Anne, Richard Fenton, and John Anne who was hanged, drawn and quartered at York, about 1588. Barbara was very proud of

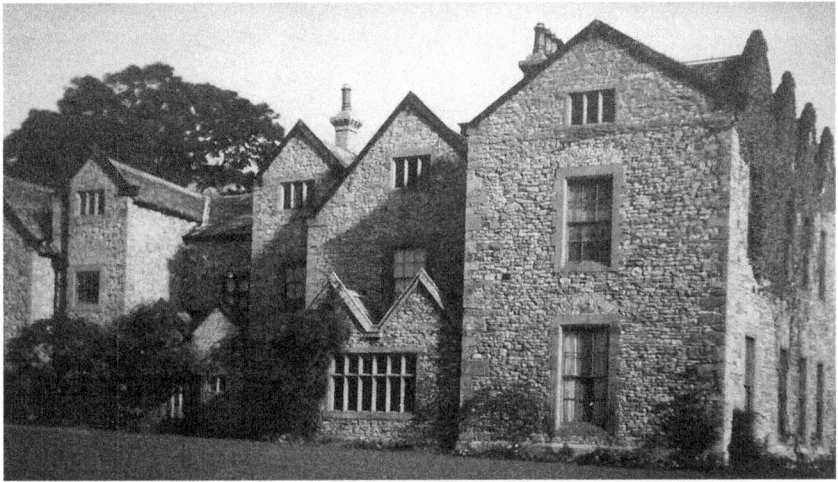

Fig. 3.1 Burghwallis Hall, c.1941. Photograph by George Anne, reproduced courtesy of Elizabeth Ellison-Anne.

these ancestors. On one occasion in the 1960s, she was exasperated with the brother-in-law of a Catholic patient she was trying to assist. He felt strongly that the patient should be helped by the Catholic community. Barbara infamously replied: 'Set your heart at rest on that point... I myself am a member of one of England's oldest Catholic families and have the blood of six martyrs in my veins, all awaiting canonisation.'[8]

Barbara knew her Anne grandparents well as she spent school holidays with them at Burghwallis. She described her grandfather Ernest Charlton Anne (Fig. 3.2) as 'a man of endless kindness who believed children should be listened to', and she recalled his words many years later:

> 'when you see somebody needing help—help him.' Then once, when I was a little girl, I got stung by nettles. He told me that wherever there were nettles there were sure to be dock leaves to cure the sting. And then he said: 'Remember that everything in life is like the nettles, there are always dock leaves if only you look hard enough' (Allen 1967).

Several formidable women in Barbara's family gave her strong female role models. Great-grandmother Barbara Charlton, Ernest's mother, was an

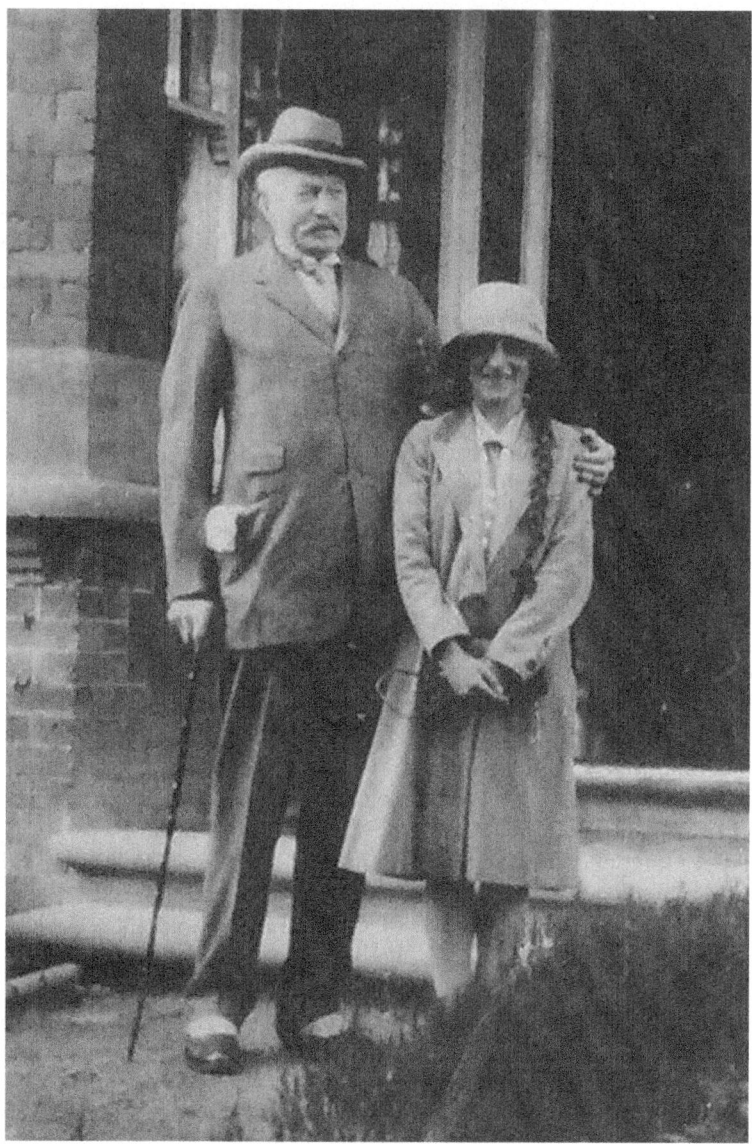

Fig. 3.2 Barbara and her grandfather, Ernest Charlton Anne, c.1922. Reproduced courtesy of Elizabeth Ellison-Anne.

acute observer and commentator on people around her and wrote her memoirs (Charlton 1949). Grandmother Edith Charlton Anne, Ernest's wife, was a professional opera singer early in life and later published novels for adults (under a nom de plume) and stories for children (Allan 1897, c.1897; Anne 1898). Another relative who inspired Barbara was her aunt Ernestine ('Missie') Anne (1887–1985). A handful of letters in the AEGIS archive reveal Barbara's lifelong, lively and affectionate relationship with her. Lacking a formal education or career, Missie had a varied life including trying to live as a Benedictine nun. Missie also 'suffered bad mental health, being liable to deep depressions',[9] sometimes requiring psychiatric treatment. Her family supported her in the face of cultural taboos towards mental illness, thus exposing Barbara at a relatively young age to a close family member suffering mental illness.[10]

Barbara had three brothers, Michael (1911–1980), Frederick John (1914–2010) and Robert (1919–1941, died on active service). Her parents had a 'ropey' marriage. They separated and moved to London, into two different houses in Kensington, but in 1935 when her mother was terminally ill with cancer,[11] they drew closer again.[12] Barbara's cousin William Charlton thought that Barbara and her siblings had a fragile relationship with their father, and Barbara's niece Elizabeth Ellison-Anne said that they did not talk to each other for years.[13] Nevertheless, Barbara paid attention to her father's health in his old age. She observed less-than-ideal care in a hospital near to his home in Brighton, which might explain why he was moved to the relatively sophisticated facilities of a teaching hospital during his last illness.[14] Personal experiences with her father may have added to Barbara's desire to improve provision for older people.

In her teens, Barbara attended the Convent of the Assumption boarding school followed by St Catherine's finishing school, both in Kensington. Her course of study included the Catholic Social Guild syllabus, which contributed to her understanding of ethics and personal responsibility. The Guild examination which she sat in 1927 included questions on the 'Manchester School' of economics, obligations of Catholics to do 'social work' and the pope's teaching on the 'Living Wage' (Catholic Social Guild 1928).[15] Barbara wanted to be a ballet dancer and danced in Verdi's *Aida*[16] with the Vic-Wells Company (Anon. 1976), the forerunner of the Royal Ballet. An ankle injury ended her dancing career, so she went to the Chelsea School of Art to study theatre stage design. At Chelsea she met Brian Fletcher Robb (1913–1979), also from Yorkshire. Barbara and Brian married in 1937 in St Helen's chapel at Burghwallis Hall. Barbara's brother Frederick was best man. Her brother Robert (Fig. 3.3) and their friend from the Chelsea School of Art, David Kenworthy, were ushers (Anon. 1937). Kenworthy became a Labour peer when he inherited the title Baron Strabolgi, and later strongly supported the AEGIS campaign.

Barbara and Brian bought a tiny cottage in Hampstead Grove, northwest London, where they would entertain family, friends, politicians and artists. She later ran AEGIS from there. The cottage was 'cabin-cruiser' size, according to one visitor: 'absolutely tiny, and spotless, and neat and rather arty'.[17] Brian, a cartoonist, illustrator and painter, had an art studio a short walk down the hill.[18]

During the Second World War, Brian was an army camouflage officer in North Africa (Robb 1944) and Barbara had various jobs. One was at St

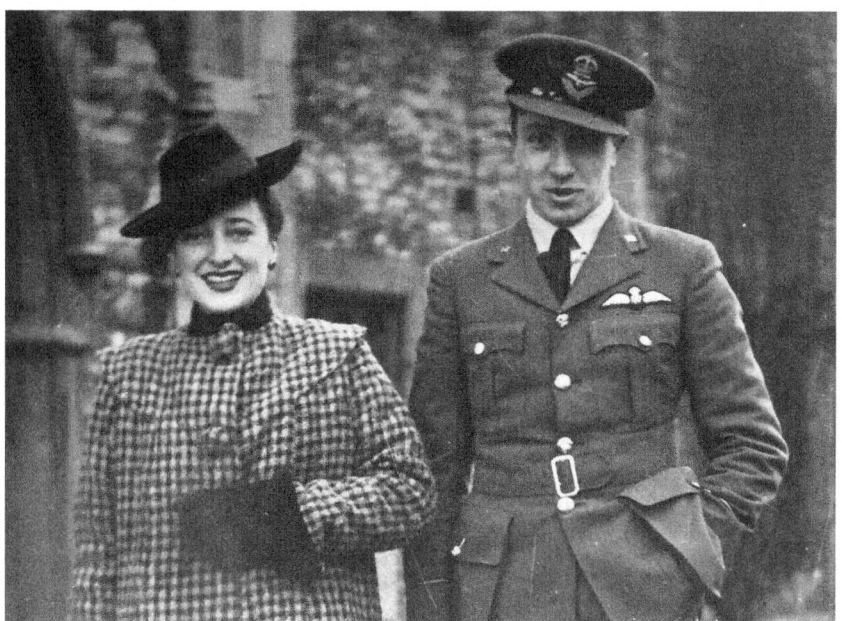

Fig. 3.3 Barbara and her brother Robert, winter 1940–1941. Reproduced courtesy of Elizabeth Ellison-Anne.

Christopher's Hostel, which nurtured and supported adolescent boys, in Hatton Garden, central London (Anon. 1939).[19] Many boys told extraordinary and distressing stories: one recounted cycling from Coventry to London after his closest pal died in a bombing raid. Others were homeless or living in poverty.[20] Barbara's experiences at St Christopher's whetted her appetite for training as a psychotherapist.[21] Despite the struggles of war time, Barbara also had time for fun. On one occasion she was a guest at Hesleyside Hall, the home of her Charlton relatives, but she did not realise they dressed for dinner and she did not have a formal outfit with her. With audacious imagination and creativity, she wore her posh silk Chinese pyjamas: the mistress of the house was not impressed, but the story lingered and the family recounted it in 2016.[22]

The Robbs had many left-wing friends, frowned on by some of Barbara's wealthy relatives. Mamie Charlton, her sister-in-law, described their friends as 'violently left wing'[23] and Barbara teased her brother Michael with favourable comments about communists. The same comments endeared her to other family members.[24] In a cartoon book (Robb 1944), Brian wrote the foreword about his future grandchildren, naming them Catherine and Nicholas, and drew himself, elderly, on the front cover with them. Barbara and Brian wanted children but Barbara had a miscarriage,[25] and parenthood was not to be.

CARL JUNG, VICTOR WHITE AND BARBARA

We know a significant amount about Barbara's personality from her interactions with Father Victor White (1902–1960) and through his long-term correspondence with Carl Jung (1875–1961), founder of analytical psychology. Victor White, son of an Anglican minister, converted to Catholicism, became a Dominican priest, a theologian and Jungian psychoanalyst. We do not know how White and Barbara met, but in early 1941 White visited his parents who were then residing at Burghwallis. Barbara was probably there at the time.[26] Barbara 'trained' in Jungian analysis under White's guidance.[27] Training at that time was often informal, a few chats with a practitioner, and without theoretical courses or personal analysis.[28] White admired Barbara's autodidactic training, including her 'remarkable self-analysis'.[29] Barbara began counselling people referred primarily through local church networks.[30] In 1943, White introduced Amy to Barbara, for psychological help (Robb 1967, p. 69). From the War until 1965, Barbara worked as a psychotherapist.[31] Practicing psychotherapy would have enhanced her insight into emotions and relationships and honed her listening and reflecting skills, all relevant to her later work.

White and Barbara had a close friendship. White recorded, in his dream diary, dreaming about her[32] and a few letters from her survive in his archive. One, in 1951, about the *I Ching*, the ancient Chinese text on divination that she was studying, indicates the breadth and depth of her interests and knowledge. The letter was also rather affectionate, opening with 'Darling V', and ending 'lovingly, B.'[33] This probably reflected her naturally demonstrative warmth to her friends. Many letters in the AEGIS archive end 'love', but those to Brian show an effervescent affection, one beginning 'Darling, Darling B' and ending 'I am so very, very, very lucky to have you.'[34]

White's correspondence with Jung began in 1945 and continued for fifteen years. Their letters explored the interface between analytical psychology and theology.[35] White first brought Barbara to Jung's attention in 1947, quoting her recent musings and dreams about Jung, for whom she prayed regularly 'that he may be all he can be'.[36] Jung answered White with interest and amusement, calling her White's 'soror mystica'—a 'mystical sister', the alchemist's female assistant,[37] a guiding collaborative partner. White replied, 'She seems to be very much more YOUR "soror mystica"!'[38] Barbara wrote out some of her dreams and her interpretations of them and sent them to White, who typed them out for Jung (Lammers and Cunningham 2007, p. 74). Jung's and White's letters about Barbara and her dreams give insights into her forceful personality and what inspired her in life, hence their inclusion here.

In one dream Barbara described having a tug-of-war with Jung but she pulled him off balance with remarkable ease, reflecting a determination to succeed even in the face of an opponent who was bigger, stronger and more famous than her. She described having bare feet, meaning having contact with the ground, the earth: 'Loving the God who had walked on the earth, I became interested in the earth itself.' For Barbara, bare feet, like ballet, implied a relationship with the ground, and signified freedom, pilgrimage and humility.[39] She wrote to White in 1947: 'I live for the Lord God who is Himself "at the service" of mankind, and it is only in so far that I am "orientated" to Him that I myself am able to serve mankind. My life is dedicated to mankind because it has first been dedicated to Him.'[40] White wrote: 'Her quite remarkable knowledge is balanced by a deeply humble and simple faith—as well as by a very earthy common-sense and gaiety—all of which I greatly envy.'[41]

Barbara met Jung in Zurich in 1951. Jung was seventy-six, Barbara was thirty-nine. They discussed older people, a subject that interested Barbara years before her campaign.[42] Barbara asked Jung what message he would give to older people: 'Tell them to live each day as if they'll be here for another 100 years. Then they really will *live* to the end' (Robb 1973). They also discussed some of Barbara's dreams, including the one the night before the 1949 Epsom Derby when she predicted the three winning horses in the correct order and instructed Brian to back them on his way to work that morning (whether he did is not recounted).[43] After meeting Barbara, Jung wrote enthusiastically to White:

> I have seen Mrs. Barbara Robb, and I assure you, she is quite an eyeful and beyond!... she is quite remarkable. If ever there was an anima,[44] it is she, and there is no doubt about it.
>
> In such cases one better crosses oneself, because the anima, particularly when she is quintessential as in this case, casts a metaphysical shadow which is long like a Hotel-bill and contains no end of items that sum up in a marvellous way. One cannot label her and put her into a drawer. She decidedly leaves you guessing. I hadn't expected anything like that. At least I understand now why she dreams of Derby winners: it just belongs to her!...
>
> It is just as well that she got all her psychology from books, as she would have busted every decent and competent analyst. I sincerely hope she is going on dreaming of winners, because such people need winners to keep them afloat.[45]

Jung's comment about needing winners to keep afloat is eerie when we find out later that Barbara used much of her personal savings to fund the AEGIS campaign, causing her supporters substantial concern.[46] White replied to Jung:

> I loved your letter—how right you are!... Barbara certainly is quite a corker, isn't she? For weal or woe I cannot see her very often these days; but it occurs to me that IF you can be moved to offer any hints about how to deal with her when I do, I'd be very grateful.[47]

Coming from two experts in psychology, Jung's and White's remarks about how to 'deal with' Barbara are extraordinary. If they floundered, then other men with less psychological understanding of people and interpersonal relationships, may well misinterpret and misunderstand her in the course of her work. The challenges of understanding Barbara fitted with Jung classifying her as an extraordinary and forceful 'intuitive introvert',[48] defined as a

> mystical dreamer and seer on the one hand, the crank and artist on the other... frequently a misunderstood genius.... The moral problem arises when he (*sic*) tries to relate himself to his vision, when he is no longer satisfied with mere perception and its æsthetic configuration and evaluation, when he confronts the questions: What does this mean for me or the world? What emerges from this vision in the way of a duty or a task, for me or the world? (Jung (1923) 1971, pp. 401–402).

Jung's characterisation of Barbara was almost prophetic. Later, she did not just ponder over her vision, but acted on it. Ann Lammers (2007, p. 258) commented that Barbara's 'verbal outpourings' in the letters created an 'atmosphere of mystical participation, tinged by Eros and hilarity, raising the temperature of the conversation and melting its formality'. These ways of interacting—in meetings, letters, interviews and phone calls—helped create her campaign style.

Jung's analysis aligned with Barbara's life story, her role models and the ethos instilled into her as a child, the uncompromising ancestral martyrs, the determined womenfolk, her wise and kindly grandfather and her education about social responsibility. A deep faith, humility, a 'grounded' security, a sense of pilgrimage and valuing her freedom all contributed to Barbara's immense drive, persistence and ability to overcome obstacles in her quest for justice.

Amy Gibbs

Amy Gibbs (1891–1967) was born and brought up in north London. In 1911 she lived in middle-class Wood Green with her parents, four sisters, a servant and her ninety-five-year-old grandmother (UK Census 1911). She did not marry. She became a clerk in the Civil Service, but left because of mental illness. She was unwell for two years before admission to Napsbury Hospital, Hertfordshire, in 1929.[49] In 1934 the authorities transferred her to the brand new Shenley Hospital, from where she was discharged eighteen months later.[50] According to Barbara:

> Her troubles arose from religious scruples. A simple soul, half-French and rather sexy, she had been taught that the devil would get her if she permitted herself any sexual sensations at all.... She responded well to my kind of

therapy, and in a few weeks was able to take a job as a seamstress with a celebrated theatrical costumier. She pursued this career until she qualified for her retirement pension.... Her religious anxieties were not too difficult to keep in check.[51]

After discharge, apart from an admission to Friern for a few months in 1941–1942, Amy remained well until 1963 (Ministry of Health (MoH) 1968, p. 28).[52] She lived alone in a rented flat in Kentish Town, northwest London. She had many talents, including writing poetry[53] and reciting and translating French verse (Robb 1967, p. 91). After Amy retired, Brian encouraged her to take up art. She created collages from foil sweet and chocolate wrappers, tinsel and milk bottle tops (Figs. 3.4 and 3.5). She sold these at art exhibitions in Hampstead and in avant-garde West End galleries.[54] Art collectors,

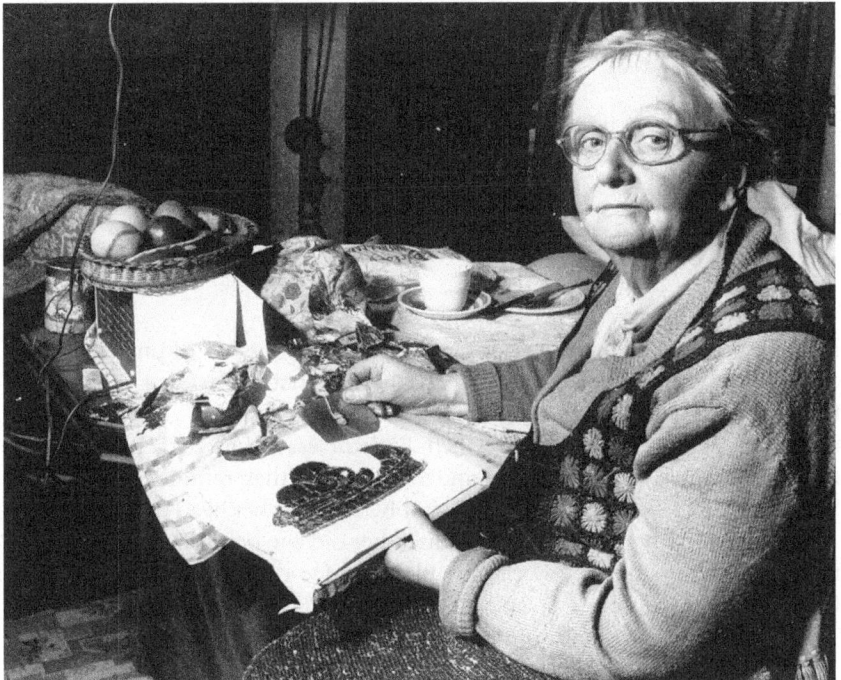

Fig. 3.4 Amy Gibbs creating a foil collage, 1961.
Source: author's collection.

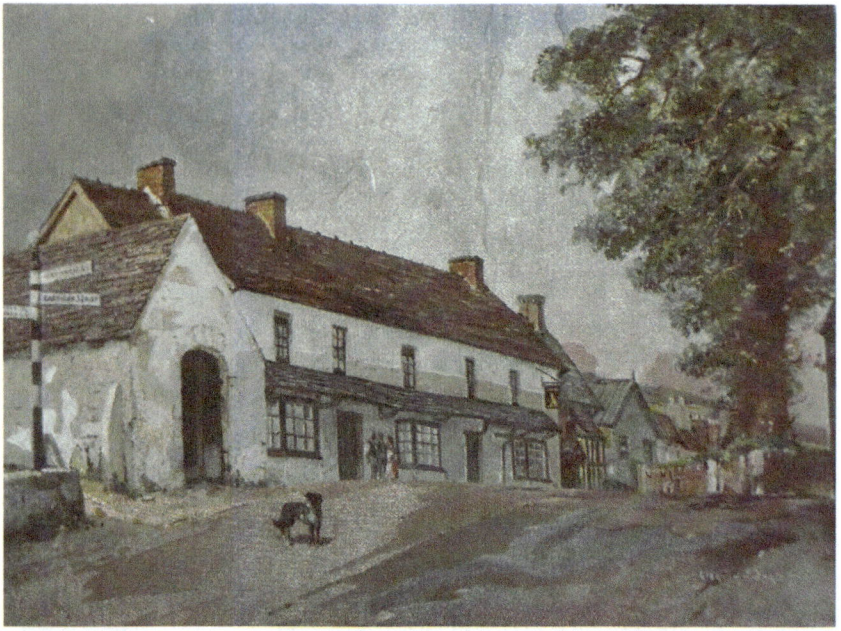

Fig. 3.5 Foil collage by Amy Gibbs.

Source: AEGIS/4/3, Library, London School of Economics. Orphan work: attempts have been made to identify copyright owner.

including professional artists, bought her work.[55] A review of one exhibition commented on her 'gift for seeing the beauty that most of us miss in the familiar things and sights of every day' (Conlay 1961). Amy gave a television interview on her work, about which Barbara commented: 'This talented, modest, sociable lady—simple minded in a way that reminded me of Sir Stanley Spencer—carried it all off admirably, and kept her head throughout'.[56] Amy's art earnings significantly subsidised her old age pension,[57] enabling her to take holidays and to pay the membership fee of the Hampstead Artists Council (HAC), 'things I can't do without'.[58] In the light of her artistic successes, her family, who shunned her after she was admitted to Napsbury, made contact again (Robb 1967, p. 86).

In 1963, Amy began to experience anxiety and other symptoms, such as spontaneous sexual sensations, which distressed her. Her GP prescribed a 'tranquiliser' which made her feel so 'muzzy' that she feared falling in the street.[59] She saw a consultant psychiatrist in an outpatients clinic who prescribed occupational therapy, and because of medication side effects, suggested an admission to Friern. Amy agreed, expecting that the admission would sort out her medication, allow her to continue with occupational therapy, and would be of short duration (Robb 1967, p. 69).

At the end of 1964, a mutual friend, Eric Buss, passed to Barbara Amy's request that she visit her in Friern. Buss was distressed by his inability to improve Amy's situation on the ward or arrange discharge. He informed Barbara that the ward doctor said Amy was 'not a mental case', even though she was in a psychiatric hospital (Robb 1967, p. 70). Because Amy was one of Barbara's psychotherapy patients, Barbara considered the ethics of visiting. She decided that because Amy was 'not a mental patient and as she kept asking to see me, it was not improper for me to visit her'.[60]

'Diary of a Nobody': Friern, Amy and Friends

Barbara was shocked when she saw Amy in ward E3 in January 1965 (Robb 1967, p. 93). In the fourteen months since they last met, Amy had changed from being plump, upright and active to being thin, stooped, frail and inactive. Her hair was cut in the uniform 'pudding bowl' style of the other patients. She wore hospital clothes, and had neither dentures nor spectacles. Most patients on the ward lacked these necessities, and hearing aids and other personal possessions, and most were apathetic 'sat as if sunk in torpor' (p. 72). Visitors were rare and staff were unfriendly and unhelpful.

Barbara usually visited Amy and attended meetings about her accompanied by Brian or a friend who would read and sign the Diary entry to confirm its accuracy. Friends included Buss and Lord and Lady Strabolgi, who knew Amy through the HAC (Cochrane 1990, pp. 29, 31) and Barbara's neighbours Audrey and Ronald Harvey. Audrey Harvey was a valuable ally. She worked with deprived people in London's East End and was an ardent citizens' rights campaigner alongside Abel-Smith and Townsend. She wrote about demeaning practices encountered by people who needed to seek welfare assistance. This helped shift the authorities' attitudes to social problems away from the culture of blaming the individual for their misfortunes, towards a more sympathetic approach, that people could fall on hard times due to an unfortunate set of circumstances (Harvey 1960, pp. 16–23; Harvey 1965b; Toynbee 1971). Harvey (1960, pp. 14–15) also understood the effects of overcrowding: 'it causes real and protracted agony, all the more painful to witness because it is so often borne with stoical patience', an observation relevant to private dwellings and to psychiatric hospital wards where resigned acceptance by patients and staff did not encourage NHS authorities to make improvements.

Barbara's twice-weekly[61] visits to the ward could not pass unnoticed. She took brandy, sweets and chocolates for the patients, offering them with the ward sister's permission (Robb 1967, p. 82).[62] Sometimes her handbag concealed a state-of-the-art pocket cassette recorder, a device available only since 1963, useful for recording meetings if she was unaccompanied[63] or to record patients' reminiscences (Harvey 1976). Amy was sometimes tearful, and Barbara was determined to find out why. Typical of psychiatric practice with older people at the time, the nurses labelled Amy as 'confused' (Robb 1967, p. 74). The label implied that Amy's comments were unreliable and should not be believed, that she could not make decisions for herself, would not get better and required passive care rather than rehabilitation. Barbara did not think Amy was confused, but Amy was nervous about complaining because she feared she would be punished for doing so (pp. 73–74). On one occasion Amy mentioned that staff threatened to put her 'out into the street' because she had complained about them (pp. 82–83). Barbara and Amy devised a code in case their conversations were overheard, such as referring to patients having a bang rather than being hit. Allegedly, the nurses slapped patients for being incontinent. Protective towards Amy, Barbara was cautious about how much she spoke to the nurses to avoid antagonising them, but noted how they responded, including their pejorative and infantilising comments towards Amy's incontinence: 'She's sometimes very dirty. She won't get out and sit on the pot' (pp. 87–90). Staff showed poor understanding of patients' emotional needs, such as telling Amy that she must not believe her friends about ever leaving Friern. Patients were generally in bed by 7 P.M. When Barbara visited one evening she found five still up, in less than dignified circumstances: 'one of the five sat on a commode; another, minus most of her clothes, was receiving treatment [personal care] nearby. No attempt was made to use screens' (p. 74).

Barbara had difficulty finding a doctor to talk to, and when she did, she received inconsistent information about Amy's diagnosis, prognosis and the possibility of discharge (Robb 1967, pp. 70, 88). Social workers also gave Barbara disconcertingly inconsistent information. The community social worker correctly informed Barbara that since Amy was not detained under the Mental Health Act, she was free to leave Friern without reference to her relatives or anyone else (p. 89). Miss Cloake, the hospital social worker, told Barbara, incorrectly (MoH 1965, pp. 3, 5) that because Amy was incontinent there was 'absolutely no possibility' of her leaving Friern (Robb 1967, p. 78), and that Amy's relatives could decide where she should live (p. 83). Amy's psychiatrist, Dr Aix, wrote to Barbara concurring with Miss Cloake that: 'Any move would have to be done with approval of her family'.[64] It was certainly important to find out where would be convenient for the family, to enable them to visit, but legally their views would not override that of a sound-minded patient. Dr Aix seemed unaware of the patient's degree of lucidity or of the legal position. Both gaps in knowledge were unacceptable and could affect care and the education of other staff, possibly influencing Miss Cloake's advice. Given the typical staff hierarchies, it is unlikely that a hospital social worker would question a consultant's opinion about discharge.

Barbara alleged that Miss Cloake was involved in dubious practices concerning clearing Amy's flat in conjunction with Miss Lovat, Amy's niece. Miss Cloake told Barbara that Amy signed the requisite form, although whether Amy had her spectacles so that she could read it, or how Miss Cloake explained it to her, is not known, and that Amy's belongings had to be disposed of as either they 'just crumbled' or were 'musty and horrible' (Robb 1967, p. 79). Those conditions were possible, because the flat was unoccupied and unheated for a year. However, neither Miss Cloake nor Miss Lovat had recently visited the flat, so it was unlikely that they knew the real condition of the property, and no evidence is given that neighbours or the landlord voiced concern. That did not prevent Miss Cloake from booking a clearance company before they visited. On the day they cleared her flat, Miss Lovat took some of the art work with her. It was neither 'musty and horrible' nor 'crumbling', which throws doubt on Miss Cloake's assessment and decision making. Later, Barbara met Miss Lovat, adding to her suspicions that Miss Cloake masterminded the sale of Amy's possessions, with Miss Lovat dutifully cooperating with, rather than challenging, her professional authority (p. 99).

Barbara was horrified by the sale of Amy's possessions. Buss wanted to buy them back for Amy, but his plan was thwarted: two weeks after the clearance, Miss Cloake said she had forgotten the name of the company and had no record or receipt (Robb 1967, pp. 84, 94), hardly a professional way to deal with a patient's property. These events coincided with Barbara hearing about antiques racketeers across the country telling relatives or officials looking after older people that their house contents were worth nothing, and then removing them (p. 100). Barbara informed the police of her suspicions. Two years later the press reported that the scam continued and that the police had difficulty tracking down the criminals (Smith 1968).

During the summer Barbara and Buss visited Amy on Sunday afternoons and took her out into the grounds where they met other patients and visitors and listened to their worries about the care provided at Friern. Some relatives complained of the long journey to visit their loved ones and others had difficulty finding the fares. About two thirds of patients on ward E3 never had visitors (Robb 1967, p. 93). Barbara and Buss also heard about staff overlooking patients' physical ailments, shouting at them and taunting them, such as a nurse offering a patient a chocolate biscuit then taking it away and eating it in front of them (pp. 99, 101).

Attempts by the hospital to arrange a care home for Amy were ineffective, so her friends took steps to find one themselves. Barbara visited St Peter's, near Vauxhall, a convent care home with 200 residents run by the Little Sisters of the Poor. The ground floor was made up of mixed communal rooms. The sleeping quarters, as at Friern, were Nightingale-type dormitories. The home had a chapel (Fig. 3.6), visits from clergy, a farmyard with chickens and turkeys (Fig. 3.7), and provided facilities for handicrafts and other activities (Fig. 3.8).[65] Barbara was impressed and they had a vacancy. To complete the necessary discharge formalities, Barbara needed to discuss Amy with Dr Giddie, the ward doctor at Friern. Buss arranged their appointment for seven o'clock that evening. Dr Giddie did not turn up. The ward Sister phoned Dr Giddie who said that she would not meet Barbara and Buss as she could not help, but Barbara should write to the medical superintendent. Dr Giddie refused to speak to Barbara on the phone. Walking through the hospital and wondering how best to find a doctor in order to expedite Amy's discharge, Barbara asked two people she thought were canteen staff. She explained the predicament, and the glance one cast at her companion inspired Barbara to ask if she was Dr Giddie. Barbara was right. The companion, another doctor, offered constructive advice, with the ambiguous remark: 'The hospital would be delighted to see your friend go' (Robb 1967, pp. 102–104).

'DIARY OF A NOBODY': FRIERN, AMY AND FRIENDS 73

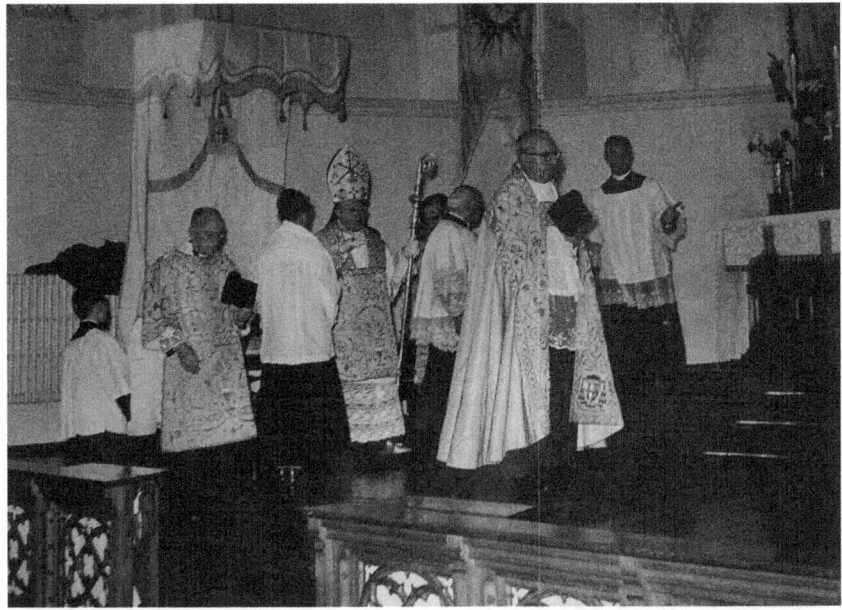

Fig. 3.6 Service in the chapel, St Peter's, 1960s. Reproduced courtesy of Sr Deirdre McCormack, Mother Superior, St Peter's.

Barbara did not trust Miss Cloake to book the ambulance to take Amy to St Peter's, so Audrey and Ronald Harvey and Barbara and Brian, took her in the Harveys' car. Amy was ready to leave when they arrived at Friern. Her outfit was hardly dignified. She was

> wearing a hideous skirt and cardigan and heavy shoes—all replacements for her own, which, we were told had worn out. At least she still had her own, decent coat... and her perky little hat. Her undies, such as they were, were on loan, and had to be returned (Robb 1967, p. 106).

At St Peter's, Amy particularly liked the food, smiling faces and having her own possessions, including a locker. She called her locker 'Vishnu'[66]—the giver and provider—more evidence of the breadth of Amy's knowledge, and her good cognitive function when she arrived there. She got stronger and more content, apart from her devastation at hearing about the

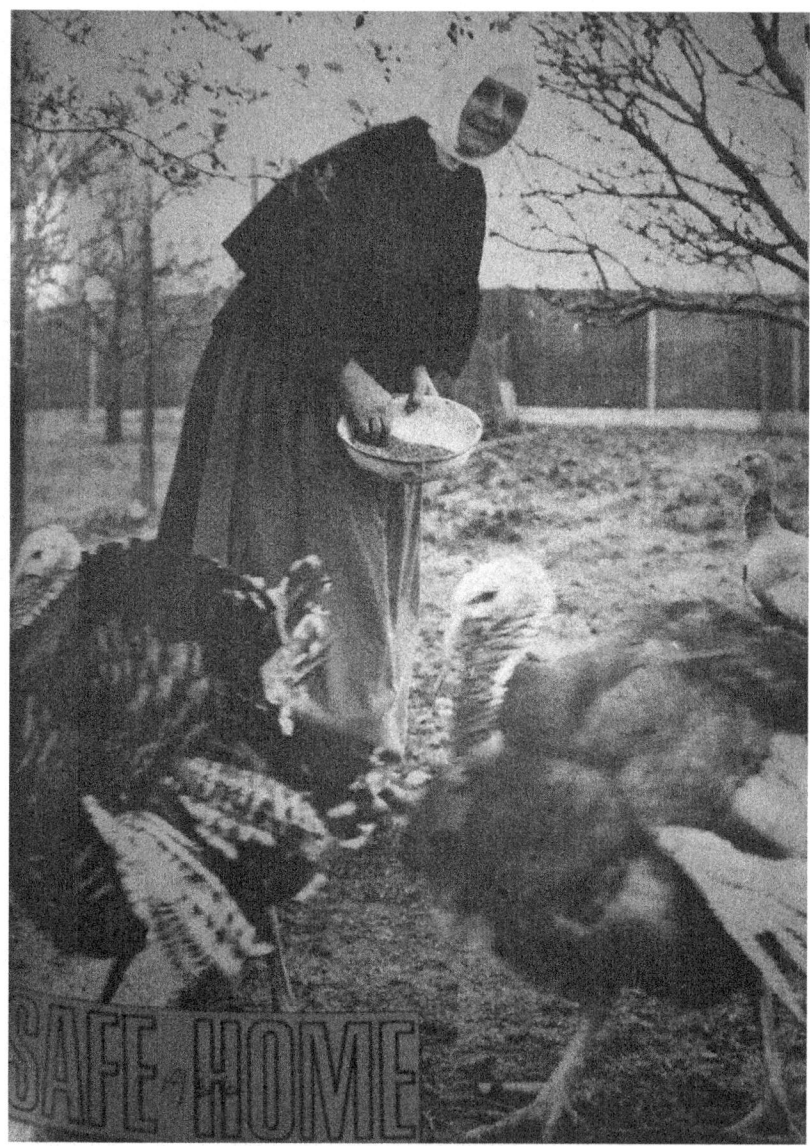

Fig. 3.7 Nun feeding turkeys in the grounds, St Peter's, 1966. Reproduced courtesy of Sr Deirdre McCormack, Mother Superior, St Peter's.

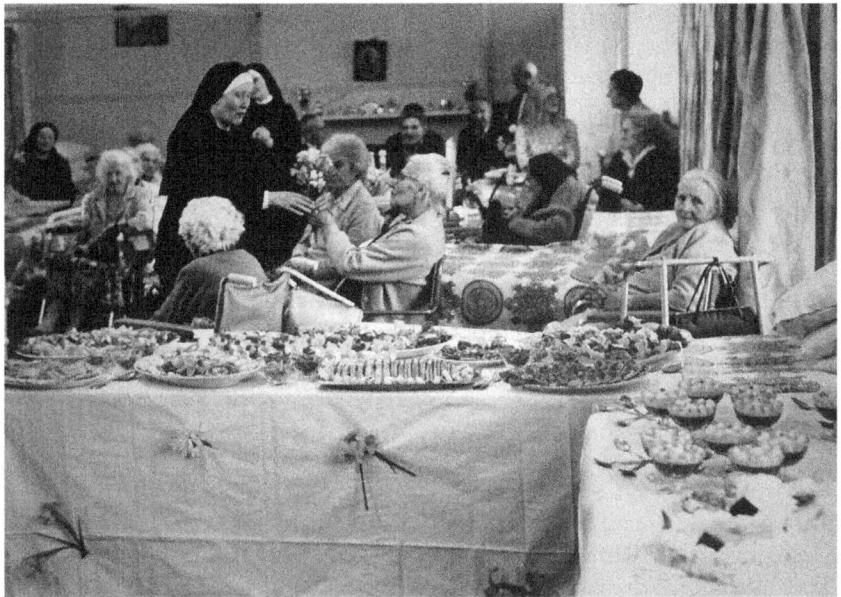

Fig. 3.8 Party on the women's ward, St Peter's, late 1960s. Reproduced courtesy of Sr Deirdre McCormack, Mother Superior, St Peter's.

disposal of her belongings (Robb 1967, p. 109). She began to write letters again. Strabolgi[67] and Missie, among others, visited her. According to Missie, Amy was in 'wonderful good health and normality' when she spent an afternoon with her.[68] Amy wrote to Barbara: 'I get kindness and sympathy here and the sisters call me pet and darling and haven't slapped my face ever, or slapped me hard on the hand which [the staff at Friern] loved to do'.[69] Despite Miss Cloake's assertion that Amy would never leave Friern, Amy lived for two years at St Peter's until her death in 1967.

Despite poor-quality care, some staff at Friern showed compassion, kindness and understanding (Robb 1967, pp. 78–79). Most poor care was not deliberately malicious but related to understaffing, overcrowding (about sixty patients on Amy's ward (p. 93)), primitive facilities, inadequate leadership, ineffective communication and staff ignorance about best practice. The stark difference between the way personal difficulties such as incontinence of urine was managed as humanely as possible in other institutions, such as Crichton Royal, Severalls or St Peter's, and the practice at Friern, where staff took few steps to minimise it and blamed patients for it, illustrates lack of knowledge or willingness to adopt practices that could improve patients' quality of life. Failure to implement best practice was also reinforced to Barbara when, on one visit to Friern, the patients and the ward looked engaging and lively, with books and sweets available, with all patients dressed and wearing their dentures. Barbara found out later that the staff were expecting an inspection (p. 89). Disturbingly, staff knew the conditions they should provide, implementing them for official visits but otherwise ignoring them. Barbara's observations also reflected her and Strabolgi's concerns about the effectiveness of planned, official inspections.

Was Amy Mentally Ill?

Retrospective diagnosis of any illness is problematic. Psychiatric conditions are especially tricky. They lack obvious physical pathology, symptoms intertwine with social and cultural understanding and expectations, and diagnostic criteria are influenced by social factors, medical knowledge and the law. In the early 1960s, many psychiatrists regarded hospital admission as integral to treating mental illness, a practice gradually challenged by research findings (Carse et al. 1958). In Amy's circumstances, a brief admission for assessment and to review medication was a reasonable option. For Amy, the main question is whether she required a *prolonged* admission. Her clinical notes do not survive.

The nature of Amy's mental illness when she was admitted in 1929[70] is unclear. However, a severe chronic disabling 'psychotic' illness such as schizophrenia was unlikely because, after discharge, she remained living independently, in employment, and with good social interactions in the years before antipsychotic medication was available. At the time of her admission in 1963, her psychiatric symptoms included anxiety and disturbing sexual sensations,[71] and an acquaintance commented that she was 'possessed of an evil spirit'.[72] These details do not permit diagnosis.

Common psychiatric diagnoses in older people include depression and dementia. Did Amy have dementia? Some episodes in the Diary suggest that she had some intermittent muddled thoughts. She might have been a little forgetful because she did not, or did not want to, remember what she had eaten at mealtimes (Robb 1967, p. 88). However, Amy's account of her fears and responses when asked questions to test her memory was compatible with anxiety more than dementia. In Barbara's words:

> when this man started asking her questions, she had thought that he might be trying to make out that she was mad, to stop her from leaving the hospital. She had been frightened and her memory had gone.
>
> He had asked her for her address. She told him she was in the old Colney Hatch. He asked for its proper name, and she hadn't been able to recall it, but had said that it might be in Middlesex. As soon as he had gone, she had remembered that it was now called Friern.
>
> Finally he had asked if she felt depressed. She had said yes, and he had asked if it was because she was 'in this place''? She had told him that it was partly that: 'Of course, it's nothing but that, really, Mrs Robb, but I didn't want to be impolite' (Robb 1967, p. 103).

Amy's recollections of the interview suggest that her memory was functioning adequately. Her improvement after discharge indicates that she did not have a progressive degenerative disorder, 'senility' or dementia, to an extent that required long-term psychiatric hospital care.

Did Amy suffer from a depressive illness? Amy did not appear to be depressed at the time of admission. She looked forward to visiting friends in Ireland who had invited her for Christmas. She was pleased with her new 'darling' home help[73] and intended to be present when her collage *The Pink Front Door* was exhibited at Kenwood in Hampstead.[74] She was optimistic that her problems would be sorted out. Her optimism changed to despair after a few weeks. She ended a letter to Barbara: 'Yours frightened'. She had no occupational therapy at Friern. She felt no better despite medication, 'a sleeping draught last thing that makes me sleep half the night and I'm awake the other half with these ghastly sensations that I can't escape'. She received a course of electroconvulsive therapy (ECT).[75] Barbara referred to ECT several times in the Diary, indicating that she was broadly disparaging about it (Robb 1967, pp. 69, 81, 99).[76] It is unlikely that she knew about the research indicating that it could be highly effective in older people with severe depression (Post 1962). More likely, she drew her knowledge from controversial, negative accounts in novels such as *One Flew over the Cuckoo's Nest* (Kesey 1962) or *The Bell Jar* (Plath 1963). Amy's symptoms did not suggest severe depression, the main indication for prescribing ECT. It is not surprising that ECT did not help, supporting the notion that assessments of her mental state were inaccurate.

Lord Amulree, a hereditary peer and high-profile pioneering geriatrician (Arie 2004), stated that 'nobody should go into a mental hospital...unless he has a disease which requires proper, skilled treatment.'[77] Amy might have had a degree of mental illness that justified her initial admission. However, evidence is lacking—from Barbara's observations and from Amy's previous independence and social adjustment, her lack of response to ECT and her well-being at St Peter's—that she suffered a severe depressive illness or schizophrenia or that she had a dementia requiring prolonged admission. This analysis cannot be conclusive. However, it supports Townsend's (1965, p. 229) observations that 'rather fewer elderly patients in psychiatric hospitals than is commonly supposed, are physically and mentally incapacitated to a severe extent.'

People and Politics

Minister of Health Kenneth Robinson had a longstanding interest in mental health. He wrote in 1958 that standards in mental hospitals fell below those of the rest of the NHS and that it was no longer reasonable to continue 'conducting our mental health services on the cheap' (Robinson 1958, p. 17). He noted that one third of mental hospital beds were occupied by people with schizophrenia, but did not mention that the same proportion were occupied by elderly people (p. 3). He was instrumental in passing the Mental Health Act 1959 and the Suicide Act 1961 (Jeger 2004). He was a Vice President of the National Association for Mental Health (NAMH)[78] and a member of the Mental Health Committee of the North West Metropolitan RHB from around 1950, resigning from that post when appointed Minister (Jones 1960, p. 178).[79]

As Minister, Robinson dealt with many competing health matters. In the 1960s, NHS spending increased in real terms and as a percentage of national income, a worry to the government. Resources were unevenly distributed, challenging the declared egalitarian objectives of the NHS (Webster 1998 p. 59). In 1965–1966, Robinson dealt effectively with the crisis in general practitioner services, which were 'in a process of disintegration' with low morale, poor recruitment and underinvestment. His carefully negotiated 'GP Charter' reversed the trend and boosted his reputation (Jeger 2004). MPs debated the needs of older people in February 1965.[80] Robinson did not speak and may not have attended. Reasons for that might have been valid, but his nonappearance was surprising for a topic for which his department had a crucial role.

A disturbing report by an anonymous consultant psychiatrist appeared in the *Guardian* in March 1965 (Anon. 1965a).[81] It corroborated Barbara's concerns: psychiatric hospitals were forbidding and prisonlike, with primitive toilet and bathing facilities, unsafe floors, high ceilings and peeling bare walls. It alleged wards of ninety people, understaffing and lack of trained social workers and that families remained silent about conditions because of stigma, or if they made a complaint, they were unlikely to take it beyond the ward to higher NHS authorities. The author wrote that his hospital probably 'compares unfavourably with the treatment of animals on our larger and more efficient farms'. Whether coincidental or conspired, a private member's ballot debate on mental health took place in the Commons the same day.[82] The consultant's article disturbed some MPs. Edwin Wainwright believed it: the consultant 'could easily be traced if necessary, so that what he says is obviously the truth'. Others, including Robinson, thought it exaggerated, except for the comments on the state of the buildings. Robinson, characteristically, praised the 'devoted staffs of these hospitals [who] maintain standards as impressively high as they are in so many cases'. Praise for staff working in poor facilities was honest and it could raise morale, but it defended existing standards and detracted from the authorities' responsibility to support staff to raise them.

Alfred Broughton MP reassured the House that although mental health services were the NHS's Cinderella, they had improved enormously and, like the rest of the NHS, were 'excellent' compared to those in other countries. However, comparisons were risky. Broughton also described the NHS as the 'best health service in the world', which, similar to saying that one is 'doing one's best under the circumstances' (Martin 1984, p. 245), implied deficits but created an impression of success and encouraged complacency. Statements of NHS superiority were also unsupported by data: comparative health outcomes were in their infancy (Scheiber 1990, pp. 159–160), and Abel-Smith did not have, but wanted to obtain, comparative economic data.[83] 'Best' was a political rather than medical or economic statement and inhibited criticism and preluded a balanced evaluation of services. Unfortunately, during the four-hour debate older people were hardly mentioned, suggesting that, despite their disproportionate occupancy of psychiatric hospital beds, their needs were easily overlooked.

Two weeks later, on 2 April 1965, Strabolgi sent Robinson a copy of the Diary signed by Barbara and the eleven people who had accompanied her on visits. Strabolgi's covering letter mentioned his 'grave disquiet' and shock at 'the atmosphere of the place and the feeling of official indifference that pervades it'. He attached a list of suggestions for improvement. Remedies included providing spectacles and hearing aids and lockers for personal possessions, dedicated units for older people who were not mentally ill, volunteers to help on the wards and better social work support (Robb 1967, p. 111). Strabolgi invited Robinson to study the Diary and expressed confidence in him: 'there is no one better to tackle the many problems' of the NHS. Strabolgi also wrote that Robinson's direct personal attention was preferable to asking a formal question in the Lords,[84] which fitted with Robinson's request for NHS problems to be raised in a low-profile way.[85] Robinson informed Strabolgi: 'I am having the case looked into and will write to you again when my investigations are complete.'[86] Strabolgi, Barbara and the other signatories waited to see the changes, for Amy and for the hospital more generally (Robb 1967, pp. 91–92).

The Ministry invited Barbara to meet with Tooth on 25 May.[87] She expected to hear the results of the investigations,[88] but it was clear at the start of their meeting that nothing had been done. The meeting was neither formally minuted nor witnessed, and it was not tape recorded by Barbara: she expected it to be a straightforward exchange of information, rather than having to fight her corner. Barbara took copious notes, which form the basis of the account here. Immediately after the meeting she went to a café and phoned Brian to say she must write it up while the details were fresh in her mind. She sent her apologies for a party at which they were expected, hosted by a professor at the Royal College of Art where Brian was head of Illustration.[89] This was an audacious act for a 1960s married woman. Sometimes Barbara's preoccupation with Amy and Friern was incomprehensible to Brian (Robb 1979).

Tooth acquainted Barbara with the term *stripping* of personal possessions and informed her that 'The Minister deplores its continued application in some hospitals, but he cannot intervene—not even in the case of patients who, far from being violent, are not even mentally ill but merely old.' Due to the Ministry delegating control of the hospitals to the RHBs and HMCs, Robinson could advise, but could not insist, that the practice be stopped. Tooth also said that the Ministry rarely received complaints from back wards, from which it inferred that care was satisfactory, although families who felt guilty at depositing their loved ones in hospital might be overly grateful, rather than critical, of staff who provided care that they themselves could not give. Barbara commented that 'many visitors were "inarticulate working class folk" who wouldn't take a complaint further than the ward', partly in the belief that those at the top '*must* know what is going on', a perspective supported by Abel-Smith (1967, p. 131) and the anonymous psychiatrist in the *Guardian* (Anon. 1965a). Tooth offered to investigate Amy's care, but 'could not recommend taking such a step, because it might lead to "something brutal" being done', echoing Amy's fears. Martin (1984, p. 150) empathised: 'It is very easy to be afraid, for a patient is always in a position of dependency, and the more closed or "total" the institution the greater the vulnerability to victimisation'. Barbara described Friern as Dickensian, 'Mrs Gamp-ery larger than life'. She ended the meeting:

> The government of my country is powerless to protect the old and helpless from un-necessary hardship and cruelty known to be inflicted upon them in its own institutions. That, Dr Tooth, is really all that you have told me.

From Private to Public

A month later, Strabolgi and Barbara still had not heard from the Ministry but with Amy safely away from feared reprisals at Friern, they could consider the next stage of their campaign. Sheila Benson, a researcher with Townsend (Townsend and Wederburn 1965), told them that stripping and the sort of treatment they observed at Friern were commonplace and that she had 'encountered other disgraces'.[90] Demeaning practices were more varied and widespread than Barbara or Strabolgi realised. This new information, together with dissatisfaction about continuing poor standards at Friern, led Strabolgi to address the House of Lords in a debate on community care.[91] Barbara listened from the gallery.

Strabolgi attributed the number of older people in psychiatric hospitals to insufficient alternatives, especially care homes that could look after 'incontinent and enfeebled' older people who were mentally well. Once in the psychiatric hospital, he said, they 'are treated worse than in the old-fashioned type of Victorian workhouses. They are treated worse because they are regarded as mentally deficient as well as merely poor.' He described stripping, lack of activities, visitors being discouraged, 'appalling' food and serving the last meal of the day as early as 3:30 P.M.

> The result of all this is an atmosphere of humiliation and neglect. The patients are...'pulped'. They lose all sense of self-respect. Worse than this, many are cowed and frightened. All just vegetate and seem lost to the world. And they are lost to the world. There is nothing more relentless than the State machine when it gets the helpless into its maw.

The national press was hot on the trail of Strabolgi's speech, to investigate the unnamed hospital (Anon. 1965b. 1965c). Strabolgi and Barbara maintained confidentiality about this, because, if the problems were widespread, naming a single hospital would detract from the broader implications of their observations. However, they encouraged the press to survey several hospitals. The *Daily Mail* obliged, promising to report in September (Anon. 1965e, 1965f).[92] The publicity brought Strabolgi a flood of corroborating letters.[93] One, from a journalist, described the 'terrible experience' of hospital care during her mother's last illness and lack of responsiveness when she challenged the authorities about it.[94] The Patients Association (PA) added to the argument that no notice was taken of complaints about hospitals and that an inspectorate was required, as existed for schools (Anon. 1965d).

Tooth gave Robinson his version of the meeting with Barbara. Based on this, Robinson wrote to Strabolgi that Barbara declined the offer of an investigation because *she* said Amy might suffer as a consequence.[95] That, however, seemed unlikely because Strabolgi and Barbara originally sent Robinson the Diary intending for him to investigate. Barbara informed Strabolgi that she would not have tried to hinder Tooth from investigating stripping if it could have prevented further suffering by older people,[96] and if it really were his duty to investigate, then her words, as a member of the public, should not have interfered with it. Differences between Barbara's and Tooth's reports might have been due to genuine misinterpretations arising from an unminuted meeting, or errors of recall, or, as Strabolgi and Barbara thought, ministerial self-justifying interpretations for doing nothing. Strabolgi replied to Robinson that because he now had evidence that stripping was more widespread, an investigation into Amy's specific predicament was obsolete. He asked Robinson what he proposed to do about stripping in NHS hospitals, if, as Tooth claimed, he deplored the practice.[97]

In August, Peter Shore MP posed a formal written question to Robinson about stripping. Shore was persuaded to do this, according to Cochrane (1990, p. 63), as part of the practice of introducing tactical, 'rigged' (Summerscales 1971; Anon. 1971), 'inspired' or 'planted' parliamentary questions 'put down by someone trustworthy'[98] at a politically convenient time.[99] It enabled the responsible minister to plan his answer. Robinson was thus able to state publicly that

> patients should be enabled to make the best use of their faculties by having proper spectacles, dentures and other aids when they need them. I deplore the practice of depriving patients of such aids which . . . is still followed in a minority

of hospitals and which can rarely be in the patient's own interest. I intend to issue guidance to hospital and local health and welfare authorities in due course.[100]

This answer informed the public that the Ministry was tackling the issue. Its timeliness paved the way for Robinson, three days later, to write to Barbara for permission to use the Diary for a RHB inquiry. In the light of 'unfavourable publicity' following Strabolgi's speech, he offered a 'full inquiry into the case of Miss Gibbs'. The inquiry would be in private and the report would not be published, and because Amy was no longer at Friern she could not be disadvantaged by it.[101]

Barbara, the Diary co-signatories, the NAMH and PA were wary of Robinson's reference to 'unfavourable publicity'. They suspected that it, rather than genuine intention to make improvements, motivated him. They feared that in a RHB investigation, the Board would deny the incidents detailed and accept the words of staff over public (a common occurrence, according to the PA[102]) and should the Diary be published, Robinson could state that it had been completely discredited to his satisfaction. Mary Applebey, general secretary of NAMH, regarded Robinson's request to investigate in private as an attempt 'to apply a well-known trick for suppressing embarrassing documents'.[103] Barbara replied to Robinson, in her 'respectful tone used when I write to ask the Pope why he has not got something done for us',[104] that he should have undertaken an inquiry when given the Diary in April, but now they knew that the problems were widespread, such an inquiry was too narrow. She also wrote that she had lost confidence in the Ministry's ability to handle complaints, and 'As for the unfavourable publicity of which you complain, may we respectfully suggest that the best way to avoid this in future is to firmly remove the faults that occasioned them.'[105]

Harvey (1965a) added to the controversy a few days later with a quarter-page article in the *Guardian*, 'The unknown prisoners'. It described Amy and her ward, without naming the hospital. Close behind, the *Daily Mail* published its survey of seven psychiatric hospitals, reportedly chosen at random, but including Friern. They found overcrowding—one had three rows of beds head to toe in the middle of the ward—and unsanitary and antiquated buildings in need of repair (Anon. 1965e). None met all the Ministry's criteria for living standards for patients, including privacy, personal lockers and clothing; regular occupation; weekly pocket money; and freedom to choose a time to go to bed (MoH 1964, p. 4). The *Mail* asked Robinson about his plans. He admitted that older people were 'an important element in the statistics' of psychiatric hospitals, that alternative care 'might have been preferable for some of them' and that he had just distributed a circular on the care of older people (Anon. 1965f; MoH 1965). A slim file at the National Archives indicates that this seven-page circular had a five-year gestation, with long periods of inactivity between discussions, and the file lacked indication of any ministerial action to achieve its recommendations. The circular reiterated proposals by Bevan[106] and in *Health and Welfare* (MoH 1963, p. iii), including that local authorities should create more small residential homes. It did not propose additional resources. Some parts of the circular related directly to concerns raised in the Diary—for example, it clarified that incontinence could be managed in care homes, contrary to what Miss Cloake told Barbara (Robb 1967, pp. 80–81; MoH 1965, pp. 3, 5). The National Archives file contains no discussion papers or drafts for the new circular,[107] suggesting, as Barbara suspected, that it was a rush job, with interest reignited so that Robinson could tell the *Mail* that something was being done.[108] The archives available do not allow definite conclusions to be drawn to corroborate this view, but the circular was timely.

Strabolgi offered during the debate in the Lords, to take Lord Taylor to visit the unnamed hospital that he described.[109] Strabolgi attempted to arrange an informal visit, with Townsend and Barbara accompanying them. However, the authorities favoured an official visit, without Barbara.[110] Strabolgi would have cooperated with an official visit if Barbara went with them, because he was confident that she was so familiar with the hospital she would 'turn something up'. He would not make an official visit without her, knowing that their itinerary would be predetermined and the patients and the wards would be smartened up for the occasion.[111] Finding his plan unachievable, Strabolgi called off the visit. The experience of trying to arrange an informal visit reinforced to Barbara and Strabolgi the farcical nature of planned, official inspection visits, under strict hospital control.[112] Other commentators on the NHS noticed this dilemma, such as Abel-Smith, who never made unannounced visits to hospitals because it would have been 'greatly resented by the administration and medical and nursing staff'.[113] Barbara wrote to the Association of Hospital Management Committees asking about established inspection processes, such as whether they had analysed the effect of staff escorting HMC visitors round the hospital and whether this might affect patients with regard to making complaints. The reply was evasive: 'the necessary reliable information is not available'.[114]

New Ideas in Psychogeriatrics

During the House of Lords debate, Taylor praised the rehabilitation and community-oriented work with older people by Russell Barton and Tony Whitehead at Severalls.[115] Giving a window of hope during an uncomfortable debate, he raised awareness of the Severalls scheme, and probably introduced Barbara to it for the first time. In September 1965, the *Lancet* published Whitehead's paper evaluating it.[116] In the aftermath of Strabolgi's speech, carrying the much sought after message that proactive psychogeriatric treatment could reduce bed use, Whitehead's paper reached the attention of the Ministry of Health. Tooth planned a meeting to discuss it. He enthusiastically suggested inviting Barton and Whitehead.[117] However, the minutes record neither their attendance nor apologies, so it is unlikely they were invited. Barton was unpopular in official circles and was known to have a volatile temperament: Tooth referred to him as the Chief Medical Officer's 'tiger'.[118] Two other eminent senior hospital consultants participated, both sympathetic to the needs of older people with mental illness, Norman Exton-Smith, a geriatrician (Irvine 2004), and Duncan Macmillan, a dynamic psychiatrist and medical superintendent in Nottingham. Macmillan was on the verge of retiring (HF 1970) and Exton-Smith did not have the creativity and dedication specifically concerning psychiatric services that Barton and Whitehead had shown. At the meeting, Tooth commented on the urgent need to improve care for older people in psychiatric hospitals. Exton-Smith and Macmillan made valid suggestions about joint psychiatric-geriatric assessment, appointing geriatricians to work in psychiatric hospitals and better training about psychiatry for nurses on geriatric wards. A second meeting was planned[119] but no further details have been traced at the National Archives. Barton and Whitehead's pioneering ways to improve older people's mental health had no direct effect on policy.

Another important event in London in 1965 was the World Psychiatric Association (WPA) three-day conference on mental illness and older people. Before this, international meetings about older people's mental health were usually single half-day sessions tagged on to broader gerontology conferences. At the WPA conference, several renowned researchers presented their findings, including Martin Roth and Felix Post, with subjects ranging from clinical practice to brain pathology (WPA 1965). For the first time, several up-and-coming young NHS psychiatrists interested in older people's mental health met each other and were inspired by established clinicians and researchers: Garry Blessed from Newcastle-upon-Tyne met Sam Robinson;[120] Klaus Bergmann, also working in Newcastle, met Post (Bergmann 2009, p. 40). Tom Arie probably met Blessed, Bergmann and Sam Robinson all for the first time.[121] The new network had the potential to shape ideas, spread good practice and support colleagues with shared interests. Barbara was working in parallel, more politically than the clinicians and researchers, but her work and the new networking created a potently fruitful conjunction of events.

COMMENT

Barbara's ancestry and early life were formative in her desire for justice. Family life, including difficulties and tragedies, and her religious education, gave her ideals that she sought to fulfil. Jung and White noted her knowledgeable, lively, determined, visionary, introverted intuitive personality: she would persist with a tug-of-war even when the odds were against her. Barbara's faith, family and friends and the financial means to dedicate herself to her task were assets that would help sustain her during the campaign years. Her humility underpinned her respect for others, and her ability to listen to them was a skill honed by her psychotherapy work. The interwoven life stories of the individual actors came together to influence the course of events: Barbara, Brian and Strabolgi at the Chelsea School of Art; White, Amy and Barbara since the 1940s; the HAC, which linked Amy, the Robbs, Strabolgi and Buss; and Barbara's neighbour Audrey Harvey, who worked with leading social rights campaigners such as Townsend and Abel-Smith.

Between January and June 1965, Barbara observed patterns of care which she and her fellow visitors to Friern found unacceptable: unkind and disrespectful nursing practices; and ignorant, unhelpful and often overworked staff in an inadequate environment. Some patients had no significant mental illness, but arranging discharge was challenging. Barbara also learnt the hard way about minuting (or tape recording) important meetings, ensuring later caution: Brian's colleague Quentin Blake, who visited the Robbs at home, was startled to hear Barbara say on the telephone: 'I should tell you I am recording this conversation, Minister'.[122]

NHS authorities did not acknowledge pitfalls of relying on planned, internal HMC inspections to assess quality of services. Their reports, together with lack of complaints, may have contributed to Robinson genuinely believing that the psychiatric hospitals functioned well, including for older people, thus fuelling his hostility to Barbara and her campaign. Her work was timely, coinciding with other revelations of unfavourable aspects of the NHS which also caused anxiety for the government. It also coincided with more interest among psychiatrists about treating mental illnesses in older people, although proactive psychogeriatric treatment in the psychiatric hospitals was still unusual, and community support as an alternative to back ward custodial care was generally insufficient. These observations corroborate Paul Bridgen's (2001) conclusions in his study of geriatric medicine and long-term care, that the slow rate of adopting active treatment for older people in the early years of the NHS was disappointing. Indifference by clinicians and NHS administrative leaders, lack of interest in unwell older people, overlooking their needs and stating that provision was adequate risked institutionalising neglect. This fits with Robinson (1958) promoting better mental health services generally but not explicitly including older people. For them, plans remained ambiguous, to the extent of lack of clarity about which hospitals or doctors—geriatric or psychiatric—should accept responsibility for their psychiatric treatment (MoH 1962, p. 5; Hilton 2016, p. 52).[123]

The rural isolation and 'total institution' (Goffman 1961) functioning of many psychiatric hospitals helped conceal deficits, and the stigma of psychiatric illness distanced the public emotionally from the happenings within them. Sheltering behind widely held beliefs about the excellence of the NHS, most hospital staff accepted established practices and acclimatised to the standards of care provided. Revelations of inhumane care were inconceivable to the public and officials who lacked experience of them. However, we must not judge the responses and attitudes existing in the 1960s by today's standards. Much that is visible today and acceptable to discuss would have been taboo in the 1960s: the Lampard Inquiry (Department of Health 2015) into the Jimmy Savile scandal exemplifies this. On the other hand, we must avoid a sense of security that all is well in the care of vulnerable people today (Panorama 2014).

Barbara made some important steps in these first few months of campaigning. She made links with the NAMH and PA and tested the waters with the Ministry. A debate in the House of Lords with much publicity, Shore's written question to Robinson, and the *Daily Mail* report highlighted concerns about standards of care. The timing of the Ministry's circular about the care of older people suggested that Barbara and Strabolgi had some influence on it. Barbara was aware of the struggle she might have to achieve her goals, including hostility, evasiveness and obstruction from the authorities. She told her plans to a 'doctor who I know well', probably Brian's brother Douglas Robb who had extensive medicolegal experience.[124] He 'turned pale green and said "For God's sake, don't do it!"' and described how hospital staff fake laboratory results, gang up and tell lies.[125]

Notes

1. Anne Robinson, interview by author, 2015.
2. Robb, 'Record of a campaign', vol. 1, 4–5, AEGIS/1/1. (AEGIS archive at London School of Economics, LSE)
3. George and Weedon Grossmith's novel *Diary of a Nobody* (1892) was adapted for television in 1964. Both the Grossmiths' and Barbara's 'diaries' use the literary device of aptronyms to describe their characters.
4. Police statement, 1969, AEGIS/A/5.
5. Robb, biographical note, 1970, AEGIS/1/10/B.
6. Anon. *Sunday Times*, 12 November 1972 (no title on cutting) AEGIS/9/1.
7. Register of Births, Wetherby, Yorkshire West Riding; a biographical note (1970, AEGIS/1/10/B) and her gravestone state 1913.
8. 'Diary of a Nobody', handwritten, 13 March 1965, AEGIS/4/8.
9. William Charlton, Barbara's cousin, email, 2015.
10. William Charlton, interview by author, 2016.
11. Mamie Charlton, Barbara's sister-in-law, interview by author, 2016.
12. Elizabeth Ellison-Anne, Barbara's niece, interview by author, 2016.
13. William Charlton, email, 2015; Elizabeth Ellison-Anne, interview by author, 2016.
14. Elizabeth Ellison-Anne, interview by author, 2016.
15. With thanks to Sr Clare Veronica, archivist of the Religious of the Assumption.
16. Information from Charlton family, 2016.
17. Anne Robinson, interview by author, 2015.
18. Note, AEGIS/1/10/D.
19. Robb, biographical note, 1970, AEGIS/1/10/B.
20. Meena Hudson, St Christopher's Fellowship, provided copies of undated newsletter pages between 1939 and 1945.
21. Robb, biographical note, AEGIS/1/10/B.
22. Elizabeth Ellison-Anne, interview by author, 2016.
23. Mamie Charlton, letter, 2015.
24. Elizabeth Ellison-Anne, interview by author, 2016; Mamie Charlton, interview by author, 2016.
25. Elizabeth Ellison-Anne, interview by author, 2016.

26. File, 'Dreams 1940–1942' 16 January 1941 (White Archive). Barbara was at Burghwallis for several weeks around Christmas 1940, see photograph album 1937–1941, in possession of Elizabeth Ellison-Anne.
27. Robb, biographical note, 1970, AEGIS/1/10/B.
28. Anne Shearer: journalist, including at the *Guardian*. Reported on Harperbury Hospital. Learning disability campaigner and Jungian analyst. Member of Davies Committee, 1971–1973. Interview by author, 2015.
29. White to Jung, 19 January 1947, in Lammers and Cunningham, *Jung-White*, 68.
30. Meeting, AEGIS, 9 November 1966, 37, AEGIS/1/20.
31. William Charlton, letter, 2016.
32. List, subjects of dreams, 1945–1946; Notes on dreams, 22 October 1951, 12 March 1953 (White Archive).
33. Letter, Robb to White, 9 November 1951 (White Archive).
34. Note, 8 November 1967, AEGIS/2/10. Corroborating this, Sir Quentin Blake (former colleague of Brian Robb: interview by author, 2016) noticed the profound affection in letters between Brian and Barbara.
35. Ann Lammers and Adrian Cunningham (2007) collected all known letters between White and Jung, publishing them in chronological order, thus dates of letters rather than page numbers are used in these notes.
36. White to Jung, 19 January 1947.
37. Jung to White, 23 January 1947.
38. White to Jung, 7 February 1947.
39. Barbara's dreams, attached to letter, White to Jung, 16 June 1947.
40. Extract of letter, Robb to White c. February 1947, sent to Jung. (Lammers and Cunningham 2007, p. 74).
41. White to Jung, 4 February 1947.
42. Barbara was enthusiastic about the writing of Ronald Firbank, especially *Valmouth* (1919), a fantasy about centenarians, with religious and sexual innuendo. William Charlton, email, 2016.
43. Competition on coincidences, *Sunday Times*, 5 May 1974, cutting in AEGIS1/10/D.
44. According to Jung, the anima is the complementary female element within a man's unconscious, representing traits that are considered female, such as gentleness, empathy and nurturing. The anima also serves as his conception of womanhood, what he considers to be the ideal woman mentally and physically.
45. Jung to White, 21 September 1951.
46. AEGIS meeting, 9 November 1966, 37, AEGIS/1/20.
47. White to Jung, 7 October 1951.
48. Jung to White, 16 October 1951.
49. Index to female patient admissions, Napsbury Hospital, c.1905–1950, H50/B/01/001–004 (London Metropolitan Archives, LMA).

50. Index to female admissions, Shenley Hospital, 1934, H49/B/07/005 (LMA).
51. 'Diary of a Nobody', draft, AEGIS/1/1.
52. Robb, 'Diary of a Nobody', draft, AEGIS/1/1.
53. 'Nature's lament on the proposed destruction of a lily pond', poem attributed to Amy Gibbs, written out by Robb. AEGIS/4/3.
54. Label, reverse of photograph of Amy Gibbs, 1961 (author's collection)
55. Strabolgi's summary about Amy Gibbs for Lord Amulree, 1965, AEGIS/2/3; Hampstead Artists' exhibition catalogue 1963–1964 (Camden Local Studies Centre).
56. Robb, chronology of events, 28 September 1960, AEGIS/4/3.
57. Letter, Gibbs to Robb, 19 September 1963, AEGIS/A/1/A.
58. Letter, Gibbs to Robb, undated, AEGIS/A/1/A.
59. Letter, Gibbs to Robb, 11 October 1963, AEGIS/A/1/A; a drop in blood pressure that could cause dizziness or muzziness was a common side effect of many tranquilisers used at this time.
60. Robb, 'Record of a campaign' vol 1, 4, AEGIS/1/1.
61. Original Diary sent to Kenneth Robinson, 2 April 1965, AEGIS/4/2.
62. Elizabeth Ellison-Anne, interview by author, 2016.
63. Instruction manuals, AEGIS/9/6; Meeting, Robb and Miss Cloake, 9 March 1965, AEGIS1/1.
64. Letter, Dr Aix (pseudonym; real name used in letter) to Robb, 16 March 1965, AEGIS/A/1/A.
65. Visit to St Peter's Residence and discussion with Sister Deirdre McCormack, Mother Superior, 2015.
66. Letters and sketches, Gibbs to Robb, 1965, AEGIS/4/5.
67. 'Community care' *Hansard* HL Deb 7 July 1965, vol 267 cc.1332–1410.
68. Note, Ernestine Anne to Robb, 1967, AEGIS/2/7/B.
69. Letter, Gibbs to Robb, December 1965, AEGIS/4/5.
70. Index to female patient admissions, Napsbury Hospital, c.1905–1950, H50/B/1/1–4 (LMA).
71. Letter, Gibbs to Robb, 11 October 1963, AEGIS/A/1/A.
72. Robb, 'Record of a campaign', vol 1, 1, AEGIS/1/1.
73. Letter, Gibbs to Robb, 1963, AEGIS/A/1/A.
74. HAC Programme, Iveagh Bequest Kenwood, 11–31 October 1964 (Camden Local Studies Centre).
75. Letters, Gibbs to Robb, November 1963, AEGIS/2/13.
76. Meeting, Robb and Ann Blofeld, 18 December 1965, AEGIS/A/1/A.
77. 'Mental health: Care of the young' *Hansard* HL Deb 13 July 1966, vol 276 cc.117–196.
78. NAMH, *Annual Report, 1958–9*, 1 (Mind Archive, Wellcome Library).
79. NWMRHB, Minutes and papers, 10 February 1964, BM 94/64 (LMA).

80. 'Needs of the elderly' *Hansard* HC Deb 19 February 1965, vol 706 cc.1508–1598.
81. In 2016, Emma Golding and Karen Jacques, archivists for the *Guardian* and the earlier *Manchester Guardian* were unable to identify the author.
82. 'Mental health service' *Hansard* HC Deb 19 March 1965, vol 708 cc.1645–1719.
83. Brian Abel-Smith, memo, May 1970, 154/3/DH/47/68 (University of Warwick Modern Records Centre).
84. Letter, Strabolgi to Robinson, 2 April 1965, AEGIS/7/8.
85. Letter, Robb to Strabolgi, 2 August 1965, AEGIS/7/12.
86. Note of exact words, Robb, enclosure 3, 76, AEGIS/1/1.
87. Meeting, Robb and Tooth, 25 May 1965, AEGIS/1/1.
88. Draft letter, Strabolgi to Robinson, July 1965, AEGIS/7/8.
89. Draft notes, meeting, Robb and Tooth, 25 May 1965, AEGIS/4/4.
90. Discussion, Robb and Sheila Benson, June 1965, 97, AEGIS/1/1.
91. 'Community care' *Hansard* HL Deb 7 July 1965 vol 267 cc.1332–1410.
92. Robb, 'Record of a campaign' vol 1, 108, AEGIS/1/1.
93. Letter, Strabolgi to Robinson, 15 July 1965, AEGIS/1/1.
94. Robb, 'Record of a campaign' vol 1, 120, AEGIS/1/1.
95. Letter, Robinson to Strabolgi, received on 12 July 1965, AEGIS/1/1.
96. Robb's report that accompanied Strabolgi's reply to Robinson, 15 July 1965, AEGIS/1/1.
97. Letter, Strabolgi to Robinson, 15 July 1965, AEGIS/1/1.
98. Memo, Robinson, about date of publication, 29 June 1968, MH159/216 (The National Archives, TNA).
99. Memo, EG Croft to Ms Hedley, 3 August 1967, MH150/350 (TNA).
100. 'Elderly and Mental Patients', *Hansard* HC Deb 2 August 1965 vol 717 cc.224–225 W.
101. Letter, Robinson to Robb, 5 August 1965, AEGIS/1/1.
102. Final report, meeting, Robb and Tooth, 25 May 1965, AEGIS/1/1.
103. Robb, 'Record of a campaign', vol 1, 147, AEGIS/1/1.
104. Letter, Robb to Strabolgi, 9 August 1965, AEGIS/7/12.
105. Letter, Robb to Robinson, 9 August 1965, AEGIS/1/1.
106. 'National Assistance Bill', *Hansard* HC Deb 24 November 1947 vol 444 cc.1603–1716.
107. 'Care of the chronic sick and elderly in hospitals and residential homes' meeting notes and papers, 1960–1965, MH160/95 (TNA).
108. Robb, 'Record of a campaign', vol 2, 10, AEGIS/1/2.
109. 'Community care' *Hansard* HL Deb 7 July 1965, vol 267 cc.1332–1410.
110. Letter, Strabolgi to Taylor, 19 July 1965, AEGIS1/1.
111. Robb, 'Record of a campaign', vol 1, 137, AEGIS1/1.
112. Robb, 'Record of a campaign', vol 1, 134, AEGIS1/1.

113. Memo, Abel-Smith to Mr Mottershead, 6 August 1969, MH159/236 (TNA).
114. Letters, Robb to AG Till, secretary of association of HMCs, 27 January 1966; reply, 11 February 1966, AEGIS/1/4.
115. 'Community care' *Hansard* HL Deb 7 July 1965, vol 267 cc.1332–1410.
116. Reprinted in Robb 1967, 115–123, and see Chapter 2, p. 33 for more details.
117. MoH, memo, probably, Tooth to Dr Boucher, 4 October 1965, MH160/486 (TNA).
118. Memo, Tooth, 30 September 1965, MH160/486 (TNA).
119. MoH, minutes, 'Provision of psychiatric services for the elderly', 12 November 1965, 1, MH160/486 (TNA).
120. Garry Blessed, discussion, January 2016.
121. Tom Arie, email, 2016.
122. Quentin Blake, interview by author, 2016.
123. MoH, 'Care of the mentally disordered', memo to Mr Dodds, 4 September 1964, D/M150/01, MH154/11 (TNA).
124. Douglas Fletcher Robb, 185, AEGIS/1/5.
125. Letter, Robb to Barton, 21 July 1966, AEGIS/1/20.

Bibliography

Abel-Smith, Brian. 1967. 'Administrative solution: a hospital commissioner?' 128–135. In Robb 1967.
Allan, Ellam Fenwicke. 1897. *A Woman of Moods*. London: Burns and Oates.
Allan, Ellam Fenwicke. c.1897. *Two Woman and a Man: A Society Sketch of Today*. London: Walter Scott Ltd.
Allen, Anne. 1967. 'One woman who refused to pass by..'. *Sunday Mirror*, 9 July.
Anne, Mrs Charlton. 1898. *One Summer Holiday: A Fairy Story*. London: John Macqueen.
Anon. 1937. 'Burghwallis Hall Wedding'. *Yorkshire Post and Leeds Intelligencer*, 22 July.
Anon. 1939. 'Radley College Mission'. *The Radleian*, 577, 5 March, 161–162.
Anon. ('A consultant psychiatrist'). 1965a. 'The scandal of the British mental hospital' *Guardian*, 19 March.
Anon. 1965b. 'Peer tells of "cowed and frightened" patients'. *Times*, 8 July.
Anon. 1965c. 'Peer says Ministry is powerless'. *Daily Telegraph*, 9 July.
Anon. 1965d. 'Patients want inspectors of hospitals'. *Daily Telegraph*, 14 July.
Anon. 1965e. 'The *Daily Mail* survey'. *Daily Mail*, 8–10 September.
Anon. 1965f. 'The minister replies to five blunt questions'. *Daily Mail*, 27 September.

Anon. 1971. 'Four ministers are 'rigging' questions in Parliament'. *Sunday Times*, 12 December.
Anon. 1976. 'The patients' campaigner'. *Hampstead and Highgate Express*, 25 June.
Arie, Tom. 2004. 'Mackenzie, Basil William Sholto, second Baron Amulree (1900–1983)'. In *Oxford Dictionary of National Biography*. http://www.oxforddnb.com, accessed 7 September 2016.
Bergmann, Klaus. 2009. In *The Development of Old Age Psychiatry in Britain 1960–1989*, (Guthrie Trust Witness Seminar 2008) ed. Claire Hilton. http://www.gla.ac.uk, accessed 18 September 2016.
Bridgen, Paul. 2001. 'Hospitals, geriatric medicine, and long-term care of elderly people 1946–1976'. *Social History of Medicine*, 14, 507–523.
Carse, Joshua. Panton, Nydia and Watt, Alexander. 1958. 'A district mental health service: the Worthing experiment'. *Lancet*, i, 39–41.
Catholic Social Guild. 1928. 'Catholic Social Guild schools examinations November 1927'. *Assumption Chronicle*, January, 20–21.
Charlton, Barbara. 1949. *The Recollections of a Northumbrian Lady 1815–1866*. London: Jonathan Cape.
Cochrane, David. 1990. 'The AEGIS campaign to improve standards of care in mental hospitals: a case study of the process of social policy change'. PhD thesis, University of London. http://etheses.lse.ac.uk, accessed 17 September 2016.
Cohen, Gerda. 1964. *What's Wrong with Hospitals?* Harmondsworth: Penguin Books.
Conlay, Iris. 1961. 'All of a glitter: the tinsel town of Amy Gibbs'. *Catholic Herald*, April.
Crossman, Richard. 1977. *The Diaries of a Cabinet Minister. Vol. 3. Secretary of State for Social Services 1968–1970*. London: Hamilton and Cape.
Department of Health. 2015. *Jimmy Savile NHS Investigations: Lessons Learned*. https://www.gov.uk/government, accessed 9 September 2016.
Goffman, Erving. 1961. *Asylums: Essays on the Social Situation of Mental Patients and Other Inmates*. New York: Anchor Books.
Grossmith, George and Grossmith, Weedon. 1892. *Diary of a Nobody*. London: J. W. Arrowsmith.
Harvey, Audrey. 1960. *Casualties of the Welfare State*. London: Fabian Society.
Harvey, Audrey. 1965a. 'The unknown prisoners'. *Guardian*, 10 August.
Harvey, Audrey. 1965b. 'Still homeless in London'. *New Statesman*, 5 November, 691–692.
Harvey, Audrey. 1976. 'Mrs Barbara Robb'. *Times*, 28 June.
HF 1970. 'D Macmillan'. *BMJ*, i, 119.
Hilton, Claire. 2016. 'Developing psychogeriatrics in England: a turning point in the 1960s?' *Contemporary British History*, 30, 40–72.
Irvine, RE. 2004. 'Smith, Arthur Norman Exton (1920–1990)'. *Oxford Dictionary of National Biography*. http://www.oxforddnb.com, accessed 10 April 2013.

Jeger, Lena. 2004. 'Robinson, Sir Kenneth (1911–1996)'. *Oxford Dictionary of National Biography.* http://www.oxforddnb.com, accessed 15 February 2016.
Jones, Kathleen. 1960. *Mental Health and Social Policy 1845–1959.* London: Routledge and Kegan Paul.
Jung, Carl. (1923) 1971. *Psychological Types* (translation: H Godwyn Baynes, revised by RFC Hull). New York: Pantheon Books.
Kesey, Ken. 1962. *One Flew over the Cuckoo's Nest.* London: Methuen.
Kingsley, Nicholas. 2016. *Landed Families of Britain and Ireland.* http://landedfamilies.blogspot.co.uk, accessed 20 September 2016.
Lammers, Ann. 2007. 'Jung and White and the god of terrible double aspect.' *Journal of Analytical Psychology*, 52, 253–274.
Lammers, Ann and Cunningham, Adrian, eds. 2007. *The Jung-White Letters.* London: Routledge.
Martin, John (with Evans, Debbie). 1984. *Hospitals in Trouble.* Oxford: Blackwell.
Ministry of Health. 1962. *A Hospital Plan for England and Wales.* Cmnd.1604. London: HMSO.
Ministry of Health. 1963. *Health and Welfare: The Development of Community Care: Plans for the Health and Welfare Services of the Local Authorities in England and Wales.* Cmnd. 1973. London: HMSO.
Ministry of Health. 1964. *Improving the Effectiveness of Hospitals for the Mentally Ill.* HM (64)45. London: HMSO.
Ministry of Health. 1965. *Care of the Elderly in Hospitals and Residential Homes.* HM (65)77. London: HMSO.
Ministry of Health. 1968. *Findings and Recommendations Following Enquiries into Allegations Concerning the Care of Elderly Patients in Certain Hospitals.* Cmnd. 3687. London: HMSO.
Panorama. 2014. *Behind Closed Doors: Elderly Care Exposed.* BBC1, 30 April.
Plath, Sylvia. 1963. *The Bell Jar.* London: William Heinemann.
Post, Felix. 1962. *The Significance of Affective Symptoms in Old Age: A Follow up Study of 100 Patients.* London: OUP.
Robb, Barbara. 1967. *Sans Everything: A Case to Answer.* London: Nelson.
Robb, Barbara. 1973. 'Jung's message to the elderly'. *Daily Telegraph*, 4 July.
Robb, Brian. 1944. *My Middle East Campaigns.* London: Collins.
Robb, Brian. 1979. *The Last of the Centaurs.* London: André Deutsch.
Robinson, Kenneth. 1958. *Policy for Mental Health.* London: Fabian Society.
Schieber, George. 1990. 'Health expenditures in major industrialized countries, 1960–87'. *Health Care Financing Review*, 11, 159–167.
Smith, Peter Gladstone. 1968. 'Antiques gangsters swindle the old'. *Sunday Telegraph*, 25 August.
Summerscales, Rowland. 1971. 'Commons row over question rigging'. *Daily Telegraph*, 13 December.

Townsend, Peter. 1965. 'A national survey of old people in psychiatric and non-psychiatric hospitals, residential homes, and nursing homes' 223–232. In *Psychiatric Hospital Care: A Symposium*, ed. Hugh Freeman. London: Baillière, Tindall and Cassell.
Townsend, Peter and Wedderburn, Dorothy, assisted by Sylvia Korte and Sheila Benson. 1965. *The Aged in the Welfare State: The Interim Report of a Survey of Persons Aged 65 and over in Britain, 1962 and 1963*. London: G Bell.
Toynbee, Polly. 1971. 'The right advice'. *Observer*, 14 November.
UK Census. 1911. http://www.ukcensusonline.com, accessed 15 March 2016.
Webster, Charles. 1998. *The National Health Service: A Political History*. Oxford: OUP.
Whitehead, Anthony. 1965. 'A comprehensive psychogeriatric service'. *Lancet*, ii, 583–586.
World Psychiatric Association. 1965. *Psychiatric Disorders in the Aged*. Manchester: Geigy.

Open Access This chapter is licensed under the terms of the Creative Commons Attribution 4.0 International License (http://creativecommons.org/licenses/by/4.0/), which permits use, sharing, adaptation, distribution and reproduction in any medium or format, as long as you give appropriate credit to the original author(s) and the source, provide a link to the Creative Commons license and indicate if changes were made.

The images or other third party material in this chapter are included in the book's Creative Commons license, unless indicated otherwise in a credit line to the material. If material is not included in the book's Creative Commons license and your intended use is not permitted by statutory regulation or exceeds the permitted use, you will need to obtain permission directly from the copyright holder.

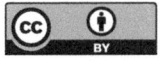

CHAPTER 4

Establishing AEGIS and Writing *Sans Everything*: 'The Case' and 'Some Answers'

Under the nom de plume 'Pertinax', Hugh Clegg, professor of industrial relations at Warwick University (Briggs 2005, p. 1472), wrote in the *BMJ*:

> More and more are responsible voices beginning to challenge many of the assumptions on which [the NHS] is based. Many must be rubbing their eyes and asking themselves why such a large carbuncle on the body politic has only just began to look so angry. The short answer is that there has been a conspiracy of silence, a conspiracy fostered by those in control and those afraid to speak (Pertinax 1967).

Barbara needed a strategy if she were to disrupt the conspiracy of silence about less favourable aspects of the NHS and succeed in improving care for older people in psychiatric hospitals. In October 1965 she established AEGIS (Aid for the Elderly in Government Institutions). The acronym occurred to her on a journey to visit Amy at St Peter's.[1] AEGIS was a snappy name, with a significant etymology. In Greek mythology, it was a shield carried by Athena and Zeus, a symbol of protection. Doing something 'under someone's aegis' means doing it under the protection of a powerful, knowledgeable or benevolent source. It was not a name for an organisation likely to admit defeat. Relating primarily to older people on the back wards, AEGIS aimed: 'to call public attention to some very serious defects that exist in the care of patients; to devise remedies for them; and to propagate modern methods of geriatric care with their strong emphasis on rehabilitation.'[2]

AEGIS adopted a role similar to the new breed of politically and media savvy health-related pressure groups emerging at the time, such as the Patients Association (PA) (Webster 1998, p. 68). AEGIS worked with the PA, whose broad remit meant that it comfortably delegated aspects of its work to enthusiasts with their own interests.[3] Working with the National Association for Mental Health (NAMH) was less straightforward. AEGIS's political and press campaign contrasted with NAMH's approach, which mainly encouraged voluntary work and maintained a successful educational programme about all psychiatric conditions, including those of older people (NAMH 1965, pp. 5, 13). NAMH was cautious about publicising the problems in mental hospitals but some NAMH staff thought it should undertake more campaigning.[4] NAMH's low-key approach related partly to its desire to keep in favour with the Ministry, which provided much of its funding.[5] Its noncontroversial standpoint was evident following the debate in the House of Lords at which Strabolgi spoke. During the debate, Baroness Elliot of Harwood, praised the work of NAMH. NAMH's report on the debate mentioned Elliot's praise but not Strabolgi's concerns, although the latter created press and public interest in the psychiatric hospitals that required a response (NAMH 1965, pp. 10–11).

AEGIS's headed notepaper reflected its professional approach. It also gave the impression of an organisation of magnitude, identifying Strabolgi as president, Barbara as chairman and Harvey as advisor. AEGIS's office was Barbara's cottage. Meetings took place there, and the shrill front door bell or Brian's footsteps on the wooden stairs would interject into the proceedings.[6] Brian took a back seat in the AEGIS campaign and would stay in the living room during meetings or make the tea.[7] AEGIS remained small and under Barbara's direct leadership. She was the voice of AEGIS and the inspiration and energy behind it, but she did not work in isolation: AEGIS expanded to include a handful of experts who could advise on specific issues.

AEGIS's early activities focussed on publicity, compiling *Sans Everything*, and planning tactically, aiming to kick-start the Ministry into action. AEGIS suffered from administrative and financial distractions integral to its story—namely, with the publisher over possible libel and with AEGIS's failure to achieve charitable status. In this chapter we also explore the disturbing comparisons made between the long-stay wards in the psychiatric hospitals and Nazi concentration camps, a theme raised by contributors to *Sans Everything*, which recurred during the formal inquiries into the allegations.

AGEIS: Supporters and Early Activities

AEGIS drafted a letter about its concerns to send to the *Times* when a suitable opportunity arose, but it needed influential people to sign it.[8] One evening Barbara saw Abel-Smith on television. She sent him the letter, and he returned it signed the next day.[9] AEGIS's goals were close to his heart: he knew from his students who worked in psychiatric hospitals for short periods 'what it was really like when the doctors weren't there' (Abel-Smith 1990, p. 259). Abel-Smith was also disappointed with the lack of impact on government policy from Townsend's study *The Last Refuge* (1962) about care for older people, which identified problems similar to those highlighted by AEGIS.[10] *The Last Refuge* initially received significant publicity, including a leader in the *Times* (Anon. 1962) emphasising government plans to close all workhouses and provide single-room longstay accommodation and greater choice for older people. Soon after, the Nursing Homes Act 1963 gave local authorities more control over maintaining standards, a first step to improving facilities. However, by 1965, for longer-term support for older people—for which financial responsibility was hotly debated between the NHS and local authorities—there was little impact (Bridgen 2001, p. 512). Thus Abel-Smith came to realise the importance of pressure groups and publicity, which he sought for his own research. *The Poor and the Poorest* (Abel-Smith and Townsend 1965), for example, was memorably launched with a press conference and television and radio broadcasts on Christmas Eve 1965. The timing ensured an immediate impact, and when linked to the Child Poverty Action Group (CPAG), had a significant longer-term effect (Thane 2015). Abel-Smith regarded a 'deliberately organised political campaign' to maintain pressure on the government as the only way for AEGIS to achieve its objectives.[11]

Abel-Smith introduced Barbara to Cecil Rolph 'Bill' Hewitt, a journalist who usually wrote under the name CH Rolph. A former police officer, in the 1960s Rolph was a left-wing political journalist at the *New Statesman* (Howard 2004). Rolph agreed to help Barbara make links with the press and manage public relations.[12] He chaired press conferences for her, gave AEGIS a platform in the pages of the *New Statesman*, 'acted in the capacity which [Barbara] was pleased to call "legal adviser"' and vetted her letters (Rolph 1987, p. 180). Vetting her letters was important because sometimes the language that best expressed her concerns was not ideal for the goals she sought. As Barbara's cousin William Charlton advised her, 'If you talk of "disgraceful negligence" and "ministerial complacency" they will think of you as an enemy, put themselves on the defensive and dig their feet in.'[13] Barbara and Rolph had a warm relationship; she characteristically ended her letters 'love from B'.[14] Rolph wrote (1987, p. 182): 'An invitation from Barbara had the same effect as a command.' Passionate and tenacious about her campaign, Barbara was 'incredibly good at seducing others to help her', according to journalist Anne Robinson.[15]

The *Times* featured an optimistic article on healthcare for older people in November 1965. In contrast to the usual pervasive negative expectation of inevitable decline, it explained that for physical and psychiatric illness, 'if Granny becomes ill and goes into hospital where there is an active geriatric unit, there is a good chance that she will be back home in a few weeks' (Special Correspondent 1965). The article provided an opportune moment for AEGIS to send its prepared letter. Barbara delivered the letter by hand to the *Times* that afternoon.[16] It appeared the following day, 10 November:

> We...have been shocked by the treatment of geriatric patients in certain mental hospitals, one of the evils being the practice of stripping them of their personal possessions. We now have sufficient evidence to suggest that this is widespread.
>
> The attitude of the Ministry of Health to complaints has merely reinforced our anxieties. In consequence, we have decided to collect evidence of ill treatment of geriatric patients in mental hospitals throughout the country, to demonstrate the need for a national investigation. We hope this will lead to the securing of effective and humane control over these hospitals by the Ministry, which seems at present to be lacking.

Signatories included Barbara, Abel-Smith, Harvey, Strabolgi, two other peers, two ministers of religion, an artist and a socialist reformer doctor, providing striking authority and prestige.[17] The letter had three messages: stripping took place, the Ministry mishandled complaints and AEGIS needed information from people 'who have encountered malpractice'. AEGIS promised confidentiality in dealing with personal data. Getting published was a breakthrough in gaining public attention. Considering stripping an unsuitable subject, the *Times* had twice refused letters about it from Charles Clark, a lawyer, publisher and active member of the PA and NAMH.[18]

Responses followed. Some people offered support, including the pioneering geriatric nurse Doreen Norton,[19] but in the main, Barbara received 'an avalanche of anguish' (Anon. 1965b). She answered every letter personally.[20] Some people asked her to visit their relatives with them, but voicing fear about complaints leading to staff reprisals against patients, they invariably asked her to keep the reason for her visit confidential.[21] The *Times* published correspondence with Maurice Hackett, then chairman of the North West Metropolitan Regional Hospital Board (NWMRHB), who had served on the Board in various capacities, including working on it alongside Kenneth Robinson. Hackett's first letter (1965a) was sanctimonious: 'We in the hospital world who are charged by the Minister to guard and protect the interest and care of patients in mental hospitals, are appalled at the irresponsibility of those who signed' the letter from AEGIS. Hackett did not state the name of the hospital implicated but implied that he knew it. He wrote that a 'public—or private independent' inquiry was offered, which Barbara and Strabolgi knew was incorrect: Robinson offered a private RHB inquiry.[22] Barbara and Strabolgi decided not to refute that publicly because if they did, the likely outcome was that the Ministry or RHB would say they offered it verbally, and the authorities, rather than AEGIS, would be believed.[23] Hackett (1965a) stated that the RHB was now conducting its own inquiry, which was accurate, although it had not informed AEGIS. Strabolgi and Barbara responded to Hackett's letter, noting that if Robinson had offered a timely inquiry when first approached, there would have been no publicity. They also queried why Hackett made no reference to stripping, AEGIS's primary concern. They blamed the difficulties of providing adequate care on a lack of finances, not on cruel staff: 'We have always recognised that the staffs of mental hospitals...work gallantly and devotedly under many difficulties...and no blame should be attached to them' (Strabolgi and Robb 1965).

Hackett's second letter to the *Times* informed the public about Strabolgi's covering letter for the Diary in April, in which he invited Robinson to 'study' it, but did not explicitly give him 'permission to make use of it' (Hackett 1965b). Hackett had a detailed knowledge of the covering letter, indicating at least some communication about it between him and Robinson, but Hackett misconstrued its meaning. It would have been pointless to send Robinson the Diary merely to peruse, and Robinson knew this, as indicated by his initial offer to investigate.[24] Hackett blamed Strabolgi's instructions for the Ministry not carrying out an inquiry. Robinson kept a low profile in the *Times* correspondence, permitting Hackett to respond on his behalf.

THE FIRST FRIERN INQUIRY

On advice from the Ministry, the RHB constituted a committee of inquiry two days before AEGIS's letter in the *Times*, and then informed Friern Hospital Management Committee (HMC):

> The Board have for some time been concerned at a number of criticisms directed towards psychiatric hospitals in general and to Friern Hospital in particular... and have now agreed to the proposal of the Minister that there would be advantage to all concerned if an enquiry were to be held by the Board.[25]

Evidence is not available to explain the timing, whether the Ministry and RHB knew about AEGIS's plan for publicity, or whether waiting until November was due to Ministry or RHB reluctance to investigate, or to multiple legitimate competing pressures. The Ministry could have been aware of AEGIS's plans because Abel-Smith was well known there (Sheard 2014, p. 187), and Robinson, Abel-Smith, Townsend, Crossman and Harvey shared other circles of activity, such as the Fabian Society.[26]

The RHB appointed Ann Blofeld to chair the committee of inquiry. Blofeld, in a voluntary capacity, had served on the RHB since 1949 and chaired its mental health committee since 1963 (Anon. 1978).[27] The committee planned to investigate the administration of Friern Hospital, the care of patients and Strabolgi's criticisms made in the House of Lords. The Diary was not included because Barbara refused permission for that in August.[28] On 2 December, Barbara and Strabolgi received identical invitations from Blofeld to attend the inquiry.[29] They were handwritten on Blofeld's personal headed notepaper from her home address, an unconventional approach for a formal inquiry, suggesting a rushed afterthought. Barbara and Strabolgi followed Blofeld's procedure: they replied with separate handwritten letters. When Barbara later asked Blofeld whether sending members of the public handwritten invitations to inquiries from private addresses was usual, she replied that she devised the procedures for the committee,[30] suggesting that the RHB lacked protocols for, and experience of, investigating complaints.

Barbara and Strabolgi were uneasy about the inquiry. In Barbara's view, because all the committee members either served on the RHB or worked in the NHS within the region, it was not a 'public—or private independent' inquiry of the sort Hackett (1965a) referred to. Barbara expected an independent inquiry to be chaired by a senior lawyer who was not a member of the RHB and for witnesses to have legal representation.[31] Strabolgi was worried that Abel-Smith, the NAMH and the PA were using them as their 'cat's-paws'.[32] The day before the meeting, the RHB asked Strabolgi to arrive at 11 A.M., and Barbara fifteen minutes later. Still cautious, they planned to arrive together at 10:45 and to refuse to be separated.[33]

At the meeting, Blofeld told Barbara 'in rather bullying tones' that she had not expected her to come. Blofeld was smug, such as announcing that she had 'many years of experience of hospital matters' and they should remember 'all the work that she had done in this field without ever having been paid anything at all for it'. The Diary, despite not being within the terms of reference, was central to the discussion. The members of the committee appeared sympathetic and interested in Barbara's points, the chairman less so.[34] Mutual distrust and antagonism seemed to characterise the meeting, hardly a recipe for a constructive outcome. Immediately after the meeting, Barbara wrote up her twelve-page account of it, which she hoped 'to publish one day'.[35]

Blofeld reported to the RHB in January 1966 with fourteen densely typed pages. The report expressed gratitude to Lord Strabolgi for helping the inquiry but was less appreciative of Barbara who was 'also present'. Despite the antagonisms, the report was surprisingly insightful, particularly regarding the care of older people. It found that some were in Friern 'merely because they are old',[36] corresponding with Townsend's research (1965, p. 229). The Friern consultant psychiatrists held divergent opinions about their older patients' potential for discharge (if alternative support and accommodation were available), ranging from 6 percent to 83 percent for women patients and 2 percent to 58 percent for the men. Each consultant had their own patients, but clinical differences between the patients were unlikely to account for these disparate expectations. More likely, expectations indicated a haphazard approach to treating older people, lagging behind best practice recommendations. Compared to similar hospitals, Friern also lacked social workers to assist with arranging discharge: it had one qualified and two unqualified social workers with high rates of staff turnover (Ministry of Health (MoH) 1968, p. 49),[37] creating an impossible workload.

The committee noted lack of activities for the patients, but thought it might be 'inhuman to attempt to stimulate the very old'. They also found an absence of dentures and hearing aids. The staff told the committee that these items were not permanently removed, but after a pair of spectacles went missing, staff collected them at night for safe keeping and handed them out the next morning. However, the committee visited during the day and saw patients without these items, incompatible with staff explanations. Possibly, staff levels did not permit them to redistribute the aids, in which case their alleged nighttime safe storage was futile, or the staff's explanation for absent aids was incorrect.[38] Bedside lockers were a logical remedy. On some wards, staffing levels were 'grave', and some staff spoke little English.[39] On the day the committee visited ward E3, where Amy had been, it had fifty-three patients, with one sister, two untrained nursing assistants, a student and a ward orderly. Staff levels were too low to provide adequate individual attention to the patients, two of whom were confined to bed with fractured femurs and many others required time-consuming physical care because of incontinence and frailty.[40]

The report condemned the twenty-four unstaffed locked wards at night, some with side rooms locked within them, because of fire and other risks: the Colney Hatch Asylum fire, which killed fifty-one patients was within living memory (Anon. 1903) (Fig. 4.1). Unequal provision of staff and resources favoured the Halliwick unit, undermining staff morale in the old building. For the hospital generally, the report described conditions unacceptable by 1960s standards: appalling 'sanitary annexes', inadequate ward heating, dismal ward environments and overcrowding. Medical care on the back wards was inadequate,[41] and poor care overall was associated with complacency and 'lack of imagination, direction and drive'.[42] Complacency of the medical superintendent, senior nurses and the HMC shocked the committee.[43] The committee concluded that Friern was a hospital 'in which progress generally is retarded', displaying unwillingness to relinquish out-of-date practices.[44] The low standards raised the possibility that the RHB was uninformed, or ignored or concealed inadequacies, patterns recognised elsewhere (Martin 1984, p. 85).[45] Friern fitted with the Ministry's descriptions of the worst psychiatric hospitals, and that 'the difference between the most and the least progressive [hospital] is greater now than ever before' (MoH 1964, p. 1). The report supported, rather than refuted, Strabolgi's and Barbara's allegations.

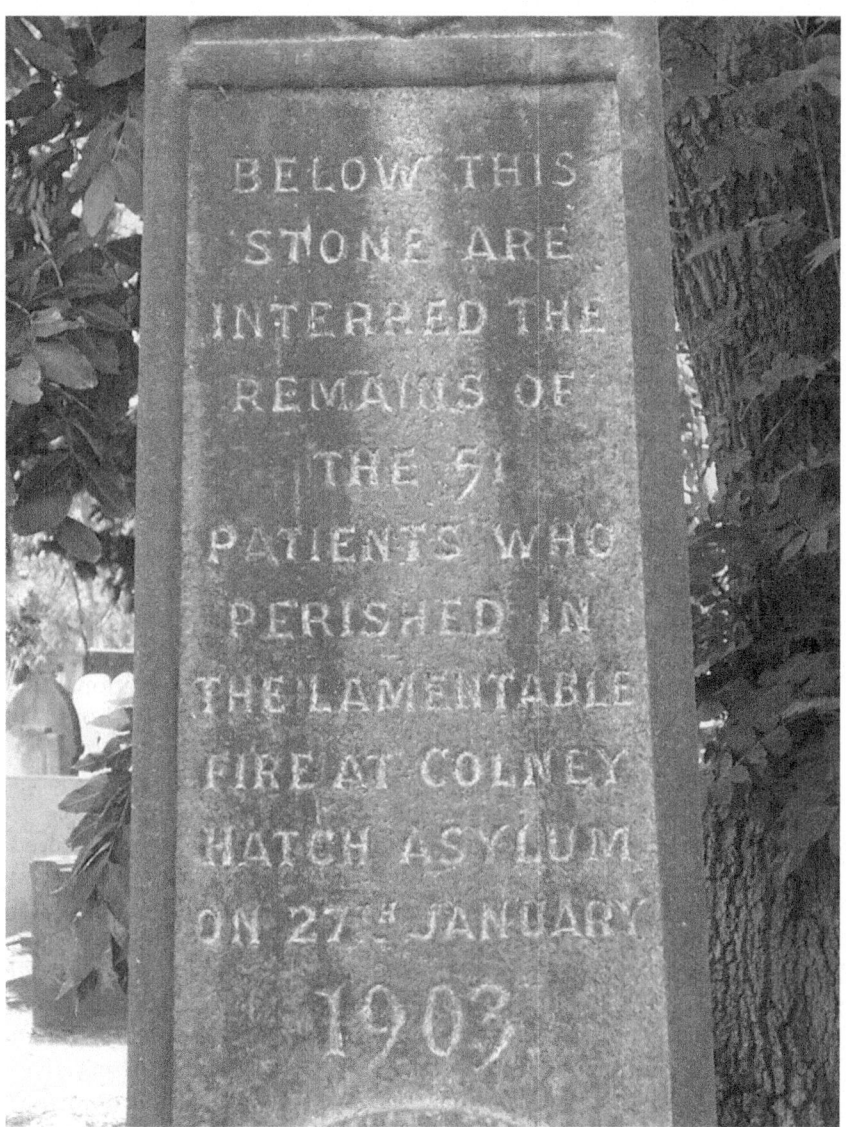

Fig. 4.1 Memorial to victims of Colney Hatch Asylum fire, New Southgate Cemetery, 1903. Photograph by author.

The Outcome of Blofeld's Report

Hackett chaired, and Blofeld attended, the RHB meeting that discussed her report. The RHB decided that the part of the report containing the most 'serious concerns must be regarded as strictly confidential', whereas the comments about limitations in day-to-day care, mainly on the back wards, were within the bounds of acceptable practice and were 'a vindication of the Hospital'. The RHB planned to discuss the report with the Friern HMC but minuted no other actions.[46] The integrity of the RHB in dealing with a private, internal inquiry that it had no commitment to publish was a stumbling block, contrasting with the honesty of the inquiry committee. Similar to Friern HMC when faced with unfavourable reports on nurse staffing,[47] the main deficits were concealed, giving no chance of the report benefitting patients. Hackett sacked Friern's clinical leaders—matron, chief male nurse and medical superintendent—because he regarded them as responsible for the deficiencies. He implied that blame lay solely with clinicians by not sacking the HMC or the 'hopeless old chairman, hopeless secretary' as Crossman described them.[48] The minutes do not document how the Board reached its conclusions and feeble plan of action, whether any Board members disagreed, or if Blofeld spoke at the meeting. After years of service on the RHB, Blofeld took on a new role in 1966 as Chairman of the Board of Governors of the Royal National Ear Nose and Throat Hospital (Anon. 1978), outside the RHB's authority. It might have indicated her dissatisfaction with the response to her report.

A later investigation at Friern criticised Hackett for the sackings and described the Board's apathy towards Blofeld's report as 'inexcusable'.[49] Strabolgi and Barbara never saw the report, but it would have shattered their doubts about Blofeld's unconventional methodology and allayed their fears about an internal inquiry inevitably being biased. Strabolgi received a brief and bland summary from Robinson, which Rolph called a 'whitewash'.[50] In December 1966, a year after Blofeld interviewed Barbara and Strabolgi, Barbara wrote to Hackett requesting a copy of the report. Hackett replied in a single line: 'I have your letter of 18th December and have no comment to make.'[51] Hackett's secretiveness was out of line with the Ministry's recent memorandum on managing hospital complaints (see below, pp. 109–112), which emphasised that explanations should be sympathetic and sufficient and 'it should be made evident to complainants that their complaints have been fully and fairly considered' (MoH 1966b, pp. 1, 3). There was no justification for the content or tone of Hackett's concluding letter to Barbara, which she described as 'short and sour'.[52] His response was pivotal to her campaign: she decided then to publish the Diary.[53]

Action on Stripping

The Ministry sent a letter to RHBs in December 1965 offering guidance on stripping, remarkably swiftly after the letter in the *Times*. The guidance also referred to personal possessions such as jewellery and watches.[54] The informal status of a letter rather than an official memorandum released the RHBs from any obligation to report back to the Ministry about the practices in their hospitals, or what was being done to improve them.[55] If, as the PA informed AEGIS, official ministerial guidance was usually ignored,[56] circulars that did not require feedback were almost worthless. The Ministry, despite claiming to deplore stripping, was half-hearted in its attempt to prevent it.

Friern HMC discussed the stripping guidance. Any action over dentures, spectacles and hearing aids to assist independence paled into insignificance compared to worries over the financial value of watches and jewellery.[57] The latter were more problematic for staff and the HMC because these objects might be stolen or given to relatives for safe keeping or not brought back after the patient went out on visits. Staff would, therefore, not know the whereabouts of belongings, leading to 'difficulties and misunderstandings'.[58] The Friern discussions also indicated the enormous control staff had over patients' lives. Staff control made life easier for the nurses but undermined confidence, independence and rehabilitation for the patients.

The Ministry's letter on stripping was unavailable to the public because of its informal status. AEGIS and the PA[59] both sought confirmation about whether it had been circulated, and to what effect. With no answer from the Ministry, in February 1966, Barbara approached Eric Lubbock MP who agreed to ask about the guidance in Parliament.[60] The press picked up the issue (Anon. 1966a), raising public awareness. One outcome was an anonymous editorial in the *Lancet*, reporting that despite the Ministry's letter, the practice continued, justified as 'the custom of the hospital' even though there was no medical reason for it, and it caused immense damage to personal pride and independence. The author stated that the quantity of an older in-patient's personal possessions indicated the effectiveness of the ward: the more the better (Anon. 1966b). Rolph backed up AEGIS with an article in the *New Statesman* on stripping and other unacceptable practices. He based it on personal experiences of visiting psychiatric hospitals and on his work as a police officer, and acerbically asked whether it was really necessary to remove spectacles, hearing aids and dentures to protect individuals:

> When the 'senile dementia' of your dormitory neighbours gets too much for you, you might break your spectacles and slash your wrists with the glass. Well, I've done my share of precautionary disarmament with people in police custody, but I never took anyone's teeth away (Rolph 1966a).

Rolph's article precipitated more letters, similar to those already received by AEGIS. In his memoir he wrote:

> I can remember the shock of misery with which I read the letters that came to me after the *New Statesman* article … despairing cries of decent, ordinary people unable to get a hearing in the hospital world. These nurses told of pitiless neglect of the helplessly old, and of the common practice of 'stripping' (Rolph 1987, p. 181).

Abel-Smith and Rolph could not fathom out why Robinson was so uncooperative about stripping. Abel-Smith commented to AEGIS that 'The moment you mentioned the word he flared up. And he doesn't flare up often,… he's been hit below the belt on it,… he is very sensitive.'[61] Barbara concluded: 'the issuing of "advice" had been no more than a feeble, face saving exercise.'[62]

Improving, Monitoring and Maintaining Standards

AEGIS proposed three ways to improve, monitor and maintain standards in the NHS: effective local complaints mechanisms; a health service commissioner or ombudsman to investigate complaints that could not be resolved any other way; and independent inspection of hospitals (Abel-Smith 1967). The PA concurred with AEGIS's strategies and noted despairingly that, especially for elderly patients, 'hospital boards and committees cannot be relied on to represent and protect patients' interests' (Hodgson 1966). Concerning complaints, no guidance for handling them was introduced at the inception of the NHS. The only formal mechanism outside the law courts was the General Medical Council, which, since 1858, managed complaints against doctors. In 1964–1965, the Ministry noted several examples of poorly managed complaints. It commented that one RHB enquiry did 'not seem to be entirely consistent with the seriousness of the matters requiring investigation'.[63] The South West Metropolitan (SWM) RHB informed the Ministry that its HMCs were inadequately acquainted with 'criticisms about their hospitals, some of which later result in quite serious complaints'.[64] Inadequate responses by RHBs to complainants left one civil servant grumbling: 'We have to spend endless time in concocting phraseology in our replies to cover this deficiency',[65] implying that the Ministry attempted to protect the RHBs rather than impartially investigate complaints. The Ministry's motivation for its method of managing complaints was partly self-preservation, to avoid 'disproportionate and damaging publicity' when, it claimed, most clinical work was carried out to a good standard.[66]

A three-page memorandum by the Ministry (1966b) about handling patients' complaints was the NHS's first official guidance on the matter (Mulcahy 2003, pp. 29, 31).[67] It had a two-year gestation, an extraordinarily long time for such a brief document, and the draft in February 1965[68] differed little from the final version in March 1966. National Archives' files do not indicate whether publication was influenced by agitation from AEGIS or the PA or whether there were genuine administrative reasons for the time lag. The Ministry based the guidance on good principles sympathetic to the complainant, but it was not binding and lacked detail. It stated, for example, that 'special arrangements may be needed in psychiatric hospitals' but did not explain what that meant. Abel-Smith illustrated his understanding of this with examples of the difficulties faced by staff, and conclusions drawn by them, when responding to complaints in psychiatric hospitals.

Complaint 1: Missing spectacles?
Response 1: Not a valid complaint, as it is inevitable if the patient has nowhere safe to put them.
Complaint 2: Patient frightened because of staff behaviour?
Response 2: Not a valid complaint as the patient is confused.
Complaint 3: Bruised patient who says she was struck by a nurse?
Response 3: Not a valid complaint: sister says it would not happen on her ward and, anyway, it would be impossible to get to the truth.

Although Abel-Smith contributed to developing the new guidance (Cochrane 1990, p. 83), in his view, it was inadequate, especially for patients in hospitals with a cultural malaise and self-protective staff loyalty that would defeat expressions of concern by patients or their representatives. The recommended processes could work well for adverse medical treatment incidents but were unlikely to succeed for a 'sick' hospital (Abel-Smith 1967, p. 132).

The new guidance did not state who would assess the complaints, nor did it propose training or the means to achieve 'adherence to a well-recognised procedure' (p. 1). It advised prompt and impartial handling of all complaints, at all degrees of seriousness, and informing the complainant of the result of the investigation and action taken. Barbara received a copy via Abel-Smith (Cochrane 1990, p. 83). In the light of her recent experiences with the Blofeld Inquiry, Barbara must have pondered over the recommendation: 'a small number of cases...so serious that they cannot be dealt with satisfactorily...should be referred for independent enquiry.' The guidance (p. 2) defined *independent* as being chaired by an independent lawyer 'or other competent person from outside the hospital service' with a committee independent of the authority concerned and that 'The complainant...should be allowed to make their own arrangements to be legally represented if they so wish', in line with Barbara's requirements.[69] Guidance on legal expenses for witnesses was not included: RHBs and lawyers held various opinions on this, from all to nothing.[70]

The Institute of Hospital Administrators (Anon. 1966c) cautiously welcomed the guidance. It criticised the recommendation that complaints that could not be dealt with by staff in a ward or hospital department had to be stated in writing, because some people lacked the skills to write or dictate a letter, and 'Perhaps that is why so many of them seem to make their complaint in the local newspaper office.' It also stated that more staff education was required, commenting that if a hospital considers it acceptable to keep older people waiting for long periods in out-patient clinics or to deprive them of dentures or spectacles, then it will 'hardly be able to satisfy people who complain'. It took up AEGIS's concerns about older people to illustrate the need for adequate complaints procedures, which was heartening for Barbara.

The complaints guidance was categorised as a 'pink' circular indicating that the Ministry required feedback on its implementation. Ben Whittaker MP for Hampstead (Barbara's constituency, another of her allies) asked

Robinson, a year after its introduction, how often the procedures for more serious complaints that could not easily be resolved had been used. Robinson replied: once.[71] Whether RHBs and HMCs publicised and implemented the guidance was therefore doubtful, a hypothesis supported by other evidence. One person wrote to Barbara about attending a recent complaint investigation:

> I feel worse than ever after the 'Committee of Investigation' last night, because I realise how utterly helpless one is against a hospital.
>
> Every so often, Dr C would pull a face and say 'Tch!' I can't really describe his facial expression or his attitude. He sat with his arms outstretched across the table, the sheaf of notes between and when he was speaking he kept his head bowed down to the papers or staring at his hands. I would call it 'shifty'. He seemed ill-at-ease, yet he could 'explain' every point at great length, so make it sound as if all he had thought of was the patient's comfort, and that I couldn't be expected to understand.[72]

The complainant requested a written report but did not receive one. Others wrote to Barbara about similar experiences. Most investigations ended in complete rebuttal of the complainant's concerns. Frequently, administrators based their analyses on the doctors' reports, without evidence of discussion with other staff, the patient, or the complainant.[73]

At Friern, HMC minutes first mentioned the guidance almost a year after publication,[74] and at the NWMRHB, it seemed to have little effect. When the *Daily Mail*, in 1967, criticised Harperbury Hospital, aligning conditions there and in other 'subnormality' hospitals with eighteenth-century slave ships, the Board sought to uncover actions of staff that might have enabled the journalist to write his report, rather than whether there was substance to the allegations.[75]

The new guidance made little impact at the Ministry which justifiably could have been expected to set an example. In 1967, a complaint submitted after a patient's relative heard of AEGIS's work, illustrated the old pattern of response. The complaint related to an elderly woman patient in a SWMRHB hospital. It described inadequate food; rude ward staff; staff insisting on bathing the patient even thought she was frightened and unaccustomed to sitting in a bath; and incontinence causing distress when the patient was unable to get out of bed.[76] The Ministry delegated the investigation to the SWMRHB, which subsequently fed back that it found no evidence of 'cruelty or neglect at any stage of her treatment'.[77] It is unlikely that a balanced investigation would have produced such a reassuring, across-the-board statement, but concluding that her care was acceptable at all stages, meant that there was no need to make improvements. The Ministry accepted the SWMRHB's assessment and wrote to the informant, criticising him: 'We are sure you will appreciate that it is helpful if matters of this sort are brought to the attention of the hospital authorities at the time, when the necessary steps to investigate can be taken immediately.'[78] With condescending responses by those in highest authority, it is hardly surprising that some complainants, like Mrs Dickens at Friern, became exhausted, demoralised and gave up.[79]

AEGIS's second proposal was for an ombudsman or commissioner to investigate apparently unresolvable NHS complaints. The Labour Party (1964) election manifesto proposed a new office of parliamentary commissioner 'with the right to investigate the grievances of the citizen'. The PA was not convinced that the government's proposal would cover complaints of the kind that they handled,[80] so wrote to the Ministry in December 1965 recommending a separate NHS appointment.[81] In a curious case of interpressure group rivalry, Hodgson (1972) claimed that a NHS ombudsman was the PA's idea, not AEGIS's. About this, Barbara commented: 'I discussed the idea of a Hospital Ombudsman with her in the Autumn of 1965—when she was being extremely kind and helpful—but she didn't *seem* to bite on.'[82] The Parliamentary Commissioner Act 1967 did not cover the NHS. Doctors' opposition contributed to that because they were concerned about interference by lay people in matters of clinical judgement, but there were also technical reasons (Anon. 1966d). These included, confusingly, that within the NHS, only the hospitals, for which the Ministry directly delegated management to the RHBs, would come under the new ombudsman, whereas the local 'autonomous bodies' which organised general practitioner and community health services, would not. The Ministry also thought it prudent to give the 1966 NHS complaints procedures a trial before introducing another scheme.[83] Reflecting ambivalence and diverse opinions on the matter, the Act was drawn up so that hospitals could be included with ease at a later stage.[84]

AEGIS's third strand was to establish a hospitals' inspectorate. However, this was not on the government's agenda in the mid-1960s. Explanations for this relate to the establishment of the NHS. The first white paper proposing a NHS (MoH 1944, pp. 10, 24) discussed ways to organise it and the possibility of an inspectorate. One organisational option for the NHS was to delegate responsibility to local authorities, as for schools. That model gave central government a supervisory role, with inspectors essential to it, to report back to assist with supervision. For hospitals, the Ministry adopted an alternative model of direct management through RHBs and HMCs. The Ministry would appoint these bodies which would be directly accountable to it, so inspection and feedback were not required. Mental hospitals, however, also had to comply with mental health legislation, so continued to undergo independent inspection by the Board of Control. Many staff appreciated these visits and the opportunity they provided to pass on information and ideas from one hospital to another and the way they could focus interest on needs long recognised by hospital staff but ignored by HMCs and RHBs (DHSS 1971, p. 1). In the course of the Royal Commission (1957) on mental illness and mental deficiency, the British Medical Association and Royal Medico-Psychological Association (later Royal College of Psychiatrists) argued for an independent inspectorate. Despite this advice, the Commission decided that 'A central Inspectorate outside the Minister's own Department is neither necessary nor desirable' (Royal Commission 1957, p. 254). Thus independent inspections of mental hospitals ceased when the Mental Health Act (1959) abolished the Board of Control. This brought mental hospitals into line with general hospitals, a far-reaching step that implemented decades-old principles of treating people with mental illness, as far as possible, under the same NHS principles as those with physical illness. It would remove independent inspections but had the potential to reduce stigma and encourage community services (Hilton 2016a). In 1964–1965 when MPs requested inspectors for hospitals, Robinson reiterated that such a system was inappropriate.[85] In July 1965, the *Daily Telegraph* reported that the PA asked the Ministry to establish an inspectorate, basing their request on evidence from its members who reported that, too often, complaints made to hospitals were ignored or insufficiently investigated (Anon. 1965a). By the time Barbara compiled *Sans Everything*, the Ministry had provided no plans for an inspectorate.

Planning *Sans Everything*

Letters to AEGIS arrived from all quarters and via unexpected routes. The Ministry of Health forwarded to AEGIS some from aggrieved relatives, including one from Miss Geraldine Richardson who petitioned the Queen on the care of older people, and another from Miss Kathleen

Gabb asking Mrs Wilson, the wife of Prime Minister Harold Wilson, to intervene on stripping.[86] It is inappropriate to discuss the hundreds of letters AEGIS received, many of which are stored in 'closed' sections of the AEGIS archive. Disclosure might be hurtful for descendants of patients or staff. For *Sans Everything*, AEGIS built its case from a few witnesses' reports selected from the many responses it received.

AEGIS planned tactically. The book was timely, according to Rolph, in the broader context of public discontent about government conspiracies, cover-ups and 'ministerial lying'. His examples included secret international dealings at the time of the Suez crisis (1956); the government inadequately handling the press concerning publication of potentially sensitive security material (1967)[87]; and 'Parliamentary question time every Tuesday, Wednesday, Thursday and Friday'. Rolph wrote to the publisher that it 'will turn out to be a seminal book and that when all the tumult has died down (which will take quite a while) there will at last be some action.'[88] He was sure that a well authenticated sensational book aimed at the general public would create a sufficient stir to provoke appropriate investigations to achieve necessary changes. He hoped at least for a public inquiry, if not a Royal Commission or a House of Commons Select Committee. His expectations linked to the recent appointment of the Mountbatten Committee on prison security in the aftermath of spy George Blake's escape from Wormwood Scrubs prison (Home Office 1966). Blake's escape received significant press attention: 'Everybody gets terribly frightened and worried and excited', Rolph said, resulting in some high profile person being appointed to investigate, followed by changes and more evaluations. Rolph wanted the same for *Sans Everything*.[89]

The title *Sans Everything* was not a given. The shortlist was scholarly and reflected the breadth of Barbara's knowledge of literature, and the depth of searching characteristic of her work. From Juvenal's Satire XI—*morte magis metuenda senectus*—she derived *More to Be Feared Than Death*. Another option was *The Last of Life* from Robert Browning's 'Rabbi Ben Ezra': 'The best is yet to be, The last of life, for which the first was made.' Another possibility was *Twice a Child*, from 'An old man is twice a child' in Shakespeare's *Hamlet*.[90] *Sans Everything* was a late addition.[91] The phrase originated in Shakespeare's *As You Like It*: 'Sans teeth, sans eyes, sans taste, sans everything.'[92] In addition, the ancestral motto from the Charlton line of Barbara's family was *Sans Varier*, meaning without changing or deviating from the path, a maxim by which she abided and that could have contributed to her final choice of title.[93]

The Witnesses and Their Statements

This section gives biographical sketches of the *Sans Everything* author-witnesses and an outline of their allegations (other than those about Friern, discussed in Chapter 3, pp. 69–76), plus some relevant contextualising material. Knowledge of the witnesses' backgrounds contributes to understanding the subsequent inquiries. It also reveals similar personality and employment characteristics, likely to have influenced staff willingness to whistle-blow, a subject relevant to the NHS in 2016 (Hilton 2016b; NHS Improvement 2016). The amount of biographical detail available for each witness varies and is drawn from several sources, including from their correspondence with Barbara and from verbatim transcripts of inquiries and, for Joyce Daniel, from information provided by her sons.

Barbara chose accounts by staff and former staff that she thought were particularly clear, convincing, factual and informed. She met each author to 'satisfy myself that they are reliable and well balanced persons' (Robb 1967, p. xiii). She continued to be meticulous about confidentiality, for the witnesses' security, because of victimisation of staff who were disobedient, or who complained or questioned hospital practices. Barbara thus gave the author-witnesses pseudonyms, except for Roger Moody who was content to use his real name. The pseudonyms derived from Barbara's ancestry, reflecting her high regard for the witnesses and creating a link with her personal commitment to the cause. Barbara took Anne family names as surnames: Osbaldeston, Isham, Swinburne, Tasberg(h), Heneage, Fenton and Cra(y)thorne. The two male nurses she called Michael and Frederick, names of several ancestors and her two surviving brothers. The women's first names linked to her aunt Louisa; grandmother Laura Adeline; great-grandmother and aunt who were both called Emily; and Elizabeth who died 'for the faith'[94] (Table 4.1).

The Witnesses, Their Names, Roles and Hospitals

None of the witnesses received payment for his or her writing or for involvement with AEGIS: they all participated to appease their consciences. As one witness, James Davie, said: 'My motives are that if I hadn't taken action as I have done here, I would never have been able to look myself in a mirror again. I was appalled. I am appalled.'[95]

Table 4.1 The *Sans Everything* witnesses

Name	Pseudonym	Role	Hospital
Dennis Moodie	Michael Osbaldeston	Assistant chief male nurse	Banstead, Surrey; Friern
Jean Biss	Laura Heneage	Ward sister	St James's, Leeds
Eileen Porter	Emily Swinburne	State enrolled nurse	Cowley Road, Oxford
Susan Skrine	Louisa Fenton	Auxiliary nurse	Cowley Road, Oxford
Joyce Daniel	Adeline Craythorne	Auxiliary nurse	St Lawrence's, Bodmin
James Davie	Frederick Isham	Auxiliary nurse	Storthes Hall, Huddersfield; Springfield, Manchester
Dorothy Crofts	Elizabeth Tasburg	Psychiatric social worker, and relative	Friern
Roger Moody	None	Trainee social worker	Friern

One of the *Sans Everything* author-witnesses was Joyce Daniel (Fig. 4.2). Born in 1911, her father, a lawyer, was Town Clerk of Devonport and later of Plymouth. She had no formal education beyond school age but in the 1930s was housekeeper for the novelist and poet Sir Arthur Quiller-Couch, then in his seventies. During the war, she had various jobs, including driving an ambulance in Southampton, a city that suffered heavy bombing. In 1945, she, her husband, and one-year-old son, settled in a cottage on a wooded smallholding outside Bodmin, Cornwall. When her husband died in 1959, Joyce went out to work to support her sons, Charles and Robin, who were then teenagers. Unusually, and resonant with the family's unconventional interests and determination, they acquired their first steam traction engine in 1962, and restored it.[96] Joyce wrote to Barbara about her family and about using their traction engine to help roll the tarmac for a local airstrip.[97] Her correspondence with Barbara, with meticulous handwriting and eloquent expressions, suggests she was an able, sociable and thoughtful person, aiming to do her best for her family and friends.[98]

In 1964, Joyce Daniel took a job as an auxiliary (untrained) nurse at St Lawrence's Hospital, Bodmin, working mainly on a long-stay female

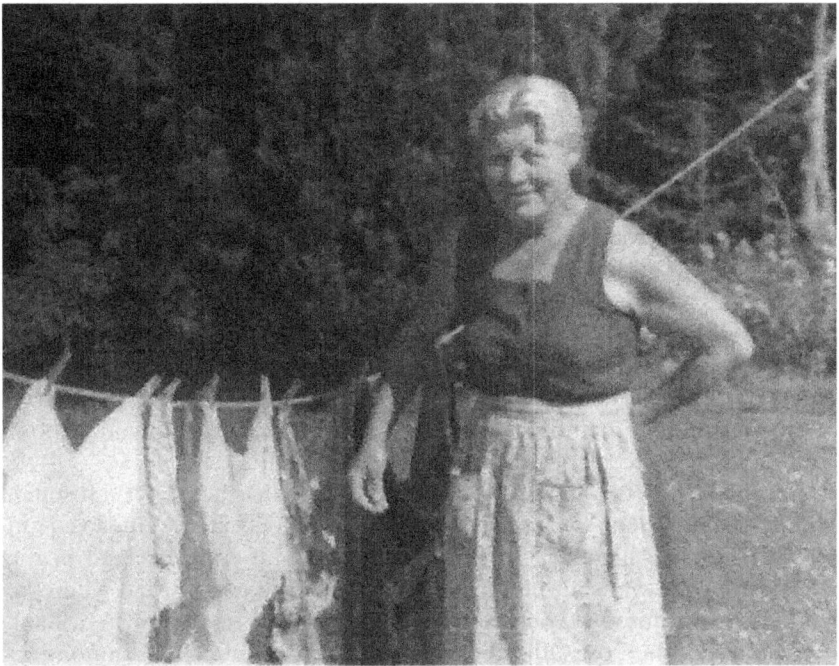

Fig. 4.2 Joyce Daniel, c.1964. Reproduced courtesy of Charles and Robin Daniel.

geriatric ward (Daniel 1967). She described, among other things: staff swearing at patients, hitting them and handling them roughly; communal bathrooms where forty-four patients were bathed in a single morning; patients 'locked in the lavatory to keep them out the way'; and staff making crude remarks about patients in their hearing. She also wrote that patients responded warmly to her interactions with them. When she complained about staff behaviours, she was taken off duties with patients and transferred to cleaning copper pipes in the ward bathroom. Her colleagues were angry with her, saying her comments created an unpleasant work atmosphere and that nurses should be loyal and unified. She resigned.

Loyalty to colleagues was central to the function of a close-knit psychiatric hospital 'total' institution. The primacy of loyalty defended staff against criticism: the critic became the unacceptable deviant. Punishing critics was common—for example, ordering them to do domestic work rather than work with patients, making life intolerable so that they resign,[99] or dismissing them (DHSS 1971). Occasionally the Ministry became involved in an appeal against dismissal on grounds of transgressing the etiquette of loyalty. The case of Mrs Glynn in 1967 illustrates this. Glynn was a nursing assistant. She received a letter from her matron: 'I feel that your disloyalty towards your colleagues and the fact that you are not happy with conditions at the Dene, leaves me with no alternative but to ask you to accept one week's notice.'[100] Glynn was subsequently reinstated and matron was reprimanded.[101] Correspondence with the Ministry does not indicate the underlying reasons for Glynn's discontent or if they were remedied. Russell Barton (1967, p. x) commented on the 'misplaced loyalty of one staff member to another.... Victimisation of anyone who is critical, whether justifiably or not, may be automatic.'

Another witness, James Davie, worked at Storthes Hall Hospital, Huddersfield, then Springfield Hospital, Manchester. He lived in Manchester with his wife, Phyllis, and their daughter. He served in the RAF during the war, but no farther afield than the Isle of Man where he worked with injured servicemen. He then worked in the Savings Bank department of the Post Office before buying a hardware and ironmongery business. He sold the business around 1964, expecting to find alternative employment, but it proved difficult.[102] At that time he was studying French at Advanced ('A') Level.[103] Davie, like Daniel, was in his fifties, had diverse life experiences but had no nurse training and sought worthwhile, secure employment.[104] He also had a life-long stammer, worse under stress, making his decision to attend the subsequent inquiries even more admirable.[105]

Davie took a job as an auxiliary nurse at Storthes Hall during a recruitment drive by the hospital (Davie 1967). He worked on several wards there, including a long-stay ward for men of all ages. His allegations included that staff hit and bruised patients or caused other injuries, then attributed the injuries to patients assaulting each another.[106] In the communal bathroom, he alleged that sometimes bathwater was not changed between patients. Sometimes, patients were punished by depriving them of food and water, nurses shoved them out of bed with a broom and he was left in charge of a ward, despite being unqualified.

In 1965, after leaving Storthes Hall, Davie went to Springfield. There, he alleged that an elderly, incontinent man was shaken 'like a rabbit' by the charge nurse, then thrown on the floor, and another was 'throttled' while being confined to bed as a punishment (Davie 1967, pp. 46–47). Senior staff were unhelpful when Davie complained, and he had the 'impression' that the doctors knew what was going on but did little to try to stop it (pp. 45, 46, 47). Davie, like Daniel, was proud of getting on well with the patients, which he attributed to patients knowing that 'no violence was forthcoming from me' (p. 44).

It is worthwhile exploring other happenings at Storthes Hall to contextualise Davie's complaints. Storthes Hall HMC minutes reveal their preoccupation with the environment and administrative matters, paying little attention to therapeutic relationships, activities for patients or rehabilitation.[107] In 1961, the minutes contained more about the piano tuner's contract, the purchase of a 'chocolate and fondant enrobing machine' and rabbit clearance on the hospital estate than about the patients.[108] The HMC made some progress in improving the environment, such as installing 'armour-plate' glass in windows in single rooms used to accommodate potentially violent patients: the new glass removed the need to close the wooden shutters, which would block out daylight, when it was necessary to protect patient and window.[109] Other problems at Storthes Hall included pilfering by staff.[110] In October 1965, police inspected the bags of staff going off-duty. Ill-gotten gains of five kitchen staff included one Bakewell tart, two pounds (weight) of cooked mutton, three loaves of bread, seven eggs and a dozen 'chocolate crunch'. The minutes reported that the staff were reprimanded[111] but did not state who tipped off the police or why at that time.

In 1962, the HMC documented only one complaint, from a mother about violence towards her teenage daughter, a patient. The single-page report of the internal investigating committee does not allow detailed analysis but indicates that it accepted unquestioningly the nurses' statement that the patient had 'never been ill-treated or harshly dealt with'. In contrast, the committee rejected all the mother's allegations. The committee concluded that the only actions needed were to thank the staff for their dedicated work and to transfer the 'difficult patient' to another hospital. The latter would avoid the HMC having to encounter the mother and grandmother 'who both indulged in bizarre, unrealistic and paranoid complaints'.[112] The process of investigation, total rejection of the complaint, criticism of the complainant, unhesitating acceptance of the staff report, and removing the patient, resembled complaint handling at Friern and by the Ministry.[113]

Storthes Hall had a custodial and paternalistic regime, a pattern seen elsewhere, such as at Friern. The Ministry knew that Storthes Hall had 'a long history of difficulty'[114] but praised the new medical superintendent, Alfred Smith, appointed in 1962, as 'courageous', a 'good' man going to work in a 'poor' hospital.[115] Smith's predecessor started at the hospital as a junior doctor in 1924 and remained there for his entire career.[116] Thirty-eight years in one traditional, custodial-style hospital, leaving a 'poor' hospital to his successor, implied a leader who made little attempt to modernise practice or who was complacent about existing standards.

Less is known about the other six author-witnesses, mainly because verbatim transcripts of the inquiries into their allegations have not been traced. Nevertheless, descriptions of their hospitals and their biographical sketches corroborate other evidence, about hospital practices, the authorities' responses towards people making complaints, and the characteristics of the whistle-blowers. Jean Biss was a ward sister for seven years at the Retreat, the Quaker-run psychiatric hospital in York, before moving to St James's, a general hospital in Leeds. There, she was appointed sister in charge of a psychiatric ward,[117] a prestigious post at a time when general hospitals were just beginning to provide psychiatric services. Biss had several concerns at St James's, including dangerously poor clinical communication between doctors and nurses; unappealing and inadequate food for patients; insufficient bed linen and towels; too few ward staff; and unsafe practices such as nurses dispensing medication from memory without using prescription charts. She raised the difficulties with matron who told her that she was 'too sensitive and felt too strongly about things' (Biss 1967, p. 27). Biss resigned after four months.[118]

Dennis Moodie was also a senior nurse who moved from hospital to hospital, frustrated by his inability to make improvements. He alleged wards being kept locked for staff convenience; violence towards patients; victimisation of staff who complained; and a HMC chairman who told him that his HMC was powerless to remedy the situation (Moodie 1967). When Barbara met Tooth she received a report about powerlessness at the Ministry, giving the impression that various tiers of NHS management could declare powerlessness, pass the buck, shrug off criticism and avoid taking initiative to make changes. This is compatible with Webster's (1998, pp. 50, 55) finding of a degree of 'ossification' of some aspects of the NHS, and an impression of inactivity by the Ministry during the 1960s. Moodie (1967, p. 14) summed up the situation for staff who wanted to improve nursing care: 'It becomes a case of "Give in—or get out". And it is always easier, in all professions, to accept the status quo.' He left Banstead Hospital in Surrey, and Friern Hospital, and at the time of *Sans Everything* worked as assistant matron at Claybury,[119] a hospital determined to make improvements for patients (Pitt 1968, p. 29).

Two of the *Sans Everything* authors, Eileen Porter and Susan Skrine, worked at Cowley Road Hospital, Oxford, the respected geriatric hospital led by Lionel Cosin. Porter looked for a job when her daughter got a place at university.[120] She was attracted to nursing, like Daniel and Davie, because the work would be 'of some use to the community' (Porter 1967, p. 27). Skrine graduated from St Anne's College, Oxford, taught for sixteen years in England and in India, worked for the Auxiliary Nursing Service in India during the war and then in Palestinian refugee camps in Jordan. She joined the staff at Cowley Road in 1958.[121] Both women, independently, reported their concerns to their superiors, including understaffing; lack of instruction; the 'almost unendurable' smell of stale urine and faeces; patients having to be in bed by 5 P.M. for the nurses' convenience; lack of respect for elderly patients, which left them frightened; and lack of dignity, such as failure to use screens for personal care (Skrine 1967; Porter 1967). Despite Skrine raising concerns to the HMC and to matron since 1964,[122] 'the only noticeable result has been to make my position in the wards more difficult' (Skrine 1967, p. 37). In Barbara's opinion, many hospitals had good and bad parts, a 'curate's egg':[123] at Cowley Road, while the leadership paid close attention to pioneering geriatric work in the acute-assessment wards, the long-stay wards were relatively neglected, as in the psychiatric hospitals.

Two social workers also contributed to *Sans Everything*. Social workers were, to some degree, outside the rigid hospital hierarchy so somewhat protected from the victimisation experienced by the nurses. Roger Moody was a trainee social worker at Friern in the early 1960s. In regard to older people, he criticised the way they were placed in mental hospitals and noted that 'society...far from honouring old age, tries to banish it completely from the mind' (Moody 1967, p. 68). The other social worker, Dorothy Crofts (1967),[124] described the care of her elderly father at Friern. Her descriptions paralleled Barbara's experiences of visiting Amy, including lack of visitors on the ward, bed time by 7 P.M., patients fearful of staff, a struggle to obtain her father's discharge and staff describing her father as confused, contrary to her perception of him.

The brief profiles of the eight witnesses make up a very small sample from which to draw conclusions. Nevertheless, some patterns emerge. Seven of the eight author-witnesses were in their forties or older, and the same number were 'new' to the hospital environment (like Montagu Lomax at Prestwich Asylum)[125] in the sense of a new job (at whatever level), as a student, or a visitor. Of the six nurses, four left jobs because of negative experiences. Skrine's Oxford education, Davie's French studies and Daniel's eloquent writing suggest that they were working in positions below their intellectual potential. Although untrained in nursing skills, the experiences of the unqualified or recently qualified nurses were diverse, including war work, bringing up children and doing jobs that required numerous interpersonal skills, which helped them interact meaningfully with patients.

The allegations were remarkably similar, including understaffing which allowed time only for basic physical care; senior staff unresponsive to concerns voiced by staff or visitors; and lack of privacy, personal respect and understanding of patients' emotional needs. Little was interpreted as deliberate cruelty. The witnesses considered it their duty to speak out, despite victimisation by doing so. Types of allegations, witness characteristics and responses by the authorities in *Sans Everything* were disturbingly consistent with those described by Virginia Beardshaw (1981, pp. 31–32) in her study of psychiatric hospital nurses fifteen years later. Similar to Martin (1984, p. 247), Beardshaw demonstrated that whistle-blowers were usually of low status in the nursing hierarchy, such as orderlies, nursing assistants and students, and that senior staff regarded them as having no business to put forward their views, because they were unsound judges, uninformed, inexperienced and immature.

AEGIS's Advisors

Nurses and doctors joined the AEGIS team of advisors. They, as Rolph, Abel-Smith, Harvey, Strabolgi and the witnesses, all worked with AEGIS unpaid.[126] The relationship between the nursing profession and AEGIS was initially fragile: some people, including Robinson, interpreted AEGIS's criticisms as a direct slur on the entire nursing profession.[127] However, AEGIS's positive statements about nurses (Strabolgi and Robb 1965; Robb 1967, p. xiv), nurses as key witnesses for *Sans Everything*, some nurse leaders supporting AEGIS, and AEGIS's actions to reduce victimisation of nurses who spoke out, did not endorse that view. AEGIS needed to build a strong relationship with the nursing profession to try to buffer any misinterpretations. This was complicated, partly because psychiatric nurses were not fully accepted into the profession. They were allowed to join the Royal College of Nursing (RCN) only in 1960, and then only if they also held a general nursing qualification. This late acceptance into the College was associated with psychiatric nursing evolving from the asylum attendants' role rather than from traditional nursing. Bill Kirkpatrick (1967, p. 48), dual trained and widely experienced, offered his support after Strabolgi's speech in the House of Lords (Cochrane 1990, p. 71). Kirkpatrick (1967, p. 49) served on the RCN's new psychiatric committee. He brought other nurses into AEGIS and, importantly, helped place AEGIS's concerns on the RCN agenda.

Kirkpatrick introduced Keith Newstead to AEGIS. He was Professional Secretary of the RCN and secretary to their psychiatric committee. At his first AEGIS meeting, he was cautious. He declared that he met with AEGIS as a private individual, not in his official RCN role.[128] Newstead was alarmed when Barbara announced that she intended to tape record the meeting, but appeared to relax when she reassured him that it was to ensure that all participants would receive an accurate copy of the minutes. By the end of the meeting Newstead seemed more confident that Barbara genuinely wished to improve nursing practice: 'Can I meet you again some time, yes?' he said before leaving.[129]

Phyllis Rowe, deputy president of the RCN and matron of St Luke's Woodside, a small psychiatric hospital in North London, also joined AEGIS.[130] She and Newstead confirmed AEGIS's suspicions that nurses at any level feared reprisals if they complained. Some would not do so even if leaving a hospital, dreading that their next employer might hear of it.[131] Most were unaware of the complaints system and had the impression that no one would listen to them anyway. Staff left rather than complain, and fear of punishment affected morale.[132] Rowe wanted to see AEGIS 'in the middle of a big campaign',[133] and she followed that up consistently.[134]

Allies within the medical profession, particularly psychiatrists, were also crucial. Psychiatrists Russell Barton, Tony Whitehead and David Enoch assisted AEGIS. Barbara first came across all three at a conference, 'Tackling Senility', at Severalls Hospital in April 1966. Whitehead said in his lecture, 'We must not sit back and say that when the Welfare Department has provided more accommodation things will be better. We must do something now.' In the panel discussion, Barbara asked him 'What can we do? What can *I* do?' Whitehead's answer included getting questions asked in Parliament and bringing pressure to bear on the Ministry, which she was doing already.[135] During an informal discussion with Whitehead, it transpired that the parliamentary question about the guidance on stripping, which Barbara requested Lubbock to ask, both inspired his answer during the panel discussion and enthused him to write the anonymous editorial on the subject in the *Lancet* (Anon. 1966b).[136]

Enoch's lecture, 'Ready for the scrapheap', a title he took from a comment written by a senior doctor on a seventy-five-year old's medical notes many years earlier,[137] also impressed Barbara. Enoch's clinical responsibilities as a consultant psychiatrist included looking after patients on eight 'chronic' wards. Accepted practices, similar to those already described, shocked him, and he struggled with the authorities to improve them. He spoke about this in an oral history interview in 2015:

> Bathing was in public...to all intents and purposes...the doctors would go in...we would see them bathing...yes...there was no privacy. That was one of the big things...I was a fresh young man, I wanted dignity, without thinking of the word...as a great word...the correct word...it just came....
>
> We had a long ward in Shelton, and that became mine. I went in through the door, there is an old picture, bent, with a rusty wire hanging, then I'd go into this long passage, dribbling men, some half naked, some badly dressed.
>
> In each of the wards, starting with one female and one male, I got carpets. The men who went out to the farm got a second suit. Then they got a narrow cupboard....And then they began to meet, with one of the staff chairing it, and to talk about the ward and what they wanted...and powerfully advocated privacy.[138]

A few months later, Barbara wrote to Barton asking for a copy of a paper he had written. The 'Dear Dr Barton...Dear Mrs Robb...Yours sincerely' style soon disappeared, and their letters ended, with 'Love from'. As Lammers (2007, p. 258) commented on the Jung-White letters, Barbara could 'melt' formality. Barton sent her wise, humorous, encouraging and cautionary letters[139] and hosted a dinner party in her honour at Claridge's, the luxury Mayfair hotel[140] (Fig. 4.3).

The AEGIS advisors contributed short essays to *Sans Everything*, which drew on their rich professional experiences and provided commentary, explanation and, importantly, 'some answers'. Whitehead's (1965) analysis of the psychogeriatric service at Severalls, reprinted from the *Lancet* provided a medical answer. Abel-Smith (1967) discussed his three-pronged 'administrative' solution—complaints procedures, inspection and ombudsman, adding that the NHS also required new buildings, more money and better recruitment and training of staff. Barton based

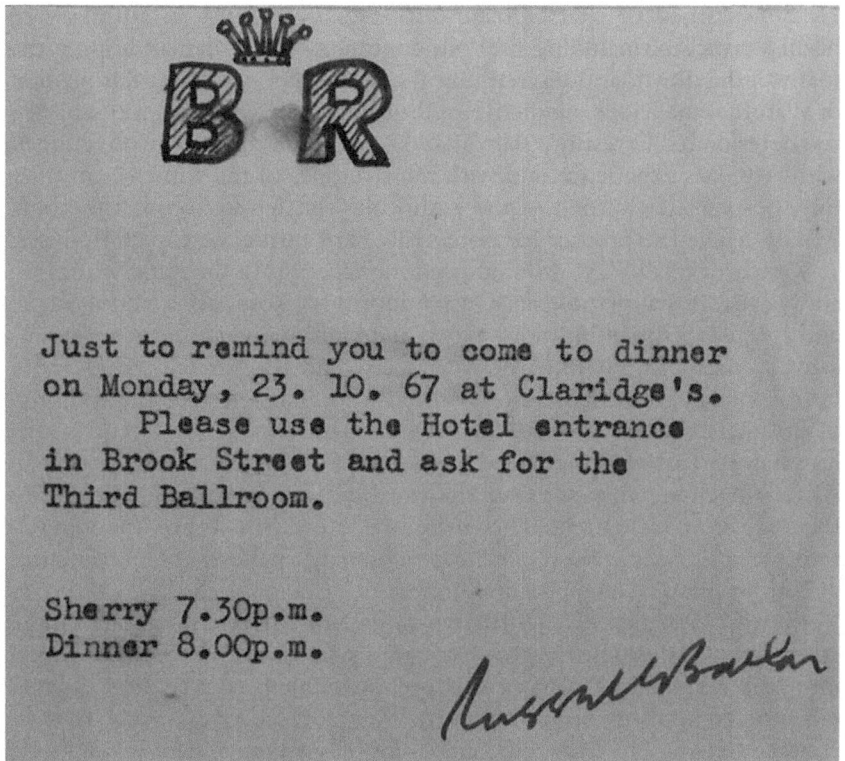

Fig. 4.3 Russell Barton's invitation to Barbara, for dinner at Claridge's, September 1967.

Source: AEGIS/1/6, Library, London School of Economics. Orphan work: attempts have been made to identify copyright owner.

his foreword on his experience of trying to change established custodial hospital practices to create humane, rehabilitative and community focussed services for patients of all ages. He knew the obstacles:

> Institutions develop powerful instruments of defence for their protection and perpetuation. Sometimes their officers or governing bodies lose sight of the primary purpose for which they were planned and their energies become deployed in rituals or personality conflicts. The purpose becomes subordinated to the personnel (Barton 1967, p. ix).

He also warned of characteristic responses from those in authority to dismiss criticism, including the 'No comment' tactic; denial; hoping the fuss will die down; and discrediting the messenger, whether staff, patient or visitor, as malicious, vindictive or disgruntled or 'too mad, too senile or too deteriorated to testify' (Barton 1967, p. ix). Barton's foreword chimed with AEGIS's experience and with the struggles of the witnesses in their own hospitals. It warned of the authorities' likely reaction to the book. AEGIS needed to prepare for potentially hard-hitting negative responses.

Kirkpatrick (1967, p. 48) endorsed the accounts of the nurse witnesses, adding that brutality took place in a 'minority' of hospitals, a tactful, vague and speculative quantification, widely used and loosely interpreted politically as meaning anything between zero and 49 percent. Abel-Smith (1967, p. 128) was dissatisfied with answers that referred to a minority of hospitals because he said that ill treatment should not occur in *any* hospital. Barbara was unprepared, however, for Newstead's response at an AEGIS meeting, when she used the word *minority* to ease the nurses into the discussion. He corrected her zealously: 'Now, Mrs Robb, I'm going to startle you by saying, for the real care of geriatric patients there are masses of bad hospitals...let's be quite honest.'[141]

Enoch (1967, pp. 136–140) wrote in *Sans Everything* about moral, ethical and legal issues. He gave examples, such as older people not fitting into 'the materialistic plan of this present affluent society' and doctors misusing compulsory orders under the Mental Health Act to achieve their rapid admission. He regarded concern for fellow human beings as a moral and religious problem, and 'the mere fact that they [the *Sans Everything* events] can occur in our so-called Christian community is appalling' (p. 136). He lay the blame for the situation on the whole of society, people who were involved in any way and those who did not want to know.

Barbara also teamed up with architect Peter Thomson to contribute plans for 'Project 70', a housing scheme on unused farmland around the psychiatric hospitals that would generate income for the NHS (Robb and Thomson 1967). It originated from Barbara's meeting with Tooth, who told her that there was no money to rebuild the psychiatric hospitals. Named because of the urgency to get it under way by 1970, it provided a financial and housing solution. Homes built on publicly owned land would be low cost. Rents from tenants could be ploughed back into NHS projects and used to finance an assortment of services and housing for older people, in small blocks and integrated into the new communities. When AEGIS first published Project 70, enthusiastic press reports supported it (AEGIS 1966; Anon. 1966e,

1966f). Rolph (1966b) wrote in the *New Statesman*: 'the staggering truth is that, until the AEGIS initiative' there were no proposals for hospital land. A *Lancet* editorial expressed disadvantages of Project 70, particularly about moving older people when they were settled in one place, stating that human relationships are more important than the physical environment (Anon. 1966g; Robb and Thomson 1966). It was also fearful about 'the danger of setting up an artificial community which will be emotionally cold and uninviting. No-one knows how long it takes a new town to become a real community.' That view was surprising, because the government built the first wave of 'new towns' immediately after the Second World War, and created more to fill the housing deficit in the 1960s.

Project 70 would help achieve government goals of providing suburban housing and closing psychiatric hospitals, both of which needed to be done economically and effectively (MoH 1966a, p. 10). Ministry indifference, even to further research on the idea, was thus unexpected. Barbara attributed it to pig-headedness: Robinson was 'in the grip of an ogre...called [Sir Arnold] France, and will just keep on saying that he thinks P. 70 stinks.'[142] Rolph and Applebey supported Project 70 and wanted it piloted. However, they agreed that Barbara should not approach Robinson about it. Rolph relished the opportunity to tell Robinson that 'a Tory Government ought not to be allowed to get the kudos for Project 70, and that its eventual fulfilment seems to me an absolute certainty.'[143] Rolph wrote to Robinson, 'an old friend', at his home address, wanting the letter to 'get straight onto his breakfast table'.[144] At their meeting, Robinson was 'affable but intransigent'. Robinson objected to Project 70 on three issues. First, like the writer of the *Lancet* editorial, he did not want to move older people from place to place unnecessarily. Second, if relatives lived with the older person in these new towns, when the older person died the relatives would be ejected from their home. Third, that placing homes for older people in hospital grounds was against NHS plans to provide accommodation closer to their previous homes. Nevertheless, Robinson said he was interested in a Project 70 plan not on hospital land, although that was troublingly inconsistent with his first two objections.[145]

Nazi Atrocities and *Sans Everything*

Extremely disparaging analogies compared the worst happenings in psychiatric hospitals with barbarities under Nazi rule during the 1930s and 1940s. Goffman (1961, pp. 24–30, 50) drew attention to common practices in psychiatric hospitals, prisons and concentration camps, including uniform haircuts, institutional clothing, stripping, depersonalisation and overcrowding as an economic way to process large numbers of people. Dickinson (2015, pp. 149–153) compared some nurses in NHS psychiatric hospitals to those in Nazi Germany who adopted unethical and inhumane practices and attributed their actions to obedience to authority. Nurses who carried out tasks in an inhumane or harmful way would try to limit any feelings of guilt and culpability. One way to do this was to ensure that they were not responsible for individual patients. This prevented a therapeutic relationship and reinforced their task-orientated work, which further dehumanised and objectified the patients. Approval from seniors encouraged and perpetuated the practices.

In *Sans Everything*, Barbara called her chapter 'Ghettos for grandparents', connecting with the ghettos into which mainly Jews were hoarded before deportation to concentration camps. Davie (1967, p. 45) compared Storthes Hall to Belsen concentration camp. Another critic of psychiatric hospitals who wrote to AEGIS, imagined collections of patients' spectacles, dentures and other belongings in the hospitals resembling stacks of personal possessions removed from prisoners at Auschwitz.[146] Similar analogies appeared in reviews of *Sans Everything*.

> Only a minority of hospitals are, of course, such Buchenwalds for elder citizens.... In this age, which we regard as one of compassion and of the responsibility of the individual, a book like this gives us a shock like the trial of Eichmann. Is group loyalty still more powerful than the conscience of the individual, and can ordinary decent human beings conform thus readily to the conventions of the institution within which they work? (Russell 1967).

Psychologists in the 1960s tried to understand how individuals carried out atrocities under the Nazi regime. They explored how detrimental and potentially murderous activities could be influenced by conforming behaviours within a group, obedience to authority and the failure of bystanders to intervene (Milgram 1963; Darley and Latane 1968; Haney et al. 1973). Understanding the psychological power of these factors makes the nurse-authors in *Sans Everything* even more remarkable for stepping 'outside' the group, evaluating working practices, and rejecting behaviours which their superiors condoned.

Barton also had strong views on the matter of concentration camps and psychiatric hospitals. In 1945, he was one of ninety-six London medical student volunteers who went to help at Belsen two weeks after liberation. Experiences there stirred him to strive for more humane psychiatric care. In 1968 he wrote about his experiences at Belsen in a widely read periodical and made controversial comparisons with psychiatric hospitals, including 'I do not believe that the German public knew about the concentration camps any more than the British knew about the way old people could be treated in mental hospitals until recently' (Barton 1968, p. 3085). Moodie made a slightly different point, that turning a blind eye to the goings-on in the psychiatric hospitals was similar to the response of German people to Nazi barbarities. He wrote: 'Most of us cannot bear too much reality. Perhaps that is why Hitler made such headway in the 'thirties: the majority of Germans—many of them good people in the accepted sense—were not prepared to admit what was happening in their midst' (Moodie 1967, p. 14).

For the Ministry, use of concentration camp imagery reinforced its criticism that AEGIS exaggerated unnecessarily. When Anne Allen (1967a), whom the Ministry 'generally regarded as a responsible journalist',[147] wrote in the *Sunday Mirror* about the back wards, a civil servant attributed her report to being 'fanned by Mrs Robb or AEGIS'.[148] In his view, Barbara exaggerated and encouraged others to do likewise, contrary to evidence that indicated Barbara was relieved when journalists did not embroider their reports.[149] The authorities assumed exaggeration when they heard about inhumanities that they could not believe (e.g., MoH 1968, pp. 22, 40, 73, 82), as happened during the Second World War with reports about Nazi atrocities (Gilbert 1984). Ignorance, disbelief and alleging exaggeration absolved the authorities from taking remedial action, especially in the face of competing priorities.

AEGIS's Distractions

In addition to campaigning, AEGIS needed a secure infrastructure. There were two main issues: finances and the publisher's concern about risk of libel. In 1966, Rolph told AEGIS that Barbara had spent '500 quid' on her campaign.[150] Barbara replied: 'Bill, I'm going to be very cross with you', but he persisted, worried that she would be 'scraping the bottom of the barrel soon'.[151] AEGIS was not a charity, but self-financed, 'out of my dress allowance' Barbara said (Anon. 1965b), although less expenditure on clothes did not stop her wearing her hallmark wide brimmed hats (Rolph 1987, p. 183).[152]

AEGIS wanted to register as a charity, which would help its financial position. However, the definition of 'charitable purposes' under the Charities Act 1960 was nebulous. In 1960 this seemed wise, as future initiatives and needs could not be predicted, but vague criteria did not help the Charity Commission decide which organisations could register (Anon. 1968). AEGIS was one of many organisations working for the public good, penalised financially by the loose definition. The *Times* reported that the British Humanist Association relinquished its charitable status, because 'If you are going in for petition-presenting, if you are going to campaign for changes in the law, if you are going to hold press conferences about national policies, you cannot, by legal definition, be a charity' (Anon. 1967). The Commission rejected the PA's application for charitable status,[153] and told AEGIS that it was 'engaging in propaganda activities' that, unless 'purely incidental', would have to cease. AEGIS appealed, as it was not a party political organisation, but the Commission stated that any activities designed to secure policy change must be ancillary to its main work rather than its raison d'être.[154] Lack of charitable status affected AEGIS's income, such as making it ineligible for some private sponsorship.[155] It could still accept donations, and Barbara's Aunt Missie was one person determined to contribute. She distributed AEGIS leaflets to her 'front-line troops' in various abbeys, organised a coffee morning and bring-and-buy in her village, and sent Barbara £45.[156] Nurses appreciating AEGIS speaking out on their behalf, also contributed. One group touchingly organised a whip-round in their nurses' home as they 'feel privileged to be able to help in some way'.[157]

Concerning libel, Barbara took legal advice. Particularly relevant to *Sans Everything* was that libel included a statement of fact that was impossible to prove. Her solicitor read her book to check for libel, and she made minor corrections.[158] The publisher also demanded affidavits (written, sworn statements of fact) from the author-witnesses.[159] They joined Barbara and a lawyer to sign them at a lunch party at 'La Gaffe', a Hampstead restaurant.[160] Barbara did not sign a contract for her book because it required her to indemnify Nelson in respect of possible libels.[161] Despite lack of a contract, in the absence of any libel action, Barbara expected to receive royalties.[162] These would, if the book sold well, contribute to AEGIS's income. Jung's comment that he hoped Barbara would continue 'dreaming of winners, because such people need winners to keep them afloat'[163] seemed prophetic.

COMMENT

Similar to other social rights campaigners tackling issues anew, such as Elizabeth Fry for prisons, William Wilberforce (1759–1833) who campaigned against slavery, and Lord Shaftesbury (1801–1885) who campaigned on child labour, factory reform and employment rights, Barbara upset many people by her frankness about unpalatable subjects most would rather have left undiscovered, and she encountered opposition from the authorities about making changes. Emphasising the inadequacies of older people's care was unwelcome in the context of widespread negativity about older people's health, within and outside the NHS (Hilton 2016c, p. 37), and economic considerations by the authorities, which perpetuated the 'human warehouses' of NHS long-stay wards (Anon. 1961). The Ministry had greater priorities, including solving the melt down of general practitioner services and creating new NHS hospital management structures (Webster 1998, p. 61).

Barbara succeeded in engaging some academics, politicians and health service professionals, but she could not break through the wall shielding the RHBs and the Ministry of Health. Robinson and Hackett ignored or defended existing hospital standards, which were often far removed from recognised best practice. Although Robinson's view might be accounted for by his official sources of information (civil servants and RHBs), evidence is lacking that he earnestly tried to verify the accuracy of the negative reports. Hackett and his RHB repeatedly dismissed complaints and provided no evidence that they tried to remedy problems at Friern. Inactivity in response to Blofeld's report, other than sacking the senior clinical staff, made Hackett's (1965a) statement in the *Times* about the RHBs' role to 'guard and protect' patients appear deceitful. NHS management gave the impression of an administrative system of concealment, complacency and fear of publicity about inadequacies, which was reinforced by stoic patients and by visitors and staff fearful of complaining and discouraged by the system from doing so. Staff, patients and relatives, with little opportunity to have their voices heard within the hospital authorities, contacted AEGIS directly. In Crossman's words (1977, p. 727),[164] Barbara was 'a kind of clearing house for all complaints about cruelty and torture in hospitals'.

The Ministry's guidance on stripping and on managing complaints was timely in the context of criticism and publicity about these matters, but because the Ministry was hostile to Barbara and AEGIS, it was unlikely to credit them with raising the concerns, and unsurprisingly, searches of official archives reveal no clues about their role. The guidance on stripping was tokenistic and created little immediate change for patients. However, it sparked discussion in the hospitals, generated press activity, and provided opportunities for doctors such as Whitehead to publicise the issue for a medical readership.

On the background of lack of interest, denial, disbelief and ignorance about marginalised and stigmatised older and mentally unwell people in hospitals, in most places change was undetectable. As Abel-Smith indicated, a sustained campaign and raised public awareness were crucial to bring it about. AEGIS had to maintain pressure to allow public, professionals and government to begin to acknowledge the genuineness of its evidence, to give it serious consideration, and then to implement improvements. AEGIS had to avoid Barbara becoming demoralised from painful and repeated rejections of the sort which deterred other complainants. Abel-Smith was an asset, with one foot in the Ministry and the other in AEGIS. The other AEGIS advisors and author-witnesses were crucial to the process and passionately supported Barbara. AEGIS's findings, proposed solutions and persistence echoed Barbara's grandfather's teaching about stinging nettles and dock leaves: if you search hard enough, you will always find the remedy (Allen 1967b).

Notes

1. Robb, 'Record of a campaign', vol 2, 15, AEGIS/1/2 (AEGIS archive, London School of Economics).
2. Robb, 'The aims of AEGIS', AEGIS/7/2.
3. PA, minutes, 1963–1967, SA/PAT/A/1/1 (Wellcome Library).
4. Notes, Robb phone call with Joyce Emerson, August 1966, AEGIS/1/3.
5. Memo, Kathleen Raven (Chief Nursing Officer) to Miss Hedley, 13 July 1967, MH150/350 (The National Archives, TNA).
6. Tape recordings of interviews at Robb's home, 11 May and 6 July 1971, AEGIS/4/27.
7. Anne Robinson, interview by author, 2015.
8. Robb, 'Record of a campaign', vol 1, 148, AEGIS/1/1.
9. Robb, 'The AEGIS Campaign: A Summary', January 1974, AEGIS/1/8.
10. AEGIS meeting, 16 March 1967, 51–52, AEGIS/1/20.
11. AEGIS meeting, 16 March 1967, 51–52, AEGIS/1/20.
12. Robb, 'Record of a Campaign', vol 2, 26, AEGIS/1/2.
13. Letter, William Charlton to Robb, 1966, AEGIS/1/18/3.
14. For example, letter, Rolph to Robb, 2 February 1967, AEGIS/1/20.

15. Anne Robinson, interview by author, 2015.
16. Robb, 'Record of a campaign', vol 2, 17, AEGIS/1/2.
17. Sheard (2014, p. 235) described Dr John Hewetson as a 'socialist reformer'.
18. Note, Charles Clark to Hodgson and Robb, 2 December 1965, AEGIS/1/1.
19. Letter, Doreen Norton to Strabolgi, 24 November 1965, AEGIS/1/5.
20. Robb, 'Record of a campaign', vol 8, 5, AEGIS/1/8.
21. Robb, 'Chapter 2', 2, AEGIS/7/10.
22. Letter, Robinson to Robb, 5 August 1965, AEGIS/1/1.
23. Robb, 'Record of a campaign', vol 2, 20, AEGIS/1/2.
24. Robb, note of exact words, enclosure 3, 76, AEGIS/1/1.
25. Letter, G Weston Secretary of RHB to CH Pearsall, New Southgate (NSG) HMC, 12 November 1965 in NSGHMC agenda papers, November–December 1965, Doc 65/110 (London Metropolitan Archives, LMA).
26. Fabian Society Archive catalogue (LSE).
27. NWMRHB, Mental Health Committee, minutes and papers, 1962–1965, October 1963 (LMA).
28. Blofeld, Ann. 1965. 'Report of the committee of inquiry on Friern Hospital' (Blofeld Report), 1 (LMA); Letter, Robb to Robinson, 9 August 1965, AEGIS/1/1.
29. Letter, Blofeld to Robb, 2 December 1965, AEGIS/2/7/B.
30. Robb, account of meeting, 102, AEGIS/A/1/A.
31. Letter, Robb to Blofeld, 2 December 1965, AEGIS/2/7/B.
32. Note, filed separately in envelope, AEGIS/3/4.
33. Robb, 'Record of a campaign', vol. 2, 3, AEGIS/1/2.
34. Robb, 'Chapter 3', AEGIS/A/1/A.
35. Robb, Chronology, 18 December 1965, AEGIS/2/14.
36. Blofeld Report, 1.
37. Joint Consultative Staffs Committee minutes, 12 September 1968, J1468, Mr Kodikara, 'Social work' (LMA).
38. Blofeld Report, 9.
39. Blofeld Report, 14.
40. Blofeld Report, 9–10.
41. Blofeld Report, 11–13.
42. Blofeld Report, 14.
43. Blofeld Report, 12–13.
44. Blofeld Report, 14.
45. Robb, 'Endpaper', 14 July 1965, AEGIS/1/1.
46. NWMRHB, Board meeting, 14 March 1966 (LMA).
47. Miss Craig, 'Loss of nursing staff', THC 65/170, July 1965, NSGHMC, agenda papers (LMA).
48. Crossman Diaries, February 1969, 156/54/69/SW (University of Warwick Modern Records Centre).

49. Lowe, Douglas. 1968. 'Report of an independent committee of enquiry into allegations concerning Friern hospital in a book entitled *Sans Everything* upon geriatric wards in that hospital and upon certain other specific complaints', NWMRHB, minutes and papers, May 1968 – November 1969, BM/283/68 (Lowe Report) 32 (LMA).
50. Letters, Robinson to Strabolgi (undated); Rolph to Robb, 8 June 1966, AEGIS/1/2.
51. Letter, Hackett to Robb, 29 December 1966, AEGIS/A/1/A.
52. Robb, 'Record of a campaign', vol 2, 71, AEGIS/1/2.
53. Robb, 'Chronology', 29 December 1965, AEGIS/2/14.
54. Letter, MoH to RHBs, 17 December 1965, about personal possessions of 'elderly or mentally disordered patients'. NWMRHB, minute book, 14 February 1966 (LMA).
55. Robb, 'Chapter 2', 11, AEGIS/7/10.
56. Final report, meeting, Robb and Tooth, 25 May 1965, AEGIS/1/1.
57. NSGHMC, 24 February 1966, minute book, 6383 (LMA).
58. NSGHMC, 24 March 1966, minute book, 6422 (LMA).
59. PA, minutes, 17 January 1966, 14 February 1966, 4.b, SA/PAT/A/1/1 (Wellcome Library).
60. Robb, 'Record of a campaign', vol 2, 160/175, AEGIS/1/2/A; 'Elderly and Mentally Disordered Patients'. *Hansard* HC Deb, 28 February 1966, vol 725 cc.184–185W.
61. AEGIS meeting, 16 March 1967, 34, AEGIS/B/2.
62. Robb, 'Chapter 2', 13, AEGIS/7/10.
63. Letter, ET Prideaux to LC Phipps, sec, North East Metropolitan RHB, 18 August 1965, MH159/24 (TNA).
64. Letter, SWMRHB to HMCs, 17 March 1964, H22/HT/A/2/16 (LMA).
65. Letter, (illegible signature), 29 December 1965, to Mr Alton (MoH) MH159/24 (TNA).
66. Letter, SWMRHB to HMCs, 17 March 1964 (LMA).
67. Letter, George Godber to Thomas Holmes Sellors, 19 March 1965, MH159/24 (TNA).
68. NHS, 'Method of dealing with hospital complaints', February 1965, MH159/24 (TNA).
69. Letter, Robb to Blofeld, 1 December 1965, AEGIS/2/7/B.
70. 'The La Vallette case: Payment of costs 19 January 1966' (unclear signature, internal document), MH159/24 (TNA).
71. 'Patients (Complaints)', *Hansard* HC Deb 10 March 1967, vol 742 c.368W.
72. Robb, letters file, 1966–1967, 34–45, Aegis/A/8.
73. Robb, letters file, 1966–1967, 96, AEGIS/A/8.
74. NSGHMC, 26 January 1967, agenda papers, 6725 (LMA).

75. NWMRHB, Board meeting, 11 December 1967, concerning *Daily Mail*, 8 November 1967, BM.556/67 (LMA).
76. Letters, R Moody to Robinson, 30 June and 18 August 1967, MH160/653 (TNA).
77. Letter, RHB to Mr Braithwaite, 14 September 1967, MH160/653 (TNA).
78. Letter, MoH to R Moody, October 1967, MH160/653 (TNA).
79. Letters: Dickens to MoH, 1 September 1967; Dickens to Robb, 5 March 1968, AEGIS/4/1/A.
80. PA, minutes, 15 November 1965, 3.iv, SA/PAT/1/1 (Wellcome Library).
81. PA, minutes, 13 December 1965, 2.b, SA/PAT/1/1 (Wellcome Library).
82. Robb, annotated press cutting, AEGIS/7/7.
83. Memo, MoH, unsigned 1967, MH150/350 (TNA).
84. 'Comments on Hospital Commissioner, Section 5 (4) of Parliamentary Commissioner for Administration', Act, undated, MH159/216 (TNA).
85. 'Hospitals (Patients' Welfare)', *Hansard* HC Deb 31 July 1964, vol 699 cc.2012–2032; 'Inspectors', *Hansard* HC Deb 31 May 1965, vol 713 c.147W.
86. Robb, 'Record of a campaign', vol 2, 149, 150, AEGIS/1/2.
87. 'D' or 'Defence' notices advised the press not to publish material which might damage national security. The row related to Harold Wilson's misjudged attack on the *Daily Express*, accusing it of breaching two D notices. A Privy Council inquiry criticised the government for its handling of the press (Bucks 2015).
88. Letter, CR Hewitt (Rolph) to Mr Baines, managing director, Nelson, 28 June 1967, Aegis/B/2.
89. AEGIS meeting, 16 March 1967, 49, 51, 53, AEGIS/1/20.
90. Act II, scene ii.
91. Letter, Robb to Rolph, 8 April 1967, AEGIS/B/2.
92. Act II, scene vii.
93. William Charlton, email, September 2015.
94. Information from Anne and Charlton families, 2016.
95. Storthes Hall transcript, 6 December 1967, 30, MH159/231 (TNA).
96. Charles Daniel, emails, 2015.
97. Letter, Daniel to Robb, c.1969, AEGIS/2/7/C.
98. Letter, Daniel to Robb, 'Good Friday', ?1969/70, AEGIS/2/11.
99. Memo, Mrs Croft to Miss Hedley, 24 January 1969, MH159/222 (TNA).
100. Letter, Matron to Mrs Glynn, 17 August 1967, MH160/653 (TNA).
101. Letter, HMC group secretary to Mrs Glynn, 15 September 1967, MH160/653 (TNA).
102. Storthes Hall transcript, 6 December 1967, 8–10, 32–34, MH159/231 (TNA).
103. Storthes Hall transcript, 7 December 1967, 48, MH159/231 (TNA).

104. Storthes Hall transcript, 6 December 1967, 9, MH159/231 (TNA).
105. Letter, Phyllis Davie to Robb, 21 January 1968, AEGIS/2/10.
106. Similar to the explanation for Bob's injuries at Friern. See Chapter 2. pp. 44–45
107. Storthes Hall HMC minutes, 1961–1965, inquiry, 17 August 1962, C416/1/184–8 (West Yorkshire Archive Service, WYAS).
108. Storthes Hall HMC minutes, 1961–1962, C416/1/184 (WYAS).
109. Storthes Hall HMC minutes, 1962–1963, inquiry, 9 August 1962, C416/1/185 (WYAS).
110. Similar at Ely Hospital. See DHSS 1969, p. 123.
111. Storthes Hall HMC minutes, 1965–1966, Management of hospital pilfering, 14 October 1965, C416/1/188 (WYAS).
112. Storthes Hall HMC minutes, 1962–1963, inquiry, 17 August 1962, C416/1/185 (WYAS).
113. Letter, MoH to R Moody, October 1967, MH160/653 (TNA).
114. Memo, Raven to Hedley, 13 July 1967, MH150/350 (TNA).
115. Comments on recommendations, O Griffiths, 30 June 1968, MH159/216 (TNA).
116. Anon. c.1962. 'Scot succeeds Scot as medical chief at Storthes Hall: prepared for a "formidable task"', local newspaper cutting, C416/add box 7 (WYAS).
117. St James's Hospital Inquiry: Part 1 Section A, 9, MH159/230 (TNA).
118. Memo, AW France to Robinson, 30 June 1967, MH150/350 (TNA).
119. MoH memo, TV programme, 30 June 1967, MH150/350 (TNA).
120. 'Report on the inquiry relating to Cowley Road Hospital', 5, MH159/234 (TNA).
121. Susan Skrine, evidence, AEGIS/A/2.
122. Susan Skrine, evidence, AEGIS/A/2.
123. Letter, Robb to Gordon Smith, *Doncaster Gazette and Chronicle*, 1 December 1966, AEGIS/1/18/2.
124. Dorothy Crofts, affidavit, AEGIS/9/16.
125. See Introduction, p. 5.
126. Robb, Plan for book: acknowledgements, AEGIS/B/1.
127. BBC2, *Man Alive*, 16 July 1968, Transcript, AEGIS/2/7/A.
128. Letter, Keith Newstead to Robb, 15 December 1966, AEGIS/1/20.
129. AEGIS meeting, 9 November 1966, 57–58, AEGIS/1/20.
130. AEGIS meeting, 16 March 1967, 1, AEGIS/B/2; Letter, Robb to Rowe, 1967, AEGIS/2/10.
131. AEGIS meeting, 9 November 1966, 49, AEGIS/1/20.
132. AEGIS meeting, 16 March 1967, 10, AEGIS/B/2.
133. AEGIS meeting, 16 March 1967, 54, AEGIS/B/2.
134. Letter, Robb to Phyllis Rowe, 1 May 1974, AEGIS/1/10/D.

135. 'Tackling Senility', conference, Severalls Hospital, 4–6 April 1966, programme and notes, AEGIS/1/2.
136. Robb, 'Record of a campaign', vol 2, 175, AEGIS/1/2; 'Elderly and Mentally Disordered Patients', *Hansard* HC Deb 28 February 1966, vol 725 cc.184–185W.
137. 'Tackling Senility', conference, Severalls Hospital, 4–6 April 1966, programme and notes, AEGIS/1/2.
138. David Enoch qualified as a doctor in 1954. Consultant psychiatrist, at Shelton Hospital in the 1960s. Interview by author, 2015.
139. Correspondence, Barton and Robb, October 1966, AEGIS/2/1/C.
140. Invitation, Barton to Barbara, September 1967, AEGIS/1/6.
141. AEGIS meeting, 16 March 1967, 25–26, AEGIS/1/19.
142. Letter, Robb to William Charlton, 20 February 1967, AEGIS/1/18/3.
143. Letter, Rolph to Robb, 2 February 1967, AEGIS/1/18/3.
144. Letter, Rolph to Robinson, February 1967, AEGIS/1/18/3.
145. Report, Rolph to Robb, February 1967, AEGIS/1/18/3.
146. Letters, Mr Leak to Robb, November 1965, AEGIS/4/5.
147. MoH memo, annotated by Mottershead, 8 February 1967, MH150/349 (TNA).
148. Memo, C Benwell, 'Condition of the elderly in mental hospitals', 10 March 1967, MH150/349 (TNA).
149. Letter, Robb to Gordon Smith, *Doncaster Gazette and Chronicle*, 1 December 1966, AEGIS/1/18/2.
150. Roughly £10,000 in 2016.
151. AEGIS meeting, 9 November 1966, 37, AEGIS/1/20.
152. Mamie Charlton, Robb's sister-in-law, interview by author, 2016.
153. PA, minutes, 11 February 1965, 3, SA/PAT/A/1/1 (Wellcome Library).
154. Letters, Charity Commission to AEGIS, 9 August and 22 September 1967, AEGIS/9/16.
155. Correspondence, Strabolgi and John Spedan Lewis Foundation, 1966, AEGIS/1/4.
156. Letters, Ernestine Anne to Robb, 11 June and 2 July 1966, AEGIS/1/18/3, approx. £800 in 2016.
157. Letter, nurses' home warden, Camarthen, to Robb, undated, AEGIS/9/16.
158. Letter, Rubenstein, Nash and Co to James Shepherd, Nelson, 17 May 1967.
159. Letter, Robb to Polson, 27 November 1967, 146, AEGIS/A/2/3.
160. St Lawrence's Inquiry, 1 November 1967, 21, MH159/228 (TNA).
161. Letter, CH Rolph (?) to Elizabeth Barber, solicitor, Society of Authors, 14 July 1967, AEGIS/B/2.
162. Letter, Robb to Bill (probably CH Rolph), 26 January 1968, AEGIS/B/3.
163. Jung to White, 21 September 1951, in Lammers and Cunningham 2007.
164. 12 November 1969.

Bibliography

Abel-Smith, Brian. 1967. 'Administrative solution: a hospital commissioner?' 128–135. In Robb 1967.
Abel-Smith, Brian. 1990. Interviewed by Hugh Freeman. *BJPsych Bulletin*. 14: 257–261.
Abel-Smith, Brian and Townsend, Peter. 1965. *The Poor and the Poorest*. London: G. Bell & Sons.
AEGIS. 1966. *Project 70*. London: AEGIS.
Allen, Anne. 1967a. 'Ghettoes for grandparents'. *Sunday Mirror*, 15 January.
Allen, Anne. 1967b. 'One woman who refused to pass by..'. *Sunday Mirror*, 9 July.
Anon. 1903. 'The Colney Hatch Asylum fire'. *Times*, 29 January.
Anon. 1961 'Human warehouses'. *BMJ*, ii, 100.
Anon. 1962. 'New deal for the old'. *Times*, 16 November.
Anon. 1965a. 'Patients want inspectors of hospitals'. *Daily Telegraph*, 14 July.
Anon. 1965b. 'The woman behind AEGIS' *Hampstead and Highgate Express*, 10 December.
Anon. 1966a. 'An "affront" to aged patients'. *Guardian*, 18 March.
Anon. 1966b. 'Sans teeth, sans eyes, sans taste, sans everything'. *Lancet*, i, 646.
Anon. 1966c. 'Pink circulars'. *Hospital*, April, 153.
Anon. 1966d. 'Top of form: should the ombudsman investigate health service complaints?' *BMJ*, ii, 1399.
Anon. 1966e. 'Hospital land for homes'. *Guardian*., 3 June
Anon. 1966f. 'Towns' in hospital grounds'. *Times*, 3 June.
Anon. 1966 g. 'Project 70'. *Lancet*, i, 1275–1276.
Anon. 1967. 'Humanists join the political fray: shedding charitable status'. *Times*, 14 January.
Anon. 1968. 'What is a charity?' *Times*, 3 January.
Anon. 1978. 'Mrs AS Blofeld'. *Times*, 22 February.
Barton, Russell. 1967. 'Foreword' ix–xi. In Robb 1967.
Barton, Russell. 1968. "Belsen' 3081–3085. In *History of the Second World War*, ed. Barrie Pitt. London: Purnell and Sons.
Beardshaw, Virginia. 1981. *Conscientious Objectors at Work*. London: Social Audit Limited.
Biss, Jean. (Laura Heneage). 1967. 'Somewhere along the line the complaints get lost' 18–26. In Robb 1967.
Bridgen, Paul. 2001. 'Hospitals, geriatric medicine, and long-term care of elderly people 1946–1976'. *Social History of Medicine*, 14, 507–523.
Briggs, Asa. 2005. *A History of the Royal College of Physicians*. Vol. 4. Oxford: OUP.
Bucks, Simon. 2015.'The D-notice is misunderstood but its collaborative spirit works'. *Guardian*, 2 August.

Cochrane, David. 1990. 'The AEGIS campaign to improve standards of care in mental hospitals: a case study of the process of social policy change'. PhD thesis, University of London. http://etheses.lse.ac.uk, accessed 17 September 2016.

Craythorne, Alice. See Daniel, Joyce.

Crofts, Dorothy (Elizabeth Tasburg). 1967. 'Not in front of the charge nurse' 58–65. In Robb 1967.

Crossman, Richard. 1977. *The Diaries of a Cabinet Minister. Vol. 3. Secretary of State for Social Services 1968–1970*. London: Hamilton and Cape.

Daniel, Joyce (Alice Craythorne). 1967. 'No-one smiles here' 37–43. In Robb 1967.

Darley, John and Latane, Bibb. 1968. 'Bystander intervention in emergencies: diffusion of responsibility'. *Journal of Personality and Social Psychology*, 8, 377–383.

Davie, James (Frederick Isham). 1967. 'Massive corruption and cruelty' 43–47. In Robb 1967.

DHSS. 1969. *Report of the Committee of Inquiry into Allegations of Ill-treatment of Patients and Other Irregularities at the Ely Hospital, Cardiff*. Cmnd. 3975. London: HMSO.

DHSS. 1971. *Report of the Farleigh Hospital Committee of Inquiry*. Cmnd. 4557. London: HMSO.

DHSS and Welsh Office. 1971. *NHS Hospital Advisory Service, Annual Report for 1969–70*. London: HMSO.

Dickinson, Tommy. 2015. *'Curing Queers': Mental Nurses and Their Patients, 1935–1974*. Manchester: Manchester University Press.

Enoch, David. 1967. 'Afterword: Ready for the scrapheap' 136–140. In Robb 1967.

Fenton, Loiusa. See Skrine, Susan.

Gilbert, Martin. 1984. *Auschwitz and the Allies: The Politics of Rescue*. London: Arro Books.

Goffman, Erving. 1961. *Asylums: Essays on the Social Situation of Mental Patients and Other Inmates*. New York: Anchor Books.

Hackett, Maurice. 1965a. 'Old people in mental hospitals'. *Times*, 18 November.

Hackett, Maurice. 1965b. 'Mental hospitals'. *Times*, 1 December.

Haney, C., Banks, C. and Zimbardo. P. 1973. 'Interpersonal dynamics in a simulated prison'. *International Journal of Criminology and Penology*, 1, 69–97.

Heneage, Laura. See Biss, Jean.

Hilton, Claire. 2016a. 'Parity of esteem for mental and physical health care in the United Kingdom: a hundred years war?' *Journal of the Royal Society of Medicine*, 109, 133–137.

Hilton, Claire. 2016b. 'Whistle-blowing in the National Health Service since the 1960s'. *History and Policy.* http://www.historyandpolicy.org, accessed 10 September 2016.

Hilton, Claire. 2016c. 'Developing psychogeriatrics in England: a turning point in the 1960s?' *Contemporary British History*, 30, 40–72.

Hodgson, Helen. 1966. 'Elderly patients'. *Guardian*, 29 March.

Hodgson, Helen. 1972. 'Management of National Health Service'. *Times*, 4 August.

Home Office. 1966. *Report of the Inquiry into Prison Escapes and Security.* Cmnd 3175. London: HMSO.

Howard, Anthony. 2004. 'Hewitt, Cecil Rolph [CH Rolph] (1901–1994)'. *Oxford Dictionary of National Biography.* http://www.oxforddnb.com, accessed 1 December 2015.

Isham, Frederick. see Davie, James.

Kirkpatrick, WJA. 1967. 'Conscience and commitment' 48–57. In Robb 1967.

Labour Party. 1964. *Manifesto.* http://www.labourmanifesto.com, accessed 1 March 2016.

Lammers, Ann. 2007. 'Jung and White and the God of terrible double aspect'. *Journal of Analytical Psychology*, 52, 253–274.

Lammers, Ann and Cunningham, Adrian, eds. 2007. *The Jung-White Letters.* London: Routledge.

Martin, John (with Evans, Debbie). 1984. *Hospitals in Trouble.* Oxford: Blackwell.

Milgram, Stanley. 1963. 'Behavioral study of obedience'. *Journal of Abnormal and Social Psychology*, 67, 371–378.

Ministry of Health. 1944. *A National Health Service.* Cmnd. 6502. London: HMSO.

Ministry of Health. 1964. *Improving the Effectiveness of Hospitals for the Mentally Ill.* HM (64)45. London: HMSO.

Ministry of Health. 1966a. *Hospital Building Programme: Revision of the Hospital Plan for England and Wales.* Cmnd. 3000. London: HMSO.

Ministry of Health. 1966b. *Methods of Dealing with Complaints of Patients.* HM (66)15. London: HMSO.

Ministry of Health. 1968. *Findings and Recommendations Following Enquiries into Allegations Concerning the Care of Elderly Patients in Certain Hospitals.* Cmnd. 3687. London: HMSO.

Moodie, Dennis (Michael Osbaldeston). 'Nobody wants to know' 13–18. In Robb 1967.

Moody, Roger. 1967. 'We haven't met one like this before' 65–68. In Robb 1967.

Mulcahy, Linda. 2003. *Disputing Doctors: The Socio-Legal Dynamics of Complaints About Medical Care.* Berkshire: Open University Press.

NAMH. 1965. *Achievements 1964–5.* London: NAMH.

NHS Improvement and NHS England. 2016. *Freedom to Speak Up: Raising Concerns (Whistleblowing) Policy for the NHS.* https://www.improvement.nhs.uk, accessed 25 September 2016.
Osbaldeston, Michael. see Moodie, Dennis.
Pertinax. 1967. 'Without prejudice'. *BMJ*, i, 755.
Pitt, Brice. 1968. 'Attempting to solve staffing problems' 29–30. In *Improving the Effectiveness of Hospitals and Services for the Mentally Ill and Mentally Subnormal: A Collection of Papers Presented at Conferences Held at the Hospital Centre in 1966 and 1967*, ed. Anthony Whitehead and D. Cortazzi. London: King's Fund.
Porter, Eileen (Emily Swinburne). 1967. 'They would rather be dead' 27–30. In Robb 1967.
Robb, Barbara. 1967. *Sans Everything: A Case to Answer.* London: Nelson.
Robb, Barbara and Thomson, Peter. 1966. 'Project 70'. *Lancet*, i, 1327.
Robb, Barbara and Thomson, Peter. 1967. 'Rehousing and financial solution: Project 70' 124–127. In Robb 1967.
Rolph, Cecil. 1987. *Further Particulars.* Oxford: OUP.
Rolph, C.H. 1966a. 'Protecting the insane'. *New Statesman*, 11 February.
Rolph, C.H. 1966b. 'London diary'. *New Statesman*, 26 August.
Royal Commission on the Law Relating to Mental Illness and Mental Deficiency 1954–1957. Cmnd. 169. 1957. London: HMSO.
Russell, Richard. 1967. 'Think on these things. Sans Everything: A Case to Answer. Presented by Barbara Robb'. *Tablet*, 19 August.
Sheard, Sally. 2014. *The Passionate Economist.* Bristol: Policy Press.
Skrine, Susan. (Louisa Fenton). 1967. 'They cannot defend themselves' 31–37. In Robb 1967.
Special Correspondent. 1965. 'Do-it-yourself health for the old'. *Times*, 9 November.
Strabolgi. Beaumont. Heytesbury. Abel-Smith, Brian. Ardizzone, Edward. Harvey, Audrey. Hewetson, John. Robb, Barbara. Sargent, Bill and Woolgar, Daniel. 1965. 'Old people in mental hospitals'. *Times*, 10 November.
Strabolgi and Robb, Barbara. 1965. 'Mental hospitals', *Times*, 24 November.
Swinburne, Emily. See Porter, Eileen.
Tasburg, Elizabeth. See Crofts, Dorothy.
Thane, Pat. 2015. 'CPAG at 50'. *Poverty*, 150, 6–8.
Townsend, Peter. 1965. 'A national survey of old people in psychiatric and non-psychiatric hospitals, residential homes, and nursing homes' 223–232. In *Psychiatric Hospital Care: A Symposium*, ed. Hugh Freeman. London: Baillière, Tindall and Cassell.
Webster, Charles. 1998. *The National Health Service: A Political History.* Oxford: OUP.
Whitehead, Anthony. 1965. 'A comprehensive psychogeriatric service'. *Lancet*, ii, 583–586.

Open Access This chapter is licensed under the terms of the Creative Commons Attribution 4.0 International License (http://creativecommons.org/licenses/by/4.0/), which permits use, sharing, adaptation, distribution and reproduction in any medium or format, as long as you give appropriate credit to the original author(s) and the source, provide a link to the Creative Commons license and indicate if changes were made.

The images or other third party material in this chapter are included in the book's Creative Commons license, unless indicated otherwise in a credit line to the material. If material is not included in the book's Creative Commons license and your intended use is not permitted by statutory regulation or exceeds the permitted use, you will need to obtain permission directly from the copyright holder.

CHAPTER 5

Reprinted Before Publication: Plotting a Route for *Sans Everything*

Barbara was belligerent with her press campaign. She enthused the press to enlighten the public and to pave the way for *Sans Everything*. Anne Robinson recalled:

> I can remember one report, one story where I didn't have the space to put in all she wanted.... The edition went at six o'clock, she turned up at the *Sunday Times* at about four to argue it in, on Saturday afternoon.[1]

In early 1967, the Ministry began to prepare for an outburst of public opinion in response to *Sans Everything* and for the fuss it anticipated that AEGIS (Aid for the Elderly in Government Institutions) would continue to make. The Ministry did not regard the allegations with the gravity that Rolph had hoped for, in terms of triggering high-level public investigations.[2] Plans emerged to hold nonstatutory, private inquiries established by Regional Hospital Boards (RHBs).

Sans Everything exploded into the headlines on 30 June 1967. The same day, *Ten O'Clock*, a BBC radio current affairs programme interviewed Barbara, and *24 Hours*, a BBC1 television news programme, featured *Sans Everything*. With anticipated high demand for the book, the publisher reprinted it before publication.[3] *Sans Everything* achieved best-seller status in the first week.[4] One reader, Mabel Franks, wrote to Barbara comparing her to Francis Chichester who returned from his solo circumnavigation of the globe in May 1967:

> I consider your achievement far more commendable than that of Chichester. Granted he is a very brave man and we all admire his courage, but your courage is of a noble kind for it will benefit humanity in the future.... You had the guts and moral fibre to pursue this matter and bring it right into the open.[5]

The Press Paves the Way

Guardian journalist Ann Shearer argued the importance of the press in publicising scandals. The press has to answer the question: 'Is it in the public interest to publish or to keep quiet?' If it is in the public interest, the press can provide information that puts people who want to see change in touch with those who are in a position to make it happen: 'the freedom of the press to put uncomfortable situations before the electorate is an essential element in the assumptions on which our societies are run. And if the media did not fulfil this role, who would?' Based on her personal experience of seeking to improve psychiatric hospitals and the responses she received from the authorities, Shearer (1976, p. 112) wrote: 'it would be naïve to leave it to "those who know best," those most involved.'

Rolph introduced Barbara to reporters and editors on several national newspapers, including the *Daily Mail, Sunday Telegraph* and *News of the World*. Barbara compiled dossiers for them, and in return they provided 'much assistance'.[6] According to Rolph (1987, p. 184) 'editors in Fleet Street... never saw manuscripts so overwhelmingly supported by authority, and never had to feel uneasy about any statement Barbara made.' Editors trusted Barbara with their, and their newspapers', futures: libel, slander or unethical information could precipitate disrepute, a legal case or a hearing by the Press Council, the public body that aimed to maintain high standards of journalism. The Press Council had no concerns about Barbara's well-backed-up allegations, but it approached Kenneth Robinson in 1966, about secretiveness and the press's poor relationship with the NHS. Despite official agreements for NHS press releases, editors complained of varying standards of information 'particularly in the matter of accidents and that sometimes there appeared to be a desire to restrict disclosure of hospital affairs beyond the point of public good'. Robinson retaliated that, on occasions, the press published 'exaggerated or distorted reports' (Press Council 1966, pp. 8–9). The Press Council complaints files were destroyed,[7] precluding chances of confirming the circumstances and evidence behind its exchange with Robinson. The Council's concerns, however, matched Richard Crossman's (1977, p. 134):[8] 'Of one thing I'm sure. The public relations of the Ministry of Health are terrible. It has an appallingly bad press office and really faulty relations with the general public.' One newspaper editor no longer sent reporters to RHB meetings because the only part of the proceedings that they witnessed was the Board operating 'simply as a rubber stamp meeting' (Fortune 1967). RHBs had the right to exclude press and public from parts of meetings for which they deemed that publicity 'would be prejudicial to the public interest'. The North West Metropolitan (NWM) RHB demonstrated this sort of exclusion when it discussed a circular from the Ministry about ill-treatment in psychiatric hospitals, although whether their exclusion was justified is unclear from the minutes.[9] Around the same time, Conservative MP Kenneth Lewis asked Robinson in Parliament how many RHBs allowed the press to attend their meetings. Robinson replied, 'All', without further explanation,[10] an emphatic but reassuring half-truth.

More reports of inadequate and custodial psychiatric care appeared in the national press and bolstered AEGIS's argument. In March 1967 the *Times* reported accidents causing the deaths of two elderly patients on an overcrowded ward of a psychiatric hospital (Leamington Spa reporter 1967). The same month, the BBC screened a documentary, *What Shall We Do with Granny*? It questioned whether any institution was an appropriate place to care for men and women who had lived independent lives for fifty or sixty years, let alone a crowded, bleak dormitory in a psychiatric hospital or former workhouse (BBC1, 1967).

Several newspapers and periodicals took up the *Sans Everything* theme before its publication. The *Sunday Times, Nursing Mirror* and *News of the World* showed particularly consistent support for the AEGIS campaign. Hugo Young was chief leader writer of the *Sunday Times*, which had a circulation of 1.5 million copies each week (Monopolies 1985). On 4 June, coinciding with Mental Health Week and three weeks before the publication of *Sans Everything*, Young cited extensively from two of the reports due to appear in the book (Young 1967). He criticised the nursing structure and the lack of training, particularly of 'people deceptively entitled "nursing assistants" whose training is only a tepid and hasty dilution' but praised the work done by nurses, 'unsung and unrewarded...among the most admirable heroes of medicine'. He alleged that complaints by staff or patients about standards of care could lead to reprisals against them. Lively debate followed in the correspondence columns, largely supporting Young's message. John Andrews (1967), nurse tutor at Claybury Hospital, wrote that psychiatric hospitals needed 'regular articles such as yours'. Applebey (1967) supported the idea of an inspectorate for all institutions where chronically ill or disabled people lived, not just for psychiatric hospitals, and if the government was unwilling to set this up, then the National Association for Mental Health (NAMH) would gladly do so if given the resources. Others added their personal knowledge about the effects of overcrowding and underfunding. A few correspondents criticised Young's article: some condemned the nurses whose accounts he cited, and one, Sir Ivor Julian (1967), chairman of the South East Metropolitan RHB, rebutted Young's argument.

The *Nursing Mirror*, read widely by nurses but not by the general public, announced *Sans Everything* two weeks before publication. The editor, Yvonne Cross, wrote that she felt privileged to have read it in advance: 'privileged in humility and shame, for we have known something of these conditions and have been powerless to do anything to help the nurses who have reported them to us.' An editorial (Anon. 1967a) invited readers' comments on three questions: Would you complain forcibly to your superior about malpractice or appalling conditions? If the complaint did not achieve its objectives, would you pursue the matter? Would you feel confident that you would survive discredit and materially alter the situation? The *Nursing Mirror* printed the first answers on 23 June (Anon. 1967c): one student nurse wrote that to go above her immediate superior, 'to pursue the matter further would be unethical, and strictly against the conduct of a good nurse', indicating her understanding of the importance of obedience in the profession. Every letter expressed fear of reprisals, and many nurses would not take that risk.

Cross also wrote directly to Robinson after the Ministry made a press release that rebutted Young's statement in the *Sunday Times* that staff and patients were fearful of speaking out:[11]

> You are mistaken in your rejection of the suggestion that reprisals are used against nurses who rebel publicly against sick administration in hospitals. There are thousands of ways in which nurses and patients can be made to pay dearly if they dare to raise their voices in criticism.... I believe this book to have created the opportunity for which thousands of people have been waiting, and... I intend to support it from the pages of the journal—and in every other way open to me.[12]

Other journalists argued similarly, that Fleet Street's support for AEGIS reflected a collective guilt about an issue of which it was distantly conscious but that had been kept under wraps (Cochrane 1990, p. 75). Concerning reprisals towards staff who spoke up, when Nigel Fisher MP asked Robinson if he would give 'protection of anonymity to anyone who comes forward with the evidence' Robinson replied: 'Yes, certainly', but he gave no clues as to how he could, or would, do that.[13] His uncertainty reflected reality when, a few months later, the Ministry nebulously instructed RHBs to try to 'dispel such apprehensions'.[14]

A third publication that offered consistent support to AEGIS was the *News of the World*, a Sunday newspaper, which, in the 1960s, had an enormous circulation of about 6 million copies a week (Rogers 2011). Their journalist, David Roxan, was familiar with mental hospitals and injustices of compulsory detention. In 1956 he worked with the National Council for Civil Liberties to secure the discharge of Peter Whitehead, who was inappropriately detained in mental hospitals for twelve years. Roxan's book, *Sentenced without Cause* (1958), described stripping Whitehead of his belongings and personal identity on admission (pp. 96–101), physical violence by staff to patients on the wards (p. 147) and difficulty securing Whitehead's discharge against the wishes of the authorities (p. 254), all detrimental processes resembling those that AEGIS uncovered. William Williams MP commented in 1958 that 'everybody' except the Ministry agreed that Peter Whitehead's detention was wrong. The Ministry, then under Conservative Party leadership, defended mental hospital practices, criticised Roxan's book as sensational and irresponsible and said that his attack on hospital practices was 'unjust' because staff, 'often under trying conditions, carry out their duties with sympathy and devotion and precious little thanks from the public'.[15] Lomax (1921), Roxan (1958) and Barbara (1967a) identified similar inhumane practices, and the Ministry rejected the allegations each time. Royal Commissions, Aneurin Bevan and others revealed difficulties in the mental hospitals, but ideas and intentions from the Ministry, Boards and hospital leadership did not match the commitment that would be necessary to ensure change. Overall, the Ministry indicated its conviction that psychiatric hospitals were fit for purpose (Rogers and Pilgrim 1996, pp. 58–71).

Roxan approached Barbara to offer his support and first cited her evidence in May 1966. Roxan (1966) also quoted COHSE, the Confederation of Health Service Employees trades union, to which many psychiatric nurses belonged.[16] Similar to the message Tooth gave to Barbara,[17] COHSE stated, according to Roxan's article: 'There are hospitals where things do happen and there is little the Ministry can do about it.' This apathetic view ignored the possibility that COHSE could improve work conditions for its members if it encouraged the Ministry to provide better patient care. Roxan also quoted Applebey: 'People may not know it but we have a major problem on our hands', and a Ministry spokesman: 'much is being done' but 'we are very much aware' that more is needed. According to Abel-Smith, the Ministry's comments were NHS jargon, similar to labelling services as 'continuously under review', all of which meant that no further action was required (Stewart and Sleeman 1967).[18] Responding to Roxan's article, a care home matron (Anon. 1966) described her difficulties of finding staff: 'The staffing in old folks' homes has never been so bad. Hours are long, pay is bad—and we superintendents and matrons have almost to accept anything on two legs as staff.' On 25 June 1967, Roxan's eye-catching report, titled 'Old folk beaten in hospital', gave details of the 'startling allegations' in *Sans Everything*, due to be published the following Friday. He also wrote that the 'usually conservative' Royal College of Nursing (RCN) upheld the allegations (Roxan 1967a).

THE MINISTRY, ROBINSON AND THE PRESS: PLANNING INQUIRIES

The independent inquiry into the Aberfan disaster, the colliery tip landslide in 1966 that killed 116 children and 28 adults, was fresh in the mind of the public. It found

> a terrifying tale of bungling ineptitude by many men charged with tasks for which they were totally unfitted, of failure to heed clear warnings and of total lack of direction from above. Not villains, but decent men, led astray by foolishness or ignorance or by both in combination, are responsible for what happened (Welsh Office 1967, p. 25).

The inquiry blamed the Coal Board, the statutory authority that ran the nationalised coal mining industry, revealing its inept management of matters for which it was responsible and accountable (Welsh Office 1967, p. 131). The broader implication was that public bodies could be negligent. The enormous publicity around Aberfan gave the public some knowledge of inquiry processes that were also relevant to the planning, procedures and disputes associated with *Sans Everything*. Inquiries are 'inquisitorial'—that is, the inquiry committee is actively involved in investigating the facts of the case, as opposed to an 'adversarial' process in which the role of the court is primarily that of an impartial referee between the prosecution and the defence. Inquiries seek to establish the facts and provide a full and fair account of what happened, especially in circumstances where evidence is disputed or the course and causation of events is unclear. Other functions include catharsis for those involved; learning in order to prevent a recurrence; and reassurance that the government is making sure the issue is fully dealt with. These aims, however, are not always entirely compatible with a single process. Public inquiries may be the best for reassurance, but an inquiry undertaken in private may be the best to determine the truth. The political need to provide reassurance that the situation will not recur drives the need to find simple causative factors, which risks blaming front-line staff, such as nurses, and diverting attention away from failures of senior management which are less visible. Finding a scapegoat can relieve rage and frustration, which is one reason witnesses need legal representation to ensure justice for themselves (Howe 1999).

The *Royal Commission on Tribunals of Inquiry* (1966) established principles for managing inquiries. It recommended that in 'circumstances which occasion a nation-wide crisis of confidence' inquiries should be established by Parliament (p. 16). For the NHS, that meant instituting an inquiry under section 70 of the NHS Act 1946. Legislation in 1967[19] brought section 70 under the jurisdiction of the Council on Tribunals, an advisory public body set up in 1958 to ensure that inquiries were run according to high standards, including being open, fair and impartial: open, for publicity of proceedings and the reasoning behind decisions; fair, through having a clear procedure, including allowing participants to present their case fully; impartial, by ensuring independence from the real or apparent influence of the authorities (Administrative Tribunals 1957, p. 10).[20] Procedures to achieve a comprehensive analysis of events included having an independent chairman who could enforce the attendance of witnesses, take evidence on oath and compel the production of documents. The Ministry identified only six instances between 1948 and 1966 when it used section 70 inquiries. All were disputes relating to employment, building works and finances.[21] None related directly to patient care or treatment. It is hard to believe that no patient-focussed serious or unresolved NHS complaints warranted section 70 inquiries during these years. One explanation for this absence was that the Ministry gave complaints only cursory attention.

In February 1967, Robinson met with Tooth and other civil servants, to plan how to investigate the *Sans Everything* allegations. He proposed that 'the desire to protect staff from allegations of brutality and cruelty might be the spur to action' and that this could stem either from a parliamentary question or a request from COHSE, which would want to protect its members.[22] Bernard Braine MP supported the concept of inquiries 'to restore public confidence',[23] which, like Robinson's aim to protect staff, implied that the allegations were false, a perspective that did not bode well for impartial committees of inquiry to approach their task open-mindedly. Robinson was also determined that Barbara should receive no credit for the outcome: 'the setting up of an Enquiry had to look convincingly spontaneous, and not as if he was being pushed into it by people such as Mrs Robb.'[24]

The Ministry was uncertain about procedures and legal matters, reinforcing the impression that it lacked experience in processing complaints. It was ambivalent about instigating inquiries because it usually delegated complaint management to the RHBs. Removing that role could be interpreted as the Ministry assuming that the RHBs lacked the necessary skills, suggesting little trust or openness for negotiation between them. The Ministry also considered how it should respond to the Mental Health Act (1959, section 126), which stated that it was a criminal offence to 'ill-treat or wilfully neglect' a patient 'receiving treatment for mental disorder' in a psychiatric hospital. That included unintentional but reckless practices. The Ministry decided to avoid mentioning the offence because it might deter witnesses from giving evidence.[25] Ignoring the law was a surprising course of action for a government department. The Ministry's legal specialist advised against using section 70, on the basis that the allegations were probably unsound rather than serious,[26] further evidence that the authorities pre-judged them. The Ministry also rejected a section 70 inquiry because the allegations related to several regions and that separate inquiries 'were no less independent but merely less cumbersome' than a single inquiry.[27] Robinson prioritised practicalities over principles, imprudent for legal processes.

In April 1967, Maurice Miller, a medically qualified Labour MP, asked Robinson an 'inspired' parliamentary question, whether 'existing methods of dealing with complaints that elderly patients, particularly in psychiatric hospitals, are ill-treated, afford adequate protection for patients and staff'. Robinson replied, reassuringly, 'Yes', referring to the complaints guidance circulated the previous year and with the implication that the Ministry could confidently deal with the issues. The parliamentary question conveniently provided Robinson with the opportunity to praise staff and to announce a loophole for not investigating *Sans Everything*: 'General unsubstantiated allegations are impossible to pursue and cast unfair suspicion on all those, doctors, nurses and others, who devote themselves to the care of these patients.'[28]

The Ministry received a prepublication copy of *Sans Everything* on 20 June. An internal memo commented: 'There is little in the book which is new' and 'It is reasonable to assume that Mrs Robb is making as damaging a case as she can from the information she has received.'[29] The first comment admitted that the Ministry knew about the problems. If that was the case, why did it try to give the impression that all was well,[30] rather than try to improve the situation? The second implied malicious intent on Barbara's part. The memo recommended that the Ministry should make a statement to refute Barbara's evidence, emphasising that she withheld permission for it to be used in 1965. However, one reason she withheld permission was because she had lost confidence in the Ministry's ability to investigate (Strabolgi et al. 1965).[31] Months of discussion at the Ministry in 1967 about how to investigate, supported Barbara's contention.

PUBLICATION DAY: 30 JUNE 1967

The presenter of *Ten O'Clock*, Mr Hunt, interviewed Barbara. He asked her, 'Which do you regard as the most brutal of your allegations?' She avoided being dragged into specific witch-hunt type questions and replied that physical brutality was scarce: 'What concerns me ... is the atmosphere in so many of the geriatric wards and the traumatic effect that this has on the patients.' When Hunt challenged her on why the nurses did not speak out, she defended them and explained their fear of reprisals. Hunt criticised her 'emotionally toned words', such as using the word *stripping*, to which she replied that she first heard it at the Ministry from a senior official, 'a very unemotional gentleman—a very charming gentleman',[32] Dr Tooth. Hunt said that emotional language might have weakened her case: the authorities did not appreciate passion or drama about a cause, or acknowledge that emotive language could indicate the complainant's desperation about the situation.

Presenters Cliff Michelmore and Kenneth Allsop probed the story on *24 Hours*.[33] Silhouettes and voices of the nurse-authors Davie, Daniel and Moodie reiterated their accounts in *Sans Everything*. Film shots taken at St Peter's showed Amy and Barbara chatting. Cross's succinct responses supported Barbara and the nurses. Cross reinforced the need to investigate hospitals rather than individuals and that nurses feared reprisals. When Michelmore challenged her about why ex-nurses did not complain, she replied: 'How much credence would you give, say, an ex-television producer, who came and said "terrible things went on in my studio when I was there five years ago"?...being an ex-anything immediately reduces your case.'

Allsop interviewed Robinson, allowing him the final word. Robinson said he would investigate if he received sufficient evidence. However, Robinson defended the NHS, and reiterated his confidence in the system: 'I am absolutely sure, that the care of our old people in our geriatric and psychiatric hospitals is as good as anything in the world.' It was ironical to make such a comment, which lacked corroboration,[34] in the context of criticising AEGIS for its unsubstantiated evidence. He said he wanted to investigate the allegations, but was concerned that, eighteen months after the events 'the trail is getting cold', indicating his concern about identifying individual wrong-doers. Allsop, reiterating Cross's point, challenged him on this focus on incidents, rather than on investigating a general malaise in the hospitals, but Robinson stuck to his plan.

The press picked up on Robinson's apparent lack of knowledge, or denial, of poor care in hospitals and his attitude to the allegations. The *Sunday Mirror* criticised Robinson, who, 'to his shame, seemed to pooh-pooh [*Sans Everything*] on Twenty-Four Hours' (Allen 1967). The BBC received a 'flood' of letters. Some people objected to the programme repeating the criticisms made in *Sans Everything*. Some complained about anonymising hospitals and silhouetting interviewees. However, many more thought the BBC was right to bring the matter into the open. Some letter writers recounted their experiences in hospitals, as patients, staff or visitors. One nurse, who wrote that her ward sister told her to 'sling' a patient in the bath even if she didn't want one, complained to matron, was ostracised by staff and left the hospital. She said: 'I was getting tough, hard-hearted, I had lost my individuality...I had lost the kindly world I belonged to.' A son wrote about his elderly mother's care. She spent the last four months of her life in hospital: she was stripped, had falls and sustained three fractures. He suspected that lack of supervision contributed to her falls, but when he enquired about whether there would be an inquest, he was told that little could be done about his concerns.[35] The *24 Hours* programme also outraged Barbara's Aunt Missie:

> When Mr Robinson said there was no truth in the 'Diary of a Nobody'... I cried out: 'He is calling *me* a liar'. I can indeed vouch that the facts... [were] told to me as they occurred. And I am ready to swear before any 'enquiry' as to Amy Gibb's wonderful good health and normality when I spent the afternoon with her at the convent.[36]

After the programme, Cross sent Robinson letters received by the *Nursing Mirror* to back up her statement about nurses fearing reprisals.[37] Robinson's private secretary replied:

> The Minister is much disturbed at the letters which report reluctance on the part of nurses to press complaints to the hospital authorities for fear of reprisals, or belief that even if they reported such things, no improvement would result. He feels that this is as much a matter for the nursing profession itself to deal with as for him, and senior officers of the Department have already discussed this with the President of the Royal College of Nursing.[38]

Robinson externalised the problem away from the authorities, towards the nurses themselves. In total, 250 nurses wrote to the *Nursing Mirror*. Many nurses would speak out if they thought it would lead to improved practice, but, as Cross reflected two years later, 'the painful truth is that, invariably, their own discredit is the only result of their efforts' (Anon. 1969).

Support for AEGIS manifest in surprising ways, such as a shift in the allegiance of the NAMH away from officialdom. Chief Nursing Officer Kathleen Raven noted a 'rather unpleasant' outcome of *Sans Everything*: Applebey sung Barbara's praises at a sherry party at the King's Fund, claiming that 'the campaign about *Sans Everything* would not have had the same effect if the NAMH had not helped to produce it.' Raven continued, that the Ministry contributed significantly to NAMH funds, '£10,000 per annum and paying expenses for health service employees to attend their annual conferences', a veiled threat of sanctions if NAMH continued side with AEGIS.[39] In October 1967 NAMH published a booklet to promote understanding of the mental health needs of older people. It opened with the words: 'When face to face with an elderly person, often sans eyes and sans ears, and nearly always sans teeth, it is tempting to wonder what this ageing man or woman might have been like as a little boy or girl' (Emery 1967, p. 1). Following so soon after *Sans Everything*, it is likely that the booklet and the words were inspired by it. AEGIS's campaign was also a factor leading to NAMH adopting a more forceful, lobbying stance (NAMH 1969, pp. 5–7; Long 2014, pp. 177–178).

After Publication: Secrecy, Privacy and Confidentiality

Barbara's concern about confidentiality and safety of witnesses was admirable. However, with the publicity given to *Sans Everything*, complete confidentiality was unrealistic. It was inevitable that people involved, and the hospitals subject to investigation, would become known locally.[40] This happened on the day of publication. Sir Arnold France, Permanent Secretary at the Ministry, noted that in Leeds 'staff at the hospital are talking amongst themselves... it may become public knowledge that Sister Biss is thought to be the nurse in question. It might get to the ears, of course, of opposition Members of Parliament.'[41] It is interesting that he centred his worries on political tactics rather than on staff or patients.

The stream of letters from staff, patients and their relatives, to AEGIS, the Ministry, Patients Association (PA), NAMH, and the press, indicated widespread hospital problems. The Ministry received 186 negative letters about the care of older people in about 100 different hospitals. A 'considerable number' of people addressed their letters personally to Robinson. The Ministry drew up 'special arrangements' to deal with the letters, to guide staff as to which required replies from the Ministry, which should be forwarded to the RHBs, and which the RHBs should investigate and then feed back to the Ministry.[42] Psychiatrists working with mentally unwell older people, such as David Enoch and Garry Blessed, trying to do their best in their own hospitals, corroborated that it was a matter of 'there but for the grace of God go I.'[43] Publicly naming the hospitals in *Sans Everything* risked scapegoating them and detracting from the wider significance of the proposed inquiries, reinforcing Barbara's stand on maintaining confidentiality for hospitals and witnesses.[44]

The Ministry lacked a clear strategy about how to define, distinguish and manage the potentially conflicting issues of 'secrecy', 'privacy' and 'confidentiality' in the context of inquiries.[45] Barbara kept the press informed about progress on these matters (Anon. 1967f, 1967g). The

Ministry's lack of clarity, however, added to Barbara's reservations about a level playing field for the proposed inquiries. In September, the Ministry apologised to her for not explaining its intentions more clearly.[46] 'Secrecy' could lead to leaks and provoke press comment,[47] antagonise the public and affect the credibility and outcome of an inquiry (Anon. 1967e). It might, for example, prevent potential witnesses from giving evidence if they did not know of an inquiry's existence. On the other hand, 'privacy' for individuals to give evidence could increase their willingness to disclose information. 'Confidentiality' was relative in government terms. The Ministry argued, 'In confidence in its widest sense would have effectively prevented the setting up of any Enquiry'[48] and that 'in confidence' had to be interpreted in the light of an inquiry's findings, including the possibility of subsequent criminal proceedings.[49] The Ministry was also under obligation to publish a report, as Patrick Gordon-Walker, minister without portfolio, had undertaken to do so during a Commons debate.[50] Robinson understood that this would include hospital names.[51] In the same debate, Robinson made an obtuse remark, probably indicating his irritation with Barbara: he praised a female MP for opening the debate 'in a way that was generally constructive and, if I may say so, unsensational'.[52]

Mr RS Matthews, Robinson's private secretary, wrote to Barbara. In a well-reasoned letter, he acknowledged her policy of publishing pseudonymously to avoid scapegoats but encouraged her to identify the complainants, patients and staff to enable a full inquiry. He pointed out that proposals made by Abel-Smith in *Sans Everything* (1967, pp. 128–135) about investigating complaints were practical only if specific incidents were identified. Alternatively, Matthews suggested, Barbara could reveal the hospital names 'in confidence', which would enable 'independent investigations' to be made into the situation at those hospitals, even if the individual incidents could not be examined. Matthews' letter ended: 'The contents of this letter are being released to the Press.' By return post, Barbara asked Matthews to define an independent investigation. He replied that *Robinson* 'would arrange for enquiries to be carried out by a legally qualified chairman from outside the National Health Service, probably assisted by other persons unconnected with the hospital concerned'.[53] Satisfied with Matthews' reply, she contacted the author-witnesses for permission to disclose details, and awaited their replies.

With consent from the author-witnesses, Barbara revealed the hospitals' names, in confidence, as the Ministry asked.[54] However, in the light of a Commons debate on 11 July, her caution was justified. Contrary to the earlier promise that Robinson would establish the inquiries, he announced that the *RHB chairmen* would undertake that task.[55] This change had huge implications. If Robinson appointed the committees, on behalf of Parliament, the inquiries would be overseen by the Council on Tribunals, but delegating the task to the RHBs removed this protection. Barbara was horrified: she revealed the names of the hospitals on the understanding that Robinson would set up inquiries. She described the change as a 'breach of faith'.[56]

Despite the RHBs appointing the committees, the author-witnesses agreed to give evidence and for their names to be disclosed to the chairmen.[57] Barbara remained concerned that RHB-appointed committees would inhibit nurses from criticising their own hospitals because of fear of reprisals,[58] and that because the RHBs were taking charge of evaluating their own performance, the committees could not be impartial. Barbara's view could be justified based on her previous experience of Blofeld's inquiry, taking into account that she never received the report. The Ministry was convinced that RHB-appointed committees would be 'completely impartial',[59] although their appointment contradicted the Council on Tribunals' principles of ensuring independence from real or apparent influences of the authorities. On this point, Barbara was particularly concerned about the Friern committee, for which the RHB proposed to appoint Isabel Graham Bryce as the lay member. Graham Bryce was chairman of Oxford RHB and therefore could not be 'lay' in the Ministry's definition of someone 'who should represent predominantly the view of the patient'.[60] More specifically, the *Oxford Mail* published a statement from the Oxford RHB, 'that the allegations made in a recent issue of a National Sunday newspaper *did not* apply to their hospitals' (Anon. 1967b). Barbara assumed that a published RHB report would have the chairman's 'knowledge and acquiescence' and that because the statement was incorrect the chairman's dishonesty would prejudice her inquiry role. The Ministry consulted Hackett about Graham Bryce's appointment. Hackett was sure that the statement in the *Oxford Mail* provided no grounds to replace her and that 'this move on the part of Mrs Robb is primarily designed to obstruct the inquiry'.[61] Crossman later described Graham Bryce as 'a mere stooge',[62] although he was also condescending towards other RHB chairmen, describing them as 'insignificant creatures trying to do a bit of public service and really entirely dominated by their officials'.[63]

The *Sunday Times* published a letter from Hackett, 'Hospitals: we are experts'. He wrote:

> A great deal of harm is being done to the Health Service by the book *Sans Everything*, with the brutal and scaring headlines in newspapers and on TV. This dreadful book will not give us one more pair of hands—what is worse, it may well cause us to lose many nurses and others, tired and disillusioned with the apparent lack of public appreciation of the work they do (Hackett 1967).

The day before Hackett's letter appeared, the *Times* published a statement made by Phyllis Rowe at a nursing conference. She said that no member of the RCN psychiatric committee denied the validity of the 'ghastly material' in *Sans Everything* and the book provided a 'wonderful opportunity for psychiatric nurses to see what could be done' (Anon. 1967d). Hackett had incorrectly assessed the nurses' mood, and his condemnation contradicted Rowe. AEGIS's careful groundwork with the RCN was bearing fruit. Like Cross,[64] Rowe reflected on a sense of guilt in the profession for not having acted sooner (Anon. 1967d). Letters in the *Sunday Times* the following week criticised Hackett and NHS managers who did not know, or try to find out, about abuse in their hospitals. Barbara's letter stated: 'In view of Mr Hackett's evident tendency to prejudge these issues, the public will surely be hoping that he is not one of the regional board chairmen being asked by the Minister to set up "independent" inquiries into circumstances in their own hospitals' (Robb 1967b).

Hackett discussed with Robinson whether any inquiry was needed at Friern because Blofeld's was 'searching' and the RHB interpreted it that 'no evidence of cruelty or ill treatment was found.'[65] Hackett and Robinson agreed that another inquiry was unnecessary but gave way to avoid the risk that they would 'be accused of having something to hide'.[66] Robinson was impatient to start the inquiries and to avoid more 'unfruitful correspondence' with Barbara.[67]

OTHER RESPONSES IN THE PUBLIC ARENA

Many people wrote to Barbara, often distraught.[68] Other letters from voluntary bodies asked for AEGIS's support or advice.[69] Supporters and admirers also wrote. Portrait sculptor Beth Jukes sent Barbara a photograph of her bronze torso sculpture of a thin, stooped, wrinkled, naked elderly woman staring down at her hands folded in her lap, called *Sans Everything*.[70] The *Nursing Mirror* reviewed *Sans Everything*, saying it was constructive despite generalisations and anonymisation and encouraged nurses to read it: nurses needed to acknowledge that bad conditions existed in some hospitals, especially where patients were the most helpless and that nurses needed to speak out (Greene 1967). A review in the Catholic paper, the *Tablet* described *Sans Everything* as 'case material for Dickens, Kingsley or Ruskin' with 'Pilate-like washing of hands at all stages in the hierarchy from nurse to member of hospital board' (Russell 1967). Allen (1967), in the *Sunday Mirror*, wrote that Barbara was 'the author of the year's most challenging book'. Allen adopted another religious analogy, the parable of the 'Good Samaritan', calling her article 'One woman who refused to pass by..'.

Some major medical journals drew attention to *Sans Everything*. Psychiatrist Tom Arie (Anon. 1967h) in the *Lancet*, did not question the validity of the reports and praised the suggestions of 'radical innovation' to improve the situation.[71] In the *BMJ*, geriatrician Eluned Woodford-Williams (1967) recognised the authenticity of the reports, and the challenges:

> Aid for the Elderly in Government Institutions has as its aim to shame the Government... into doing something about the cruelty and neglect which is the lot of many of our aged citizens.... The danger is that the lack of facts may enable it to be too easily dismissed, for those who have worked with the aged know that there is some truth in the accusations.

James Mathers (1968), a psychiatrist in Birmingham, wrote: 'let us not pretend that we think that *Sans Everything* (even if exaggerated) was an unjustified publication and that anyway it is no responsibility of the doctors.'

The *British Journal of Psychiatry* did not publish a review, despite the book's emphasis on psychiatric hospitals. Neither did *Gerontologia Clinica*, a leading journal of geriatric medicine that Woodford-Williams edited. The absence of reviews in both of these was surprising. Reasons for their absence could have been because the journals were not offered the book to review or it might relate to difficulties finding a reviewer, taking into account lack of interest of many geriatricians in the goings-on of mental hospitals (Denham 2004) and of many psychiatrists in undertaking clinical work with older people (Fine 1963). Some psychiatrists also objected to Barbara, as an outsider, interfering in service-related matters, and some geriatricians objected to the lack of mention in *Sans Everything* about good geriatric services that increasingly existed in general hospitals (Felstein 1969, pp. 9–11).[72]

Some RHBs had good intentions about improving conditions for older people. Manchester RHB (Mackay and Ruck 1967) investigated their needs. Its report, published internally, was logical and innovative such as proposing 'that long stay patients should have the best accommodation in a hospital rather than the worst' because, as their permanent home, it should be as pleasant as possible and favourable conditions promoted older people's independence and reduced disability (p. 9). The RHB proposed to address the report's concerns 'as opportunity occurs' and 'as their resources permit' (pp. 5–6), but an open-ended promise, amid competing priorities, was unlikely to succeed. The laissez-faire approach risked neglecting the report in the same way as the wards and people it sought to assist: 'dumping grounds, the patients becoming chronic discards' (p. 19). SK Ruck, one of the researchers, wrote to Barbara, attributing renewed interest in his work to *Sans Everything*: 'I'm half inclined to wonder whether it would have seen the light of day but for your book, since it has lain "incommunicado" with the RHB for more than a year since it was written.'[73] The *Times* commented that the Manchester report: 'confirms, in rather more official language, many of the more startling disclosures' in *Sans Everything* (Northern Correspondent 1967). Commissioned by the NHS, the Manchester study had respectability and authority, but lacking priority it risked neglect, reinforcing the need for dedicated pressure groups for unpopular social issues.

The media, according to Hackett, failed to provide the statutory authorities with an opportunity to present their side of the *Sans Everything* argument to the public, even though Robinson was prominent on *24 Hours* on 30 June. Hackett wanted a second *24 Hours* programme in which he could 'confront Mrs Robb'. He approached the BBC to arrange it.[74] Whether Hackett's request contributed to the BBC's decision to produce a second programme is unclear, but the BBC enlisted him and Abel-Smith as the 'experts' for the programme.

The programme began with Allsop recapping on the *Sans Everything* issues, then interviewing people who had witnessed abuse, this time facing the cameras. The interviewees included a nurse and three relatives whose reports were uncomfortably close to the allegations described in *Sans Everything*: uncooperative staff, unkindness to patients and an elderly woman who was slapped for being incontinent. Abel-Smith commented on how to improve NHS complaints procedures, especially the need for independent inquiries. Allsop then asked Hackett for his comments, in the context of his recent *Sunday Times* letter, 'Hospitals: we are experts'. Hackett overlooked the essence of the question and answered by finding fault with the *Sunday Times* editor and promoting his own skills: 'the headline you just quote about being experts wasn't mine. The one I put was a much better one but the papers altered it.' With prompting by Allsop to achieve a relevant answer, Hackett was unhesitant: there was no need to change the complaints procedures, of course the RHBs would investigate properly, 'we are on the side of the patient. That is what we are there for.' Abel-Smith retorted: 'You might as well say that the Chairman of the Coal Board should be appointed to investigate the Aberfan Disaster.' Hackett followed the plan Robinson stated in the previous *24 Hours*, aiming to find individuals at fault. With names of the hospitals, he said, 'we can investigate the cases of cruelty'. In contrast, Abel-Smith focused on principles and had the last word: 'Mrs Robb is fighting for a principle, the principle of totally independent inquiries and she is going to win the battle. What she wants is an inquiry set up right outside the hospital service and we don't normally get it.'[75]

'SMOULDERING DISCONTENT' ELSEWHERE

Just before publication of *Sans Everything*, the Ministry wrote to chairmen of all RHBs instructing senior staff to make 'searching enquiries' to ensure that there were no grounds for complaints in their hospitals. The letter was worded to prompt the reply that all was well.[76] RHBs obtained data from HMCs and fed back to the Ministry, but not all reports were positive. Clare Turquet and Stella Brain[77] wrote about provision in the South West Metropolitan region. They doubted that 'physical cruelty could go long unchecked', but 'harsh and unsympathetic treatment, and some lessening of the dignity of the individual elderly patients, may well be accepted in the wards'. They noted other problems, including boredom, and patients not encouraged or allowed to wear spectacles, hearing aids or dentures, from which they might benefit. They concluded: 'Whether the distressing incidents [*Sans Everything*] sets out are substantiated, or not...we all know in our hearts that there are still very bad conditions in some of our hospitals.'[78]

Other HMCs reassured their RHBs that malpractice did not happen in their hospitals (DHSS 1972, p. 8).[79] However, as a direct result of the publicity around *Sans Everything*, a staff member at Ely Hospital in Cardiff and nursing students at Whittingham Hospital in Lancashire, revealed discontent and concerns about standards of care in their hospitals (DHSS 1972, pp. 7–8).[80]

When the Welsh Hospital Board (WHB, with the iconic address 'Temple of Peace and Health', Cardiff) sought feedback from its HMCs, the HMC responsible for Ely Hospital replied:

> We are, of course, assured by the senior officers...that there is no inhumanity in the treatment of patients, particularly elderly patients, and if the number of complaints which are made direct to the Committee or myself is a yardstick, we can feel assured that this is so.... We have a system of monthly rota visits by members.... All these reports state that there were no complaints from the patients or staff.[81]

By the time the HMC sent this summary to the WHB, Roxan had forwarded to the Ministry a report about scandalous practices at Ely that he received following his article about *Sans Everything* in the *News of the World* (Roxan 1967a).[82] This report was one of five sent to Roxan, all of which outlined situations similar to those in *Sans Everything*. Each report gave the informant's name and address and identified the hospital. With the authors' agreement, Roxan sent the reports to the Ministry. For the Ministry, the report from Michael Pantelides, an assistant nurse at Ely, stood out. Allegations included violence towards patients, lies by staff about injuries, and pilfering of patients' food (also found at Storthes Hall).[83] The Ministry cautiously criticised the informant but did not deny the contents. An official wrote:

> This is an astonishing document and quotes names lavishly. Moreover it gives the names of 3 other nurses willing to give evidence.... There is a danger that Mr Pantelides is a man with a grievance making reckless allegations and that his 3 witnesses will not support him but nevertheless I do not think that anything but an independent enquiry would be satisfactory.[84]

The Ministry feared that if it neglected the reports, Roxan would put pen to paper and discredit Robinson's sincerity about seeking improvements. The Ministry sought guidance from its legal advisors on how to proceed.[85]

In August, the *News of the World* published anonymised summaries of the reports (Roxan 1967a, 1967b). Because this was during the parliamentary summer recess, there could be no anticipatory Commons discussion or conveniently planted or inspired questions to minimise their impact.

Ely, a hospital for 'mentally subnormal' people, rather than for psychiatric illness, had wards for children and adults. The HMC inspection reports were usually brief, about half a page, and suggest cursory scrutiny, particularly focused on the physical environment and lacking discussion with staff or patients, as was typical of that sort of inspection (Barton 1959, p. 48). Nevertheless, the reports changed markedly after 1960. In the early 1960s, the HMC generally approved of what they saw and praised the staff, including how the nurses cared for patients. The positive became interspersed with minor criticisms and then, with a marked change in tone, to clear concern. In March 1965, one report noted that 'Every effort should be made to reduce the overcrowding in this hospital, urgently.' In October 1965, 'The staffing situation is deteriorating and calls for urgent attention' and gave suggestions how to ameliorate it. The HMC visitors also noted, on one ward, one toilet for forty-five patients. In 1967, attempts were made to upgrade the wards, but planning was poor and did not meet needs: 'The day rooms are very small and some ambulant patients must remain in bed until after dinner as there is not sufficient space for them to sit and eat.'[86] Shockingly, around 1965, the Ministry inspected Ely and found scandalous conditions: a deplorable report 'had gone on file' at the Ministry without any intervention (Crossman 1977, p. 411).[87] The Ely HMC did not respond to early warnings of dysfunction in the hospital, similar to responses at Friern and Storthes Hall.

The events at Ely matched AEGIS's concern that planned inspections were ineffective and that number of complaints as a measure of quality was inaccurate. Pantelides left Ely having 'found the atmosphere uncomfortable' because colleagues were hostile towards him.[88] An inquiry into the happenings there followed the *Sans Everything* inquiries but had significantly different outcomes. This is taken up again in Chapter 7 (pp. 214–222), after discussion of the *Sans Everything* inquiries.

As at Ely, events at Whittingham Hospital unfolded because of *Sans Everything*. In July 1967, 'smouldering discontent among the student nurses caught alight' when forty-five student nurses met with the senior nursing tutor (DHSS 1972, p. 7). The tutor proposed to discuss patient care 'in relation to recent Press statements... arising from the publication *Sans Everything*' (p. 52). The students alleged dangerous and demeaning practices: patients struck with a key strap, put to bed too early in the evenings, locked in the coal-house or bathroom, tormented for the amusement of staff and bathed with long mops when incontinent. Although there was some safety in numbers, as punishing all the students would draw attention to problems at the hospital, the students feared retribution, especially if they reported individuals and specific incidents (pp. 52–53).

The tutor informed the chief male nurse about the allegations, and he called a second meeting, with the students, the tutor, matron and himself. Still fearful of victimisation, the students refused to particularise allegations (pp. 52–53). Subsequently, the three senior nurses met with the HMC chairman, to help answer the Ministry's letter about malpractice in their hospital, but they did not mention the students' complaints. The senior nurses made a few more attempts to obtain precise details of the students' allegations, but the students 'piped down'. The HMC was not informed of their concerns (p. 8). These events supported the notion that juniors feared making complaints and took their concerns only to their immediate seniors and that HMCs and RHBs could genuinely be unaware of the extent of problems in their hospitals.

In 1970, Barbara received more information about events at Whittingham, indicating long-term failure to deal with concerns, similar to Ely, Storthes Hall and Friern. Barton, for example, raised concerns there in 1965, but to no avail.[89] After the conviction of a nurse for manslaughter of a patient kicked to death at Whittingham, Barton's conclusion was brief: 'Belsen had similar episodes.'[90]

A committee of inquiry was appointed at Whittingham in 1971, under section 70 of the NHS Act (DHSS 1972, p. 1). Somebody—Barbara did not know who—sent her a copy of the report before publication. She ensured that summaries appeared in several national newspapers, pressing for publication of the full report and paving the way for more publicity to ensure improvements at Whittingham.[91] The inquiry report found unacceptable practices mainly on long-stay back wards, the rest of the hospital practicing more therapeutically (DHSS 1972, pp. 1, 26). This underlined earlier concern about the two-tier, double standards in hospitals, providing better quality, rehabilitation-focussed psychiatric treatment, usually for younger people. Sir Keith Joseph (Secretary of State for Social Services, 1970–1974; Conservative government under Edward Heath) admitted after the Whittingham Inquiry that the government was not 'sufficiently alive to this danger' and was 'grappling' with it (Joseph

1972, p. iii). Joseph's comment was surprising, suggesting ignorance at government level about long-standing discriminatory patterns of resourcing, staffing and facilities, such as at Claybury, Friern/Halliwick, and elsewhere (Jones and Sidebotham 1962, p. 62).[92]

Comment

Sans Everything stimulated more revelations of ill-treatment, indicated by the many letters sent to AEGIS, the Ministry, the NAMH, PA and BBC, and the press. AEGIS's links with the national press enabled timely and often prominent reports that highlighted the problems and indicated the value of investigative journalism in a campaign context. *Sans Everything* also stimulated established bodies, such as the RCN and NAMH, to become more involved with AEGIS's objectives and helped bring the constructive Manchester RHB study into the open.

AEGIS recognised common patterns of NHS dysfunction, including that deficits in care could be long-standing and that numbers of complaints and planned inspection visits were of dubious value in determining quality of provision. It also found that junior, new or inexperienced staff were often the whistle-blowers, and seniors and their peers generally responded unconstructively to their concerns. How to achieve a NHS culture that responds constructively to whistle-blowing remains a problem in the twenty-first century.

AEGIS masterminded the production of *Sans Everything*. It distributed copies of the book to significant people prepublication and enthused the press to announce when it would be available to the public. *Sans Everything* set out to shock. It did not just rant against the system, but proposed ways to make improvements, authoritatively backed by experts. The Ministry, however, grasped only the rant and repeatedly scapegoated Barbara for unnecessary, inappropriate and damaging publicity and time-consuming intrusions for which it had little patience. No evidence has come to light that the Ministry made any attempt to resolve AEGIS's concerns by face-to-face meetings or that it considered changing its tactics in the light of mounting evidence. Enoch thought the NHS leadership 'didn't want to know, they didn't want to believe it. Nobody wanted to believe it.'[93] Ralph added that any serious inquiry 'won't be set off by Kenneth, you can bet your life on that'.[94] Labour MP Dennis Hobden wrote to Barbara: 'I long ago gave up [on] Kenneth Robinson. There has been nothing but evasion and covering up by Hospital Management Committees from top to bottom.'[95] Hobden, Rolph, Cross and 'Pertinax' (1967) all alleged government coverups and lying and that a culture of fear encouraged the silence of hospital nurses. The Ministry's filing of a damning inspection report about Ely and the sequence of events at Whittingham reinforced the notion that coverups happened at all levels of psychiatric hospital administration. Suspicion that the NHS sought to conceal its inadequacies was consistent with the Press Council's complaint in 1966, and with Robinson's and Hackett's defensiveness of the NHS and their hostility towards AEGIS, although their responses did not blind the press or public.

Robinson sometimes sounded genuinely incredulous that practices happened as described in *Sans Everything* or that staff and patients feared reprisals if they complained. To believe the allegations he said, 'would be to accept that there is…a conspiracy against the patients, and especially the weakest and most helpless patients. Does anyone, do the authors of *Sans Everything*, does the editor of the *Nursing Mirror*, really believe this?'[96] He appeared unaware of the many who did. The Ministry's failure to deal dispassionately with complaints, its lack of knowledge about establishing inquiries and the absence of patient-focussed section 70 inquiries during the NHS's first eighteen years, reinforced impressions of the Ministry's disregard for patients and its institutional self-justification and defensiveness, if not a conspiracy.

Robinson stated his expectations of the proposed inquiries into the *Sans Everything* allegations when interviewed on *24 Hours*. When asked, 'Are you satisfied that [poor care] has been reduced, now, almost to non-existence?' Robinson replied, 'That is my belief and I hope that any enquiries we can make will bear that out.'[97] Incredulity in the upper echelons of government about the allegations remained the dominant mind-set: it would not encourage impartial inquiries. From the Aberfan Inquiry it was clear that statutory authorities could mismanage services and neglect their responsibilities to the point of disregard for human life. Whether committees of inquiry into the *Sans Everything* allegations could disengage from establishment self-righteousness and preconceptions about the excellence of the NHS remained to be seen.

Notes

1. Anne Robinson, interview by author, 2015.
2. AEGIS meeting, 16 March 1967, 49, 53, AEGIS/1/20 (AEGIS archive, London School of Economics).
3. Frontmatter, *Sans Everything*, Robb 1967a.

4. Robb, note, AEGIS/B/2.
5. Letter, Mabel Franks to Robb, July 1967, AEGIS/2/10.
6. Robb, 'Record of a campaign', vol 2, 84, AEGIS/1/2/A.
7. Tonia Milton, Independent Press Standards Organisation (IPSO), email to author January 2016.
8. 14 July 1968.
9. NWMRHB minutes, 17 July 1967, BM.354–5/67 (London Metropolitan Archives, LMA).
10. 'Regional Hospital Boards (The Press)', *Hansard* HC Deb 8 May 1967, vol 746 c.143W.
11. Ministry of Health (MoH) press service, 'Conditions of the elderly in hospitals'. 6 June 1967, MH150/349 (The National Archives, TNA).
12. Letter, Cross to Robinson, 9 June 1967, MH150/350 (TNA).
13. 'Mental Hospitals (Conditions)'. *Hansard* HC Deb 26 June 1967, vol 749 cc.69–70.
14. Letter, A France to RHBs, 28 June 1967, MH150/350 (TNA).
15. 'Rampton Hospital (Peter Whitehead)', *Hansard* HC Deb 14 March 1958, vol 584 cc.875–886.
16. They belonged to COHSE rather than the Royal College of Nursing (RCN), the nursing trades union and professional body, because of the restrictions on mental nurses joining the RCN. COHSE merged with other unions 1993 to form UNISON.
17. Meeting, Robb and Tooth, 25 May 1965, AEGIS/1/1.
18. AEGIS meeting, 16 March 1967, AEGIS/B/2.
19. Tribunals and Inquiries (Discretionary Inquiries) Order 1967.
20. Other standards were being efficient, timely and accessible.
21. MoH, c.1966. list of section 70 inquiries, MH159/213 (TNA).
22. MoH, 'Meeting with the Minister', 21 February 1967, MH150/349 (TNA).
23. 'Mental Hospitals (Conditions)', *Hansard* HC Deb 26 June 1967, vol 749 cc.69–70.
24. MoH, 'Meeting with the Minister', 21 February 1967, MH150/349 (TNA).
25. Memo (illegible signature) to RS Matthews, 27 June 1967, MH150/350 (TNA).
26. Memo, JC Hales to 'Secretary' 4 July 1967, MH150/350 (TNA).
27. MoH, Some notes in dealing with press inquiries, c. June 1968, para 4; 'Formal inquiries under S 70', c.1967, MH159/213 (TNA).
28. 'Elderly Patients (Complaints)', *Hansard* HC Deb 11 April 1967, vol 744 cc.172–173W.
29. Memo, Benwell to Hedley, 20 June 1967, MH150/350 (TNA).

30. MoH, 'Meeting with the Minister', 21 February 1967, MH150/349 (TNA).
31. Letter, Robb to Strabolgi, 9 August 1965, AEGIS/7/12.
32. BBC Home Service, *Ten O'Clock Programme of News and Current Affairs*, 30 June 1967, transcript, AEGIS/1/6.
33. BBC1, *24 Hours*, 30 June 1967, transcript, AEGIS/1/6.
34. See Chapter 3, p. 80.
35. BBC1, *24 Hours*, 28 July 1967, transcript, AEGIS/1/6.
36. Signed statement, Ernestine Anne, 1967, AEGIS/2/7/B.
37. Letter, Cross to Matthews, 5 July 1967, MH150/350 (TNA).
38. Letter, Matthews to Cross, 12 July 1967, MH150/350 (TNA).
39. Memo, Kathleen Raven to Hedley, 13 July 1967, MH150/350 (TNA).
40. Letter, Matthews to Robb, 17 August 1967, MH159/220 (TNA).
41. Memo, France to Robinson, 30 June 1967, MH150/350 (TNA).
42. Memos, 'Complaints about care of the elderly in hospital', July 1967, MH150/350; Giddon to FDK Williams, November 1967, MH159/220 (TNA).
43. Garry Blessed, letter, to author; David Enoch, interview by author, 2015.
44. Letter, Robb to Miss Nevin, South West Metropolitan (SWM) RHB, 22 August 1967, AEGIS/2/10.
45. Letters, Fanklyn Williams, Welsh Hospital Board to Croft, 27 September 1967; Geoffrey Howe to Robinson, 22 October 1967, MH159/221 (TNA).
46. Draft reply, Ministry to AEGIS's solicitors, 29 September 1967, MH159/220 (TNA).
47. Letters, Howe to Robinson, 22 October 1968, and reply, 6 November 1968, MH96/2198 (TNA).
48. Memo, Croft, 23 October 1967, MH159/220 (TNA).
49. Letter, LR Warner to AEGIS's solicitor, 8 September 1967, AEGIS/A/1.
50. 'Care of the elderly', *Hansard* HC Deb 11 July 1967, vol 750 cc.431–554.
51. Note, Robinson, 3 October 1967, MH159/220 (TNA).
52. 'Care of the elderly', *Hansard* HC Deb 11 July 1967, vol 750 cc.431–554.
53. Letters, Matthews and Robb, 29–30 June 1967, MH159/220 (TNA).
54. Letter, Robb to Robinson, 3 July 1967, MH150/350 (TNA).
55. 'Care of the elderly', *Hansard* HC Deb 11 July 1967, vol 750 cc.431–554.
56. Letter, Robb to Matthews, 19 July 1967, MH159/220 (TNA).
57. Letter, Robb to Robinson, 11 August 1967, MH159/220 (TNA).
58. Letter, Robb to Matthews, 19 July 1967, MH159/220 (TNA).
59. Letter, FDK Williams to Council on Tribunals, 4 August 1967, MH159/213 (TNA).
60. Memo, Croft to Hedley, 1 August 1967, MH159/213 (TNA).
61. Memo, Poole to Hedley, 17 October 1967, MH159/213 (TNA).

62. Crossman Diaries, March 1969, 178/69/SW (University of Warwick Modern Records Centre, UWMRC).
63. Crossman Diaries, 30 April 1969, CD1162-3 (UWMRC).
64. Letter, Cross to Robinson, 9 June 1967, MH150/350 (TNA).
65. NWMRHB minutes, 17 July 1967, BM.354-5/67 (LMA).
66. Memo, (illegible signature) to Robinson, 4 July 1967, MH150/350 (TNA).
67. '*Sans Everything* (Investigation of Complaints)', *Hansard* HC Deb 26 July 1967, vol 751 cc.175–176W.
68. See mainly AEGIS files /5 /6 /8.
69. From 'Help – The Community Publications Group', AEGIS/1/3.
70. Letter and photo, Beth Jukes to Robb, 1967, AEGIS/1/3.
71. Tom Arie identified this as his writing.
72. Anon. psychiatrist, interview by author, 2016.
73. Letter, SK Ruck to Robb, 4 August 1967, AEGIS/1/3.
74. NWMRHB minutes, 17 July 1967, BM.353/67 (LMA).
75. BBC1, *24 Hours*, 28 July 1967, transcript, AEGIS/1/6.
76. Letter, France to RHB chairmen, 28 June 1967, MH150/350 (TNA).
77. Stella Brain: Granddaughter of Dr John Langdon-Down who gave his name to 'Down's Syndrome', and married to the neurologist Walter Russell, Baron Brain of Eynsham (Pickering 2004).
78. Stella Brain and Clare Turquet, 'Care of the Elderly in Hospital', SWMRHB, 4 October 1967, MH160/653 (TNA).
79. Letter, Thomas to WHB, 29 August 1967, BD18/816 (TNA).
80. Letter, with statements, Roxan to MoH chief press officer, 26 July 1967, MH150/350 (TNA).
81. Letter, Thomas to WHB, 29 August 1967, BD18/816 (TNA).
82. Memo, MoH press office to Croft, 27 July 1967, MH150/350 (TNA).
83. Storthes Hall HMC minutes with index, 1965–1966, Management of hospital pilfering, 14 October 1965, C416/1/188 (West Yorkshire Archive Service).
84. Comments by Croft about Mr Pantelides statement, received 27 July 1967, MH159/215 (TNA).
85. Memo, MoH press office to Croft, 27 July 1967, MH50/350 (TNA).
86. Visiting book, Ely Hospital HMC, DHE/1/6/1 (Glamorgan Archives, Cardiff).
87. 12 March 1969.
88. Memo, Croft to Hedley, 24 January 1969, MH159/222 (TNA).
89. Letter, André Masters to Barton, 12 December 1970, AEGIS1/10/B.
90. Letter, Barton to Robb, 18 December 1970, AEGIS/1/10/B.
91. Letter, Robb to 'Dearest Sister' (Convent), 1971, AEGIS/1/9/2.
92. See Powick Hospital, Chapter 7, pp. 205–206.

93. David Enoch, interview by author, 2015.
94. AEGIS meeting, 16 March 1967, 49, Aegis/B/2.
95. Letter, Dennis Hobden to Robb, 25 April 1967, AEGIS/2/3.
96. 'Care of the elderly', *Hansard* HC Deb 11 July 1967, vol 750 cc.431–554.
97. BBC1, *24 Hours*, 28 July 1967, transcript, AEGIS/1/6.

Bibliography

Abel-Smith, Brian. 1967. 'Administrative solution: a hospital commissioner?' 128–135. In Robb 1967a.
Administrative Tribunals and Inquiries, Report of Committee. 1957. Cmnd. 218. London: HMSO.
Allen, Anne. 1967. 'One woman who refused to pass by..'. *Sunday Mirror*, 9 July.
Andrews, John. 1967. In 'Public apathy to blame'. *Sunday Times*, 18 June.
Anon. 1966. 'Old folk'. *News of the World*, 8 May.
Anon. 1967a. 'Editorial'. *Nursing Mirror*, 16 June.
Anon. 1967b. 'Report of Board meeting, Oxford RHB'. *Oxford Mail*, 17 June.
Anon. 1967c. 'First response to last week's editorial'. *Nursing Mirror*, 23 June.
Anon. 1967d. 'We know such things go on'. *Times*, 22 July.
Anon. 1967e. 'MP condemns secret inquiry on hospital'. *Daily Sketch*, 2 October.
Anon. 1967f. 'Legal threat on naming hospitals'. *Times*, 24 October.
Anon. 1967g. 'How long does a confidence stay confidential'. *Daily Mirror*, 24 October.
Anon. 1967h. 'AEGIS'. *Lancet*, ii, 85–86.
Anon. 1969. 'Editorial'. *Nursing Mirror*, 24 January.
Applebey, Mary. 1967. In '*Sans Everything*: a misfortune to grow old today'. *Sunday Times*, 11 June.
Barton, Russell. 1959. *Institutional Neurosis*. Bristol: John Wright and Sons.
BBC1. 1967. 'What shall we do with granny?'. *Scrutiny*, 31 March, http://genome.ch.bbc.co.uk/, accessed 26 September 2016.
Cochrane, David. 1990. 'The AEGIS campaign to improve standards of care in mental hospitals: a case study of the process of social policy change'. PhD thesis, University of London. http://etheses.lse.ac.uk, accessed 17 September 2016.
Crossman, Richard. 1977. *The Diaries of a Cabinet Minister, Vol. 3. Secretary of State for Social Services 1968–1970*. London: Hamilton and Cape.
Denham, Michael. 2004. 'The history of geriatric medicine and hospital care of the elderly in England between 1929 and the 1970s'. PhD thesis, University College London. http://www.discovery.ucl.ac.uk, accessed 17 September 2016.
DHSS. 1972. *Report of the Committee of Inquiry into Whittingham Hospital*. Cmnd. 4861. London: HMSO.

Emery, Ralph. 1967. *Understanding Old Age*. London: NAMH.
Felstein, Ivor. 1969. *Later Life: Geriatrics Today and Tomorrow*. Harmondsworth: Penguin Books.
Fine, Wilfred. 1963. 'Care of the elderly disturbed patient'. *Lancet*, i, 557.
Fortune. John. 1967. 'Hospital management'. *Times*, 16 May.
Greene, John. 1967. 'Review: *Sans Everything*'. *Nursing Mirror*, 30 June.
Hackett, Maurice. 1967. 'Hospitals: we are experts'. *Sunday Times*, 23 July.
Howe. Geoffrey. 1999. 'The management of public inquiries'. *Political Quarterly*, 70, 295–304.
Jones, Kathleen and Sidebotham, Roy. 1962. *Mental Hospitals at Work*. London: Routledge and Kegan Paul.
Joseph, Keith. 1972. 'Foreword' iii–v. In DHSS, 1972.
Julian, Ivor. 1967. In '*Sans Everything*: a misfortune to grow old today'. *Sunday Times*, 11 June.
Leamington Spa reporter. 1967. 'Call for action over crowded hospitals'. *Times*, 18 March.
Lomax, Montagu. 1921. *The Experiences of an Asylum Doctor: With Suggestions for Asylum and Lunacy Law Reform*. London: G Allen and Unwin.
Long, Vicky. 2014. *Destigmatising Mental Illness? Professional Politics and Public Education in Britain, 1870–1970*. Manchester: Manchester University Press.
Mackay, JSB and Ruck, SK. 1967. *The Care of the Aged in the Manchester Hospital Board Area*. Manchester: RHB.
Mathers, James. 1968. 'Old people in hospital'. *BMJ*, iii, 374.
Monopolies and Mergers Commission. 1985. *United Newspapers PLC and Fleet Holdings PLC*, 5–16. http://web.archive.org/web/20070928073311/http://www.mmc.gov.uk/rep_pub/reports/1985/fulltext/190c02.pdf, accessed 25 September 2016.
NAMH. 1969. *Annual Report, 1968–9*. London: NAMH.
Northern Correspondent. 1967. 'Disclosures are confirmed'. *Times*, 20 July.
Pertinax. 1967. 'Without prejudice'. *BMJ*, i, 755.
Pickering, George. 2004. 'Brain, Walter Russell, first Baron Brain (1895–1966)'. *Oxford Dictionary of National Biography*. http://www.oxforddnb.com, accessed 4 March 2016.
Press Council. 1966. *Press and the People*. London: Press Council.
Robb, Barbara. 1967a. *Sans Everything: A Case to Answer*. London: Nelson.
Robb, Barbara. 1967b. 'Don't let him judge'. *Sunday Times*, 30 July.
Rogers, Anne and Pilgrim, David. 1996. *Mental Health Policy in Britain: A Critical Introduction*. Basingstoke: Macmillan Press.
Rogers, Simon. 2011. 'News of the World circulation data: who read it and how many bought it?' *Guardian*, 8 July.
Rolph, Cecil. 1987. *Further Particulars*. Oxford: OUP.
Roxan, David. 1958. *Sentenced without Cause*. London: Muller.

Roxan, David. 1966. 'Brutality to old folk: it's happening now in some of our hospitals'. *News of the World*, 1 May.
Roxan, David. 1967a. '"Old folk beaten in hospital" allegation'. *News of the World*, 25 June.
Roxan, David. 1967b. 'Heartbreak hospitals'. *News of the World*, 20 August.
Roxan, David. 1967c. 'I saw patients being treated like dogs'. *News of the World*, 27 August.
Royal Commission on Tribunals of Inquiry. 1966. Cmnd. 3121. London: HMSO.
Russell, Richard. 1967. 'Think on these things. *Sans Everything: A Case to Answer*. Presented by Barbara Robb'. *Tablet*, 19 August.
Shearer, Ann. 1976. 'The news media' 109–118. In *Changing Patterns of Residential Services for the Mentally Retarded*, ed. Robert Kugel and Ann Shearer. Washington, DC: President's Committee on Mental Retardation.
Stewart, Rosemary and Sleeman, Janet. 1967. *Continuously under Review: A Study of the Management of Out-patient Departments*. London: Bell.
Strabolgi. Beaumont. Heytesbury. Abel-Smith, Brian. Ardizzone, Edward. Harvey, Audrey. Hewetson, John. Robb, Barbara. Sargent, Bill and Woolgar, Daniel. 1965. 'Old people in mental hospitals'. *Times*, 10 November.
Welsh Office. 1967. *Report of the Tribunal Appointed to Inquire into the Disaster at Aberfan on October 21st 1966*. HL 316, HC 553. London: HMSO.
Woodford-Williams, Eluned. 1967. 'Misery in our midst'. *BMJ*, iii, 484–485.
Young, Hugo. 1967. 'The old in hospital'. *Sunday Times*, 4 June.

Open Access This chapter is licensed under the terms of the Creative Commons Attribution 4.0 International License (http://creativecommons.org/licenses/by/4.0/), which permits use, sharing, adaptation, distribution and reproduction in any medium or format, as long as you give appropriate credit to the original author(s) and the source, provide a link to the Creative Commons license and indicate if changes were made.

The images or other third party material in this chapter are included in the book's Creative Commons license, unless indicated otherwise in a credit line to the material. If material is not included in the book's Creative Commons license and your intended use is not permitted by statutory regulation or exceeds the permitted use, you will need to obtain permission directly from the copyright holder.

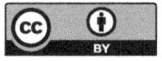

CHAPTER 6

The Inquiries: A Lion's Den

Barbara's personal experience of inquiries was limited to the brief, informal discussion chaired by Ann Blofeld. From that experience, she may not have realised the ordeal through which she was about to put her author-witnesses. The *Sans Everything* inquiries, between August 1967 and February 1968 (Ministry of Health (MoH) 1968, pp. 4, 54), were disturbing and unpleasant, to say the least. Each inquiry committee was made up of a chairman who was a QC (Queen's Counsel, senior barrister), a lay person, a nurse and a doctor. The medical and nursing members were needed to comply with the Ministry's recommendations to include 'a person or persons competent to advise on any professional or technical matters' (MoH 1966). Two of the medical members were geriatricians and the other four were psychiatrists (MoH 1968, pp. 5, 10, 21, 54, 58, 82). All were specialists in their field, but none was experienced in modern treatment and rehabilitation practices of both geriatric medicine and psychiatry, and stereotypical beliefs affected perceptions of each other's patients, roles and specialties (Hilton 2014, pp. 1072–1074). These features risked limiting the clinical guidance that medical members might provide to the chairmen and the lawyers.

All committees had the same terms of reference: to investigate the allegations 'so far as available evidence permits'; to examine the geriatric/psychiatric wards at the time of the inquiry; and to make recommendations (MoH 1968, p. 21). The loose criteria meant that each chairman could decide on the process of his inquiry and on definitions of standards of care to underpin his committee's judgements.[1] This increased the chance of the committees producing different answers to similar questions, which would make overall conclusions hard to draw. Loosely defined protocols would also affect how the committees interpreted the Ministry's instructions to produce two reports for each inquiry, a full report and a summary with recommendations for publication. The brevity of some of the published reports belied the duration of the hearings, between four and seventeen days each.

Archive sources available for each inquiry vary substantially, so not all can be explored in a similar way or to the same depth. I have therefore focussed on three: Friern, St Lawrence's and Storthes Hall. Friern is particularly important because its story was at the heart of the AEGIS (Aid for the Elderly in Government Institutions) campaign, and St Lawrence's and Storthes Hall have the most comprehensive records, including verbatim transcripts of proceedings.[2] The other inquiries are included where they contribute fresh insights. The Ministry's and Regional Hospital Boards' (RHBs) prepublication handling of the inquiry reports and the critique of inquiry procedures by the Council on Tribunals shed additional light on their processes and outcomes.

Friern

The Friern Inquiry focussed mainly on 'Diary of a Nobody' (Robb 1967). It also covered the accounts in *Sans Everything* by Moodie, Moody and Crofts and four additional complaints that members of the public raised with the Ministry around the time the book was published.[3] All the *Sans Everything* witnesses were willing to give evidence. Douglas Lowe QC[4] chaired the committee, which included Isabel Graham Bryce as lay member. The inquiry took place at the North West Metropolitan (NWM) RHB headquarters, several miles from the hospital.[5] That, sensibly, would reduce prying and speculation by Friern staff about their colleagues attending. However, in addition to Lowe's formal briefing by the RHB, the location would facilitate informal communication between the inquiry committee and senior members of the RHB, including Hackett, who vehemently and openly denied AEGIS's allegations, risking weakening the committee's impartiality.

Noting that the hospital would be legally represented at public expense, Barbara requested Lowe to allow the *Sans Everything* witnesses representation, at her personal expense, in case of publicity.[6] She also asked that the dates for the inquiry be set to give her lawyer sufficient time to prepare the case.[7] These requests were consistent with the principles of the Royal Commission on Tribunals of Inquiry (1966), that a witness 'should be given an adequate opportunity of preparing his case and of being assisted by his legal advisers'. Barbara did not argue over the Commission's other point, that, for witnesses who help inquiries in the public interest, 'legal expenses should normally be met out of public funds' (p. 44). Lowe refused to allow the *Sans Everything* witnesses to have legal representation because, in a private inquiry, 'There ought not...be publicity.'[8] He overlooked, or had not been informed, that the Ministry intended to publish the findings.[9] AEGIS's lawyer advised the witnesses not to attend without representation.[10] During these negotiations, Lowe informed Barbara that the committee 'consists of busy people', implying that she was wasting their time.[11] Lowe's condescending attitude to Barbara, AEGIS's absence from the inquiry and the committee's principle that where a 'complaint cannot be investigated [it] must be dismissed' (MoH 1968, p. 26) had the potential to prejudice the inquiry.

Lowe's committee described the *Sans Everything* allegations as 'wild', 'unsubstantiated' and 'probably exaggerated' (MoH 1968, p. 23). It deemed the *Sans Everything* witnesses as irrational, incompetent and unqualified to criticise: 'none of them possesses a medical qualification' (p. 27). It was 'unprepared to accept any statement by Mrs Robb that has not been admitted or corroborated either in evidence given or in documents placed before them' (p. 27). Verbal corroboration was unlikely because evidence was not taken on oath and staff would not voluntarily incriminate themselves. Written confirmation was also unlikely: undignified practices, such as chastising or hitting a patient would not be documented and information that should have been recorded was not, such as the name of the firm that Miss Cloake hired to clear Amy's flat (Robb 1967, p. 84). The committee deduced incorrectly that because Barbara did not complain during Amy's admission (she did: the Diary went to the Ministry, and she met Tooth) 'the explanation is simple', the allegations 'are basically false' (MoH 1968, p. 31). How the Ministry allowed this inaccuracy to appear in the final published report under their authority is unclear.

In contrast to its approach to AEGIS, the committee was sympathetic to hospital staff who gave evidence and it had 'naturally borne in mind the effect on people's memory' of the time since the events (MoH 1968, pp. 21–22). If staff members declared that they could not recall an event, or denied it, the committee concluded that the allegation was false. Overall, it believed staff rather than complainants (p. 25) much as the Patients Association (PA) warned in 1965.[12] The report used the word *distortion* to describe evidence only from complainants, not from staff. For example, it described Crofts' evidence: 'The discrepancies, distortions and omissions of vital facts may be due to the highly emotional state in which Miss Tasburg [Crofts] seems to have been' (p. 24). Her evidence was: 'a gross distortion of many of the facts, a suppression of other facts, and a remarkable inability... to perceive or accept the truth' (p. 26). Because the committee never met the *Sans Everything* witnesses, its conclusion about their characters was speculative, based on perceptions gleaned from the contents of the book, which they disbelieved, or on reports from hospital staff who were defending their practices.

The committee demonstrated misunderstandings and lack of knowledge about subjects on which it was expected to make judgements. For example, it concluded that many elderly patients desire 'nothing more than just to sit or loaf around owing to their mental condition [and] they are often incapable of animation' (MoH 1968, p. 22), that 'Neither spectacles nor hearing aids... would have been of much use to most of them' and that most were 'very old and senile' (p. 30). These descriptions were incompatible with other observations by the committee. For example, the committee reported that patients were sufficiently well for one in ten of them 'selected at random among those who had been in those wards in 1965' to be interviewed in 1967 (p. 42). How many this included is not stated, but if they were chronically mentally incapacitated to the extent of being 'incapable of animation' in 1965, it is unlikely that they would have been well enough to give meaningful answers two years later. If they had chronic schizophrenia, a common diagnosis of long-stay patients, they would not have improved. If they were 'senile' in 1965, it is unlikely that they would have remembered the events at that time in order to describe them accurately. If they were well enough to be interviewed in 1967, they would almost certainly have benefitted from spectacles and hearing aids two years earlier. The committee made other assumptions about older people, such as that it was acceptable for them to go to bed at 7 P.M. as 'owing to their age many would wish to do so' (p. 31). It allowed contradictory evidence to pass without comment, such as that Amy, 'as an informal patient, was of course, free to leave the hospital at any time' (p. 31) but also that 'her family would have to approve any arrangements for her transfer' (p. 32): only one was correct. It commented that many older people had 'not uncommon predatory proclivities' (p. 31), which meant that they tended to steal. It ignored the fact that most patients never left the ward and they lacked lockers or any other place in which to hide their allegedly ill-found gains. Whether staff might steal was not mentioned, although it happened in other hospitals (DHSS 1969, p. 123).[13]

Some of the committee's judgements were based on standards incompatible with known good practice. There is no evidence that the medical member of the committee provided specialist guidance about this, thus allowing erroneous or outdated views to influence deliberations. For example, concerning locking ward doors, the committee wrote that they were locked to ensure the safety of patients: 'What is not brought out [in *Sans Everything*] is the undoubted necessity to keep many, if not all, wards locked because of the propensity of many patients to wander and the clear risk of their being lost or even injured on the near-by highway' (MoH 1968, p. 22). This was illogical, not least because the so-called near-by highway was a suburban street with one lane of traffic in each direction, about 200 metres from the hospital building and through a gate with an adjacent porter's lodge. Also, research by Mandelbrote (1964) and others (e.g., Martin 1962, pp. 18, 82), about the low risk of leaving ward doors unlocked, and Malcolm Campbell's observation that institutionalised patients at Friern were usually too frightened to go very far,[14] clashed with the committee's view. In an understaffed custodial regime lacking rehabilitation goals, Moodie's allegation (1967, p. 15) that the doors were locked 'for the sisters' convenience' seemed apt (MoH 1968, p. 22).

The committee accepted that some of the events in *Sans Everything* might have happened, such as shouting at or pushing patients, and unkindness, intolerance and teasing (MoH 1968, pp. 38, 45–46), but it dismissed allegations of cruelty towards Amy and other patients (p. 41). The committee justified staff behaviours that patients or onlookers could perceive as cruel and frightening as 'the result of long hours and overstrain' (pp. 45–46).

The committee investigated four unrelated complaints. These were only documented in the unpublished inquiry report. They shed more light on the inquiry process. Even though the witnesses gave evidence in person, the committee rejected all their allegations. It rejected one as 'ill-founded or fictitious'[15] and a second as 'worthless',[16] without giving details about how it reached these conclusions. It rejected a third, Mrs Dickens' complaint on behalf of her brother, 'in toto'.[17] Dickens wrote to Barbara about the committee's hostility: her daughter was not allowed to accompany her into the inquiry room, and Mrs Dickens could not 'speak freely without being side-tracked and what I did say was at times twisted'.[18]

A fourth complaint was from Rosemary Thomas, a psychology student on placement at Friern in 1965. Her allegations included forced feeding of a patient held down by four nurses, a patient 'dragged around' by a nurse (which the committee attributed to the patient's recalcitrance) and a nurse who 'thumped' a patient (who the committee regarded as 'merely being restrained'). The committee did 'not think that such treatment of patients was frequent, or indeed would be tolerated by sisters or matrons'. Thoughts were flimsy grounds on which to base conclusions, and it is dubious whether frequency could be a satisfactory argument concerning harsh behaviours (Abel-Smith 1967, p. 128). The committee agreed that some older patients were slapped to get them out of bed in the morning, but there were 'legitimate reasons for this, provided of course that the slap was not too severe'. The committee regarded demeaning practices only in terms of physical harm. It ignored undignified, psychologically damaging and untherapeutic methods, revealing little awareness of current knowledge (e.g., Barton 1959; Goffman 1961, Martin 1962, Mandelbrote 1964). The committee implied that patients were at fault, that nurses behaved appropriately and that slapping older people could be legitimate. It dismissed the student's allegations, describing her as 'an immature, idealistic, young woman.... Her attempts to describe conditions were a sincere reflection of what she thought she had witnessed.'[19]

As Cohen wrote (1964, p. 24), hospitals worked as a caste system, with patients at the bottom. Genuine concern of individuals outside, or at the foot of, the NHS hierarchy appeared automatically rejected from serious consideration. It is possible that *all* the complainants at Friern were dishonest troublemakers, but taking into account the risk of victimisation to which they exposed themselves or their relatives, that was unlikely. Instead, rejecting their allegations was underpinned by arguments about their personal integrity and was in keeping with assumptions of NHS excellence, as expressed by Hackett and Robinson. In summary, evaluating the allegations at Friern linked to beliefs that staff would not permit malpractice; that patients could be treated harshly; and that patients, relatives, friends and vocational students were too muddled, emotional, ignorant or immature to interpret accurately what they saw and heard.

It was harder for the committee to refute what it witnessed directly when it inspected Friern. It was shocked by low ward temperatures (MoH 1968, p. 43), wards unattended at night (p. 48) and 'gravely inadequate' staff levels (p. 43). It found that 'indifferent communication' between staff, and 'the relatively bad name that Friern has got' (p. 49), contributed to understaffing. Visiting times were too short, evening meals served too early, wards 'too large and overcrowded' and local authorities provided insufficient accommodation and support for those well enough to leave hospital (pp. 47–48). Social work provision was inadequate, and the 'Committee are amazed by the antiquated arrangement whereby only one external telephone exists for the whole of the female side of the hospital' (p. 50).

Blofeld raised many of the same concerns two years earlier, but the RHB took no action to remedy them. Lowe's committee criticised the RHB and HMC for ignoring her report and the reports into nursing shortages. It condemned the RHB, which 'at times discounted if not disregarded' the HMC's requests to help them make changes (MoH 1968 p. 51). In contrast with Robinson blaming *Sans Everything* for lowering morale,[20] the committee attributed poor morale to ineffective management and defeatist attitudes of the RHB and HMC. The committee was 'far from convinced that Friern has had its fair share of even the limited amount of money available to the Regional Board' (p. 51). The report made twenty-three recommendations, mainly directed towards the HMC and RHB, and linked largely to their inspection rather than to the investigation of the complaints. Recommendations included acting on the reports about nurse staffing; negotiating with the local authorities for more social care; providing more occupational therapy; improving wards, patients' clothing and toilets; and noting that the RHB 'should allocate more funds to Friern' (pp. 52–53). The committee, however, wondered whether the relationship between the RHB and HMC 'was such as to enable them to work together to achieve a solution'.[21]

The report directly criticised Hackett who 'presumably reflecting on the collective view of the Board...was remarkably complacent'.[22] It also criticised his response to Blofeld's report, especially the

> so-called resignations of the Chief Male Nurse and of the Matron.... neither was given any reason for what was in effect dismissal—Mr Hackett had said

that he caused them to resign, together with Dr Sutton—because he regarded them as responsible for the inefficiencies disclosed in the Report.

The committee received no criticisms about these senior people (although that could have been an artefact of hospital protocol about criticising one's superiors) but it left the committee with 'an uneasy feeling that their treatment was arbitrary and possibly unjust'.[23] The committee summed up Hackett's approach, which 'betrays, we think, the superficial instead of searching approach to the shortcomings then revealed'.

The RHB discussed these criticisms. It resolved to

> unanimously record their continued and complete confidence in their Chairman [Hackett] who, by his untiring personal efforts during his three years of office, has done more than anyone to raise the standard of psychiatric hospitals in the region; ... the Minister of Health to be informed accordingly.[24]

The RHB removed the offending passages from the report after Lowe's committee signed it, but before publication. Dame Muriel Powell, the nursing member of the inquiry committee, was furious.[25] Despite the censoring, numerous indictments of the RHB and HMC remained in the published version (MoH 1968, pp. 47–51). The hospital hardly received a clean bill of health. We can only guess at what Barbara would have thought had she known the full extent of the committee's criticisms, especially of Hackett.

St Lawrence's Hospital, Bodmin

The St Lawrence's Inquiry took seventeen days, in three separate weeks, between September and November 1967.[26] George Polson QC chaired it (MoH 1968, p. 58), and it was the only inquiry to have a 'true' lay member from outside the NHS, a former secretary of a manufacturing company. In contrast to the Friern Inquiry, it took place in the hospital to which the allegations related,[27] which could raise rumours about staff who entered the committee room. The local MP, Peter Bessell, created additional publicity,[28] further undermining the myth of a 'confidential' inquiry. He also, reasonably, remarked on the social damage such an inquiry could inflict on a stable rural community.[29]

As at Friern and in Leeds,[30] other investigations were tagged-on. At St Lawrence's, the first week of the inquiry included the case of Sister W, suspended in July 1967, accused of hitting patients and swearing at them.[31] Sister W worked with older people and was implicated by Joyce Daniel in *Sans Everything*. Daniel planned to attend this part of the inquiry, in line with the Ministry's (1966) guidance that a complainant, and those who were the subject of a complaint, should have the 'opportunity' to be present throughout the hearing and of cross-examining witnesses. However, on the morning the inquiry was due to begin, she received a letter from Polson advising her that she should be accompanied by a lawyer.[32] This took time to arrange. Polson did not tell the committee *why* Daniel was absent, merely that she 'will not be able to assist the tribunal'.[33]

Much during the first week related to Daniel's allegations, and the committee handed copies of her account to hospital staff and questioned them about it. For example, the committee asked Nurse X whether he had heard patients say 'Don't hit me, will you, nurse. Don't drag me' (Daniel 1967, p. 38). He conceded that he had, but attributed it to the patient being 'rather confused and misunderstanding' and that it was 'in the context where there has been no suggestion of any ill treatment at all' (MoH 1968, pp. 63–64).[34] Polson probed neither how Nurse X ascertained the context nor how he assessed the confusion. Polson also used leading questions implying a negative response, such as, 'You have never seen anything like that at all, have you?'[35] His style of questioning raises issues about biases during the investigation and their effect on the outcome.

The committee reviewed the hospital's internal investigations about Sister W's suspension, which, creditably, included senior staff asking patients about her behaviours, an uncommon practice at the time (Cohen 1964, pp. 9, 39–40). One patient saw Sister W: 'hit Sarah J in the face and left finger marks'. Another said: 'the sister uses bad language.... To the patients'.[36] The inquiry transcript illustrates Nurse Y's discomfort at witnessing Sister W's practices and being asked about them:

Polson: What has sister referred to patients as from time to time?
Nurse Y: 'Bitch' sometimes.
Polson: Do not have any inhibitions.
Nurse Y: Or 'bloody bitch', not often; I remember that because it was one particular occasion... I cannot really remember what gave rise to it...
Polson: And that was to the patient?

Nurse Y: That was to the patient.
Polson: Apart from language used have you seen any other kind of bullying behaviour...something you would recoil from and say 'This ought not be done'?
Nurse Y: Yes, I suppose...in the long run from my point of view, rightly or wrongly, it is as well to let certain things that I do not like pass.

Nurse Z said she witnessed Sister W slap a patient punitively 'across the face', telling the patient that she 'had had enough of this silly nonsense', and the patient was then 'dragged to the toilet in tears'. Nurse Z challenged Sister W about this incident, and Sister W allegedly responded: 'you don't understand you have got to be hard with them.'[37] Sister W brushed off Nurse Z's criticism, supporting the notion that seniors disregarded statements from staff of lower ranks. Another ward sister commented: 'I believe it is fairly well known amongst staff that Sister W is rather noisy and gesticulating, and she frightens patients, and that I would call irregular treatment.'[38]

The committee of inquiry exonerated and reinstated Sister W. It justified its decision:

> Due to pressure of work and shortage of nursing staff Sister W had to work under circumstances which in our view would have tested the patience of a saint. She has certain temperamental weaknesses in that she tends to shout at and bustle people along in order to get things done. She tends to lose her patience under stress and strain, and she has got into the habit of swearing at patients...we do not think she would ever deliberately ill-treat [any patient].[39]

Descriptions of her behaviour—bustling and shouting—were imprecise. Stating that they did not 'think' her actions were deliberate, was, similar to the inquiry at Friern, arbitrary and subjective. Their conclusion implied that undignified and disrespectful behaviour towards patients was acceptable if it occurred under pressure due to daily routines or was unintentional.

During the week, the committee examined other aspects of St Lawrence's, including having locked unstaffed wards at night, a hazard also identified at Friern (MoH 1968, p. 48). The committee at St Lawrence's chillingly highlighted disrespect for patients' lives when it asked the nursing superintendent what would happen in an emergency on a locked, unstaffed ward: 'Assistance has been summoned in the case of one upstairs ward and a night nurse down in the ward below with a patient banging on the floor. Apart from that we are dependent upon a patient in the ward being able to use the telephone.'[40]

In October, at the beginning of the second week, Mr S, the lawyer representing staff who were members of the Confederation of Health Service Employees union said: 'quite frankly I anticipate that some of the allegations in the book may very well not be quite so impressive after cross examination.'[41] Against that proposition, the committee and the lawyers defending the hospital and its staff, laid into Daniel, starting with the validity of her affidavit. Barbara had changed some of the authors' personal details, with their agreement, such as dates of hospital employment, to help conceal their identities (Robb 1967, front matter). Polson interpreted the discrepancies between the information in *Sans Everything* and the hospital staff records as indicating that Daniel's entire report was a pack of lies: 'And, to put it more forcibly, it is a lie, is it not, sworn on the bible?' The entire contents of *Sans Everything* were similarly tainted, he said, since Barbara encouraged the authors to sign and knew the details were untrue. It was unfortunate that the affidavits were signed at the restaurant with the extraordinary name 'La Gaffe', the mistake,[42] and that the committee was unaware of Barbara's rationale for anonymity. It was even more unfortunate that Polson used the affidavit to distract from the main issues.

Mr S discredited Daniel for discrepancies between her report and the hospital records, such about the number of patients on the ward. Daniel (1967, p. 39) wrote seventies, the hospital records stated sixties, and Mr S commented: 'Well, it is a little artistic licence. She is a poet, after all.'[43] Daniel's meaning, that the ward was severely overcrowded, was lost. Another lawyer, Mr T, representing the HMC, described Daniel as 'sentimental and sloppy and perhaps soft, this has had an influence on her which it would not have had and has not had on other people'.[44] At the end of the first day Daniel wrote to Barbara: 'I cannot convey the air of hostility.'[45]

Daniel, like Barbara, *did* misunderstand some things. So did the committee and the lawyers, which could lead to poorly framed questions and incorrect conclusions. However, the medical member of the committee gave little clinical guidance. For example, he offered no clarification when the committee disbelieved Daniel's allegation (1967, p. 41) that a patient became animated and spoke after months of being mute. The committee did not know that beginning to speak could be a response to kindly social interaction (Roland 1948; Barton 1959).[46] When a qualified nurse described the patient as 'incapable' of responding as Daniel described (MoH 1968, p. 73), the committee rejected Daniel's observation: the opinion of the hospital's senior staff, rather than independent clinical knowledge, guided the committee's decisions.

Another example of the committee's inaccurate knowledge concerned distress and depression. Daniel (1967, p. 40) wrote: 'Many patients moaned and wrung their hands.... The general air of cringing and weeping was beyond bearing.' Polson asked a ward sister: 'No doubt with a lot of old ladies of this character you do get them wringing their hands?' She replied that she would have been concerned if one patient had stopped doing so.[47] A lawyer explained that 'acute depression' was normal for older people in long-stay hospitals.[48] However, it was out-of-date to accept depression as understandable or normal and not to treat it (Roth 1955; Post 1962). Psychiatrists at another hospital in 1967 illustrated this. They reflected on their embarrassment, and the tragedy, of underdiagnosing depression:

> We felt very humiliated... when a woman who had been there for 30 years suddenly started to talk.... It was found that a mistake had been made six weeks' previously when she had been given tofranil [an antidepressant] instead of her usual largactil [a sedative]! Surely there is a moral in that?[49]

The moral was that adequate assessment and treatment of depression, regardless of duration of admission, age or other factors, could improve well-being.

Daniel (1967, p. 38) described an undignified process for bathing, with up to eight naked patients in the bathroom at once. This allegation was inconsistently supported and dismissed by staff during the inquiry.[50] Hair washing, done in the bath, was traumatic for some patients. Daniel (p. 38) alleged that bowls of water were 'thrown over nervous patients' heads.' Sister W told the committee that water was 'poured' over their heads in the course of hair washing as there were no alternatives, like showers or large basins into which patients could lean backwards. When asked 'Was it done with any malice?' Sister W answered 'No.' We do not know whether Daniel exaggerated ('thrown') or Sister W minimised ('poured'),[51] or if the truth lay somewhere in between. Nevertheless, staff attributed patients' fears and flinching to them not understanding why certain things were done to them,[52] rather than to inadequate explanation from staff, or slapdash or uncaring nursing practices that were not modified to accommodate patients' needs.

The committee also rejected Daniel's complaint about lack of 'scented soap' for bathing patients. That seemed minor, until explored in the context of Sister W's comment that staff washed patients with the same Lifebuoy soap as they used to scrub the floors.[53] Allowing that to happen, objectified rather than humanised the patients. Daniel also alleged that patients drank from the lavatory pans, but senior staff took the view: 'there are always in every psychiatric hospital patients who drink from toilet pans.'[54] Opinions from senior staff, that demeaning and disrespectful practices and attitudes were acceptable, normal or justifiable, ignored their detrimental effects on patients, visitors and staff and reinforced the continuation of the practices. The committee's obsequiousness to the hierarchical system of hospital management, and ignorance of current good practice, precluded candid scrutiny.

The committee did not attribute harsh nursing to malice and therefore did not consider it to be cruel. The contrast between their sympathetic reinstatement of Sister W and their hostility towards Daniel was startling. In his summing up, one lawyer said: 'The question arises as to whether we should dismiss this book as a tissue of lies or whether it is founded on some basis of fact. Of course we must admit that there is some foundation of fact upon which the whole thing is based.' To support his argument, he gave examples of 'dirty and smelly floorboards and chamber pots and slippers in odd places', patients dragged and an outbreak of scabies. 'We have the evidence, we cannot deny it' he said. Nevertheless, he concluded, 'The actual care of the staff for these geriatric cases is quite out of this world.'[55]

After the inquiry the Ministry criticised 'the extraordinary way' in which the committee interpreted its terms of reference,[56] alluding to the duration of the inquiry, its 120-page report and the time spent on minute points and technicalities such as Daniel's affidavit. Polson criticised the South Western RHB, but the Ministry rejected his criticisms for two reasons. First, the Board did not appear before the committee[57] (although the Ministry did not apply the same criteria to AEGIS's witnesses who were absent from the Friern Inquiry and during the first week at St Lawrence's). Second, perhaps more justified, the subject fell outside the committee's terms of reference[58] in the context of the Lord Chancellor's advice advising to 'keep this kind of inquiry narrow' (Crossman 1977, p. 426).

Polson wanted the entire report published, but he did not fight when the Ministry refused.[59] He declined to summarise it for publication, so the Ministry delegated that task to the RHB.[60] The published version noted that the RHB allocated insufficient revenue to St Lawrence's (MoH 1968, pp. 80–81), but otherwise, unsurprisingly, it did not criticise itself.

The published report made eleven bland general recommendations, such as the hospital needing more staff with better communication between them, better supervision by senior nurses at weekends and improved food (MoH 1968, pp. 78–80). Five of the nine paragraphs in the 'summary of findings' praised staff for high standards of work, the other four attacked Daniel personally. That alone justified Barbara's concern about anonymity for her witnesses. The report accused Daniel of misinterpreting, misunderstanding and distorting her observations, that her judgements were 'manifestly unsound' and her 'sentimental approach' conflicted with the 'objective attitudes' of other staff. It described Daniel as 'rather a solitary person with a somewhat simple mind' (p. 78). Daniel's correspondence with Barbara and the reports from her sons do not bear this out, instead suggesting that she was a colourful and socially integrated character.[61] The report concluded, demonstrating acceptance of low standards for older people, that 'we have no hesitation to say that in our unanimous opinion there is no substance whatever in the allegations of cruelty by staff' (p. 78) and that the hospital standards 'might well be emulated by the rest of the country' (p. 81).

Daniel wrote to Barbara. Staff who she thought would support her let her down, and her 'old terrible nightmares' returned since she had seen again the 'ministering angels', her former colleagues.[62] Daniel received threatening phone calls.[63] Her sons and her friends feared for her physical safety and suggested that she moved out of the area until the anger died down. She decided to remain because she had things to do at home, and 'I feel going away would look as if I am afraid.'[64] Afterwards, Daniel spoke little about the events to her sons, although Charles recollected in 2015 that 'I think in herself she was angry that the enquiry was a "whitewash".'[65] Daniel was concerned that Barbara might have 'lost faith' in her because of her mistakes,[66] but that worry was allayed, and Daniel continued to support AEGIS.[67] Daniel wrote, at the end of 1967, 'God bless you Barbara for all the wonderful work you are doing.'[68] In 1971, Daniel sent Barbara a newspaper cutting: 'St. Lawrence's to get another £750,000: plans include new geriatric unit'.[69] The plans included up-grading the building which contained four of the five wards where Daniel had worked (Anon. 1971).

Storthes Hall and Springfield

Davie's allegations in *Sans Everything* concerned two hospitals, Storthes Hall and Springfield (Davie 1967, pp. 43–47). At Storthes Hall, as at St Lawrence's, the inquiry took place in the hospital, and evidence was presented in front of the staff being criticised.[70] Confidentiality was impossible due to Storthes Hall's 'jungle telegraph'.[71]

Davie faced a barrage of 799 questions on the first day. The committee questioned, and lawyers cross-questioned, his motivation for contributing to *Sans Everything*, suggesting that he wanted to be the centre of attention, which he emphatically denied.[72] Potentially incriminating documents went missing, and the chairman could not 'understand why a book, the size of a London telephone directory, could be missing as easily as that'.[73] Lack of written evidence[74] meant that one person was pitched against another, hardly ideal for the proper conduct of an inquiry.

The committee took every opportunity to nitpick minutiae of language in Davie's *Sans Everything* report. This detracted from the main argument and aimed to show his ignorance to discredit his evidence. They quibbled, for example, over his use of the word *bestiality* (Davie 1967, p. 43). Mr U, a lawyer, cross-questioned Davie about the idea that bestiality meant only sexual intercourse between a person and an animal:

Mr U: Did you use it without knowing what it actually meant?
Davie: I have used it in the sense in which I am quite sure [it] can be used.
Mr U: Is this your sense of responsibility, to use this term about the psychiatric hospitals for the public to read; to destroy public confidence in the treatment in hospitals... by using this term?
Davie: I considered it a perfectly fair word to use. It means other things apart from what you describe.[75]

Davie used the broader, and primary, meaning: 'The nature or qualities of a beast; want of intelligence, irrationality, stupidity, brutality' (*Oxford English Dictionary*, *OED*) but the lawyer did not accept that usage. In response to Davie's (1967, p. 44) comment that staff had little appreciation of psychological principles (which one nurse demonstrated when discussing 'punishment' and 'treatment'[76]), another lawyer quizzed him on his understanding of the term *psychological*, which he answered competently.[77] A punitive, repressive approach to patients' socially unacceptable behaviour was common in psychiatric hospitals where custodial attitudes dominated (Martin 1962, p. 14). It could maintain discipline and help staff control patients, but it was not therapeutic.

Davie challenged the value of HMC or RHB inspections and highlighted barriers faced by patients who wanted to make complaints: 'anyone who has worked here knows that as soon as the visiting committee gets to the front gate, somebody is on the 'phone, and all wards know, and everything is very quickly put in order. And what they see is not a true picture.' Cross-examining, Mr V asked about patients raising concerns during inspections: 'Those witnesses who are capable of giving a logical account of themselves, are they spirited away, then?' Davie replied: 'No; they are there, and very often they feel that they would like to say something—maybe indeed they have. They would like to say something, but with one eye on the charge nurse, who will exact reprisals.'[78] The committee interviewed, Mr G, a patient deemed to have capacity to answer the questions put to him. Mr G was alleged to have been assaulted. He kept 'one eye on the charge nurse':

> we questioned [Mr G] in a side room in the presence of a few immediately-interested persons. Mr G described an assault by a Charge Nurse (one blow on the back of the head) of a wholly different character from the assault described by Mr Davie (very many blows with open hand on the *face*—*not* the head): he could not or would not name the Charge Nurse: he did not identify... his assailant although he saw him present in the room. There is no casualty report with the Case Notes of Mr G, nor is there any relevant entry in his case notes.[79]

Disinclination of a patient to directly criticise a staff member who would potentially be his nurse again, illustrates the obstacles a patient could face in getting his voice fairly heard. Lack of corroborative clinical notes and discrepancies between the verbal reports were interpreted as evidence that there was no assault. This fitted with Davie's observations that when families and friends complained based on what the patient told them, staff responded: 'Well, the patient is insane in any case, and he is not to be relied upon.... We are really not brutes here, you know.'[80] Attributing patients' complaints to their illnesses[81] was similar to the response Mrs Dickens received about her brother at Friern.[82] Abel-Smith noted:

> Anything [patients] say to visitors or others may be too readily dismissed as a consequence of their confusion.... We have also to allow for relatives who

are frightened of being told to take the patient home and look after him or her themselves,... they may be silenced by the threat of the return of the patient.[83]

Davie also wrote in *Sans Everything* (p. 46) that cruelties 'took place not at Belsen, but in the north of England.' Asked about this at the inquiry, he explained his rationale for the analogy: 'The hospital was a "hell-hole": it was like Belsen because Belsen means a place which is brutal, bestial and beastly, and those epithets applied to the hospital.'[84] That fitted with the definition in the *OED*: '"Belsen" may be used hyperbolically to describe any very unpleasant place.' The committee would accept only the historical definition of the Nazi concentration camp. Their unrelenting questioning made Davie back down,[85] allowing them to conclude that he exaggerated. The committee also described him as 'consumed by malice towards the hospital, and towards nearly all who worked in it'. Such statements justified their approach of not seriously evaluating his evidence, while giving the impression that their inquiry process was valid. The committee wrote: 'if somewhere in his evidence there lurked some grains of truth, such grains are so deeply buried, and so obscured by distortion, falsehood and exaggeration that they are either quite undiscoverable, or unrecognisable as the truth.'[86]

The final report on Storthes Hall stated: 'we were quite unable to give any credence to his evidence; and, accordingly found none of his allegations... to have been proved' (MoH 1968, p. 56). This contrasted with the response of a separate committee at Springfield Hospital which also evaluated Davie's evidence. It

> formed the impression... that while his evidence was confused, exaggerated and emotional, there was some basic sincerity about the man. He certainly did not invent his stories out of whole cloth. We conclude that he certainly witnessed one assault upon a patient.[87]

Davie wrote one account in *Sans Everything* about his experiences in the two hospitals. Allegations were similar at both and staff at both denied malpractice. It is unlikely that Davie changed in personality, trustworthiness or motivation between working at the hospitals, writing about them and attending the inquiries. The committees and lawyers were the major difference between the two inquiries, and their conclusions diverged, about him and his evidence.[88] The Springfield Report surprised the

Ministry. It was the only one to accept that a *Sans Everything* witness was genuine in his concerns, and the only one to uphold 'findings of ill-treatment'.[89] The best explanation is that the committees' assumptions about Davie and the hospital staff affected the evaluation of evidence and therefore also their conclusions. Notably, and in contrast to the other inquiries, at Springfield, there is also ample evidence that the medical member of the committee advised the chairman and lawyers about hospital and clinical matters.[90]

THE OTHER WITNESSES

Davie,[91] Daniel,[92] and Susan Skrine and Eileen Porter at Cowley Road Hospital,[93] all refused Barbara's offer to pay their lawyers' fees: the witnesses considered it part of their contribution to the AEGIS campaign. Similar to Davie and Daniel, other public-spirited witnesses had distressing experiences: Jean Biss described her experience of the St James's Inquiry as 'like being crucified'.[94] Dorothy Hurley, whose report to the *News of the World* was investigated tagged-on at Leeds, received a phone call 'telling me to be careful if I went into town as some of the staff were gunning for me'.[95] Moodie's former supporters at Banstead deserted him when faced with a formal inquiry. They were 'hostile towards me, and for me to attend the enquiry without witnesses, would enable them to prove quite easily, that black was in fact white.... When I do go into battle, I prefer at least a small chance of winning.' Most of those staff lived in tied accommodation, which Moodie, and others (Martin 1962, p. 9) linked to their reluctance to criticise openly.[96] Despite the unpleasant experiences at the inquiries, the witnesses continued to support Barbara and her work. Mabel Franks wrote to Barbara: 'Mrs Biss informed me that those nurses who are your disciples in this fight against wanton neglect and cruelty will never never let you down.'[97]

THE MINISTRY PREPARES THE WHITE PAPER

The Ministry decided to publish all the inquiry reports about *Sans Everything* as a single white paper. This would 'soften the impact of the bad report and discourage accusations of "white-washing" in the good reports'.[98] The brief, negative one-and-a-half-page report about Springfield was tucked away at the back of the book. The reports included forty-eight recommendations for general improvements, including staffing levels, nurse education, communication within the hospitals, reducing overcrowding and working with local authorities to increase support and accommodation for older people in the community. Robinson ignored the Springfield Report, the criticisms of the Friern committee about the hospital and RHB, and the forty-eight recommendations. In a letter to Crossman he asserted that 'generally speaking the hospitals come out of the enquiries well'.[99] Robinson also told Crossman that the white paper 'would be completely uncontroversial because it would simply demolish Mrs Robb'.[100] He underestimated her.

The Ministry published abridged reports, partly because that was usual practice.[101] Shorter reports were more likely to be read, although they also carried the risk of inviting criticism by their exclusions.[102] It was therefore important that the committees, rather than the Ministry, made the summaries so the Ministry could not be accused of deliberately editing out controversial material. That did not stop the Ministry delegating the editing to at least one RHB, and condoning another changing a committee's report, to minimise criticism of the Boards in the published version.

The Ministry produced guidance notes to assist its staff when dealing with press inquiries after publication.[103] Aiming to reassure the public, the guidance stated: 'The depth of investigation made into matters alleged to have occurred years ago was only possible because of the quality of the records kept of the treatment and progress of patients.' With examples of poor-quality documentation at Friern and missing records at Storthes Hall, it was hard to justify that statement. The notes also informed the Ministry's staff that none of the solutions in the second part of *Sans Everything* was original, which begged the question that if they were known, why had none been implemented? It described Whitehead's 'medical solution' in *Sans Everything* as 'widely practiced', which was inaccurate when only a handful of such schemes existed nationally (Hilton 2016). The Ministry's advice to its staff was unconvincing, verging on dishonest.

Between Inquiries and White Paper: Barbara's Activities and the Council on Tribunals

During the brief hiatus after the inquiries and before publication of the white paper, Barbara chaired symposia,[104] lectured and wrote. At a five-day geriatric medicine conference for doctors, *Sans Everything*, mental illness and 'care of the dying' were allocated the 'graveyard slot'—after lunch on the final day.[105] However, Barbara incorporated her audiences' views into a letter to the *Times*: that the allegations in *Sans Everything* were 'an indictment of every one of us who knew these things were happening and did nothing about it' (Robb 1968), a broad collective responsibility, resembling Roxan's view about journalists (Cochrane 1990. p. 75) and Cross's[106] and Rowe's views about nurses (Anon. 1967).

Barbara informed the Council on Tribunals of her concerns about the conduct of the inquiries. The Council criticised: Robinson's decision not to establish them under section 70; the lack of common procedures for conducting them; and lack of uniform criteria for making judgements, such as about ill-treatment or standards for personal care that could be ethically complex to determine (Council on Tribunals 1969, pp. 13–14).[107] Supporting the view about ethics, Townsend stated that it could be difficult to draw the dividing line between deprivation and cruelty,[108] and the Springfield committee recognised that 'it is often extremely difficult to distinguish between cruelty and necessary constraint'.[109]

The Council wrote to Robinson about his choice of procedure for *Sans Everything*, and informed him that section 70 should be used as widely as possible. Robinson replied to the Council in a patronising way, irritating them by giving 'elementary information which he might have assumed we would already know'.[110] He ignored the Council's criticism that he had not observed NHS guidance on handling complaints. He explained that he could only instigate a section 70 inquiry in 'exceptional circumstances', but he did not clarify the principles which would underpin that decision. Greater rigour and uniformity and Council oversight, would have enabled more equitable and balanced treatment of witnesses and allegations that could have affected the conclusions.

The Council particularly criticised Lowe for his conduct of the Friern Inquiry, including lack of compliance with NHS complaints guidance and ignoring the Royal Commission's recommendations about witnesses having legal representation, on which point the Ministry concurred with the Council.[111] The Council also criticised the report on Friern: because the committee 'heard no evidence from the witnesses whom AEGIS proposed to call, the tone of it struck us as being intemperate'.[112] The unrestrained language in Lowe's report was ironic considering that his committee deplored Barbara's 'flamboyant and exaggerated style' and stated that the Diary (Robb 1967) would have been 'more impressive if stated factually without adjectival adornment' (MoH 1968, p. 27).

The Council wrote directly to Barbara, supporting her criticisms and giving her permission to publish its letters. It thanked her for her input and stated that it would use her material when considering NHS plans for establishing an ombudsman and for creating procedures for inquiries that would come under their supervision. Barbara was delighted with this outcome.[113] AEGIS's press statement led to articles in national papers about Robinson mishandling the *Sans Everything* complaints (Anon. 1969a, 1969b; Prince 1969). The *New Law Journal* (Anon. 1969c) congratulated the Council for their stance, which made 'trenchant criticism' of Robinson. Personal letters congratulating Barbara included one from the editor of *New Scientist*: 'you have dented the bureaucratic shell'.[114]

COMMENT

Numerous difficulties underpinned the inquiries and hindered dispassionate evaluation, influencing the committees' deliberations and conclusions. The effect of the RHBs appointing the committees was probably less problematic than the nonuniform inquiry procedures each adopted and the RHBs altering the committees' reports to remove criticisms about themselves. The terms of reference centred on investigating the specific allegations in *Sans Everything* and examining the situation on the relevant wards. In the event, attempts to identify and prove specific incidents such as hitting, teasing or harsh handling proved virtually pointless, as Cross and Abel-Smith warned.[115] The truth did not emerge about anecdotal events: unkindnesses were unlikely to be documented in hospital records, some potentially relevant documents were 'lost' and staff, fearful of retribution, were not questioned under oath. James Loring, director of the Spastics Society[116] said: 'It is difficult to prove anecdotes of the sort contained in Mrs Robb's book—they concern ephemeral events. But we know of many similar cases. We couldn't prove them legally but we still know them to be true' (Anon. 1968).

The committees held stereotypic views of the excellence of the NHS and its staff, and less favourable views about older people for whom they accepted particularly low standards of care. The chairmen lacked experience of inquiries into public sector administration, and their unfamiliarity with internal NHS politics and protocols, at local, regional and national levels,[117] affected inquiry outcomes. For example, the committees ignored, or did not comprehend, the effects of the rigid, hierarchical nursing regimes that resisted change and inhibited honest, and potentially constructive, criticism (Dickinson 2015, pp. 145,171). The committees' questioning indicated their paternalistic attitudes towards the patients, their relatives, vocational students, and staff without formal qualifications. By contrast, gender discrimination was less overt, unexpected at a time when it was commonplace in the public arena and when the women's movement was in its infancy (McCarthy 2010, p. 105). This could be accounted for by each committee having at least one female member, usually a nurse at the top of their career, reducing gender bias but reinforcing acceptance of the soundness of the nursing hierarchy.

Lacking understanding of modern, proactive clinical practice in psychiatry and geriatric medicine, committees erroneously set standards according to the opinions of the senior staff they investigated rather than using independently derived criteria. If senior staff advocated a harsh, undignified or out-of-date approach, committees naïvely accepted it, despite similar behaviours being considered inhumane or disrespectful in more progressive hospitals. Too often, the committees qualified their judgements according to what they *thought* rather than what they *knew*. The committees employed recognised tactics and logical fallacies to protect their assumptions. These included criticising the complainants personally rather than evaluating their evidence impartially; describing controversial allegations as exaggerations that could be dismissed automatically; and using leading questions and ambiguous, vague language.

Historical analysis of the *Sans Everything* inquiries is in keeping with Crossman's opinion that the committees were 'fairly well rigged',[118] and the view of Max Beloff, Professor of Government and Public Administration at Oxford. Beloff (1967) wrote: 'the danger with our close-knit political-administrative network is that most inquiries are so manned that they turn out to be nothing but the system looking at itself, and finding more to admire than to blame'. These opinions corroborated the view of AEGIS's lawyer at the Leeds Inquiry who stated that an ordinary member of the public might 'think that the Committee was sitting merely as a stooge of the Minister to whitewash the accusations which have been made'.[119] Concerning giving evidence, Mr Cumming, Davie's lawyer, wrote to Barbara:

> I feel most strongly that the truth never did have a chance of emerging from people who were having to speak in front of a QC, a Physician, Matron, Chairman of a Bench of Magistrates, a Medical Superintendent, the Chief Male Nurse and the so-called accused Male Nurses, backed up by their Trade Union officials straining at the leash.[120]

Imagery of 'straining at the leash' conveyed the inquiry's hostile atmosphere. The array of senior staff, legal professionals and local dignitaries, intimidated staff and patients who wanted to speak up, and precluded honesty, much as the style of official hospital inspections inhibited patients and ward staff from complaining. The structures and expectations of the committees of inquiry humiliated the AEGIS author-witnesses and gave them little chance of validating the *Sans Everything* case. These witnesses showed extraordinary dedication to AEGIS's cause and remarkable ability to remain dignified under pressure.

Notes

1. Discussion with Daphne Loebl, barrister, 2015.
2. St Lawrence's transcript, about 1,000 pages, MH159/225–9; Storthes Hall transcript, about 600 pages, MH159/231 (the National Archive, TNA).
3. Lowe, Douglas. 1968. 'Report of an independent committee of enquiry into allegations concerning Friern hospital in a book entitled *Sans Everything* upon geriatric wards in that hospital and upon certain other specific complaints', NWMRHB, (Lowe Report) 32. Minutes and papers, May 1968–November 1969, BM/283/68 (London Metropolitan Archive, LMA). 'Lowe Report' refers to the full, unpublished report. The shorter published report is referenced MoH 1968.
4. Memo, Hales to Hedley, 4 April 1967, MH150/349 (TNA).
5. Invitation, HMC to Ronald and Audrey Harvey, 18 November 1967, AEGIS/A/4 (AEGIS archive, London School of Economics).
6. Letter, Robb to Lowe, 16 October 1967, AEGIS/A/4.
7. Lowe Report, 2.
8. Letter, Lowe to Robb, 17 October 1967, AEGIS/A/1/A.
9. 'Note, Robinson, 3 October 1967, MH159/220 (TNA).
10. Robb, 'Chapter 2', 41, AEGIS/A/1/A.
11. Letter, Lowe to Robb, 17 October 1967, AEGIS/A/1/A.
12. Meeting, Robb and Tooth, final report, 25 May 1965, AEGIS/1/1.
13. Storthes Hall HMC minutes with index, 1965–1966, Management of hospital pilfering, 14 October 1965, C416/1/188 (West Yorkshire Archive Service).
14. Malcolm Campbell, interview by author, 2015.
15. Lowe Report, 64.
16. Lowe Report, 65.
17. Lowe Report, 62.
18. Letter, Dickens to Robb, 5 March 1968, AEGIS/4/1/A.
19. Lowe Report, 67.

20. BBC2, *Man Alive*, 16 July 1968, transcript,18, AEGIS/2/7/A.
21. Lowe Report, 32 (removed from MoH 1968, p. 51).
22. Lowe Report, 29 (removed from MoH 1968, p. 49).
23. Lowe Report, 32 (entire paragraph absent in MoH 1968).
24. Attached to page 36 inside Lowe Report.
25. AEGIS meeting, Charing Cross Hotel, 7 May 1970, AEGIS/2/6/A.
26. St Lawrence's transcript, MH159/225–9 (TNA).
27. Letter, Daniel to Robb, 6 December 1967, AEGIS/2/10.
28. Anon. 'Hospital Union men attack MP: Bessell's behaviour 'unfortunate', *Western Morning News*, 17 October 1967.
29. Letter, Peter Bessell to Robinson, 2 October 1967, MH160/651 (TNA).
30. Letter, Mr Cobb to Dorothy Hurley, re: her *News of the World* complaint, 18 September 1967, AEGIS/A/2.
31. St Lawrence's HMC, minutes, HC1/1/1/38, 31 July 1967 (8), (Cornwall Record Office); 'Interim report of the committee of inquiry into allegations made in the book *Sans Everything*', to the South Western (SW) RHB, October 1967, MH159/225; interviews by Mr Ely and Dr Donovan, July 1967, MH160/651 (TNA).
32. Letter, Polson to Daniel, 22 September 1967, AEGIS/2/10.
33. St Lawrence's transcript, 26 September 1967, 2, MH159/226 (TNA).
34. St Lawrence's transcript, 25 September 1967, 79, MH159/226 (TNA).
35. St Lawrence's transcript, 26 September 1967, 65–66, MH159/226 (TNA).
36. Interviews by Mr Ely and Dr Donovan, July 1967, MH160/651 (TNA).
37. Interview, Mrs Z by Mr Smith, Mr Ely, Mr James, 7 July 1967, MH160/651 (TNA).
38. Interview, Mr Mullis, July 1967, MH160/651 (TNA).
39. SWRHB. 1968. 'Report of the committee of inquiry into allegations made in the book *Sans Everything* concerning St Lawrence's Hospital Bodmin', 9, MH159/227 (TNA).
40. St Lawrence's transcript, 15 September 1967, 44, MH159/226 (TNA).
41. St Lawrence's transcript, 30 October 1967, 54, MH159/228 (TNA).
42. St Lawrence's transcript, 1 November 1967, 20–22, MH159/228 (TNA). The name arose from the reasoning that for a Cypriot and an Italian to open a French restaurant in north-west London could only be a 'Gaffe'. http://www.lagaffe.co.uk, accessed 12 February 2016.
43. St Lawrence's transcript, 19 November 1967, 8–9, MH159/229 (TNA).
44. St Lawrence's transcript, 22 November 1967, 7, 92, MH159/229 (TNA).
45. Letter, Daniel to Robb, 'Wednesday', AEGIS/2/10.
46. David Enoch, interview by author, 2015.
47. St Lawrence's transcript, 19 November 1967, 9, MH159/229 (TNA).
48. St Lawrence's transcript, 22 November 1967, 14, MH159/229 (TNA).

49. JC Barker, Mabel Miller, 'The problem of the chronic psychiatric patients', Shelton Hospital, post graduate education programme, 14 December 1967, 31, AEGIS/2/3.
50. St Lawrence's transcript, 25 September 1967, 66, 74, MH159/226 (TNA).
51. St Lawrence's transcript, 19 November 1967, 23–24, MH159/229 (TNA).
52. St Lawrence's transcript, 31 October 1967, 12, MH159/227 (TNA).
53. St Lawrence's transcript, 19 November 1967, 20, MH159/229 (TNA).
54. St Lawrence's transcript, 25 September 1967, 83, MH159/226 (TNA).
55. St Lawrence's transcript, 22 November 1967, 87–88, MH159/229 (TNA).
56. Memo, Hedley to Mottershead, 5 March 1968, MH159/225 (TNA).
57. 'Note for the file', Mr Hewitt, 12 March 1968, MH159/225 (TNA).
58. Memo, Hewitt to Miss Hauff, 11 March 1968, MH159/225 (TNA).
59. Memo, Hales to Hewitt, 15 February 1968, MH159/225 (TNA).
60. Memo, Hewitt to Croft, 26 March 1968, MH159/225 (TNA).
61. Letter, Daniel to Robb, c.1972, Aegis/2/7/C. See Chapter 4, p. 116.
62. Letter, Daniel to Robb, 10 November 1967, AEGIS/2/10.
63. Letter, Robb to solicitor, 1 July 1968, AEGIS/2/7/A.
64. Letter, Daniel to Robb, 6 December 1967, AEGIS/2/10.
65. Charles Daniel, email to author, 2015.
66. Letter, Daniel to Robb, 6 December 1967, AEGIS/2/10.
67. e.g. BBC2, *Man Alive*, 16 July 1968, AEGIS/2/7/A.
68. Letter, Daniel to Robb, 6 December 1967, AEGIS/2/10.
69. About £11 million in 2016.
70. Letter, Davie to Robb, 18 January 1968, AEGIS/2/10.
71. Storthes Hall transcript, 8 December 1967, 29, MH159/231 (TNA).
72. Storthes Hall transcript, 6 December 1967, 30, 41, 76, MH159/231 (TNA).
73. Storthes Hall transcript, 7 December 1967, 1, MH159/231(TNA).
74. Storthes Hall Report part 1B, 19, MH159/230 (TNA).
75. Storthes Hall transcript, 7 December 1967, 34, MH159/231 (TNA).
76. Storthes Hall transcript, 18 December 1967, 12, MH159/231 (TNA).
77. Storthes Hall transcript, 7 December 1967, 25, MH 159/231 (TNA).
78. Storthes Hall transcript, 6 December 1967, 44, MH159/231 (TNA).
79. Storthes Hall Report, part 1, B, 17, MH159/230 (TNA).
80. Storthes Hall transcript, 6 December 1967, 45, MH159/231 (TNA).
81. Storthes Hall transcript, 3 January 1968, 6, 61, MH159/231 (TNA).
82. Letter, BS Lord to Dickens, 24 September 1964, AEGIS/4/1/A.
83. Memo, Abel-Smith to Mottershead, 6 August 1969, MH159/236 (TNA).
84. Storthes Hall Report, part 1, B, 16, MH159/230 (TNA).
85. Storthes Hall transcript, 7 December 1967, 34, MH159/231 (TNA).
86. Storthes Hall Report, part 1, 20, MH159/230 (TNA).

87. Springfield Report, part 1, 2, MH159/233 (TNA).
88. Storthes Hall transcript, 6 December 1967, 30, MH159/231; Memo, Hedley to Matthews, 2 April 1968, MH159/233 (TNA).
89. Memo, Hedley to Matthews, 22 April 1968, MH159/233 (TNA).
90. Springfield Inquiry, Professor WH Trethowan, appendix A, MH159/233 (TNA).
91. Storthes Hall transcript, 6 December 1967, 4, MH159/231 (TNA).
92. Letter, Daniel to Robb, 'Tuesday', AEGIS/2/10.
93. Letter, Skrine to Robb, 25 May 1968, AEGIS/6/15.
94. Letter, Daniel to Robb, 6 December 1967, AEGIS/2/10.
95. Letter, Hurley to Robb, undated, AEGIS/A/2.
96. Letter, Moodie to Robb, 6 January 1968, AEGIS/2/10.
97. Letter, Franks to Robb, 3 November 1967, AEGIS/2/10.
98. Memo, Croft to Hauff, 16 May 1968, MH 159/216 (TNA).
99. Letter, Robinson to Crossman, 12 June 1968, MH159/216 (TNA).
100. Crossman Diaries, 16 July 1968, 151/68/SW (University of Warwick Modern Records Centre, UWMRC).
101. MoH, 'Some notes in dealing with press inquiries', c. June 1968, MH159/216 (TNA).
102. Letter, Gibbens to Hauff, 9 May 1968, and reply, 13 May 1968, MH159/234 (TNA).
103. MoH, 'Some notes in dealing with press inquiries', c. June 1968, MH159/216 (TNA).
104. Three day study symposium at Severalls, April 1968, AEGIS/1/10/A.
105. Programme, 'Course in Geriatrics', 18–22 March 1968, University of Cambridge, AEGIS/B/3.
106. Letter, Cross to Robinson, 9 June 1967, MH150/350 (TNA).
107. Letter, Baroness Burton to Crossman, 26 March 1969, MH159/217 (TNA).
108. Peter Townsend, speech at Annual Conference, NAMH, 20 February 1969, AEGIS/2/8.
109. Springfield Report, part 1, 3, MH159/233 (TNA).
110. Letter, Robinson to Burton, 30 July 1968; 'Comments by Mrs Bell on the Minister's reply of 30th July 1968', Annex B. BL2/862 (TNA).
111. Memo, Croft to Matthews, 24 May 1968, MH159/216 (TNA).
112. Letter, Burton to Crossman, 26 March 1969, MH159/217 (TNA).
113. Letters, Alistair Macdonald and Robb, 13 and 17 January 1969, AEGIS/2/9.
114. Letter, Donald Gould to Robb, 3 February 1969, 3, AEGIS/2/9.
115. BBC1, *24 Hours*, 30 June and 28 July 1967, transcript, AEGIS/1/6.
116. A charity, founded with the aim of improving and expanding services for people with cerebral palsy. Now called 'Scope'.

117. Memo, Hales to Hedley, 4 April 1967, MH150/349 (TNA).
118. Crossman Diaries, 12 November 1969, JH/69/39 (UWMRC).
119. Concluding speech, St James's, Leeds, 14 January 1968, AEGIS/2/7/C.
120. Letter, Mr Cumming to Robb, 13 August 1968, AEGIS/2/7/A.

Bibliography

Abel-Smith, Brian. 1967. 'Administrative solution: a hospital commissioner?' 128–135. In Robb 1967.
Anon. 1967. 'We know such things go on'. *Times*, 22 July.
Anon. 1968. 'Minister under fire on 'cruel hospitals' probe'. *Observer*, 14 July.
Anon. 1969a. 'Allegations against hospitals "mishandled"'. *Guardian*, 7 January.
Anon. 1969b. 'Short note'. *New Society*, 23 January.
Anon. 1969c. 'Sans everything'. *New Law Journal*, 17 July.
Anon. 1971. 'St. Lawrence's to get another £750,000: plans include new geriatric unit'. *Cornish Guardian*, 5 May.
Barton, Russell. 1959. *Institutional Neurosis*. Bristol: John Wright and Sons.
Beloff, Max. 1967. 'Defining the limits of official responsibility'. *Times*, 11 September.
Cochrane, David. 1990. 'The AEGIS campaign to improve standards of care in mental hospitals: A case study of the process of social policy change'. PhD thesis, University of London. http://etheses.lse.ac.uk, accessed 17 September 2016.
Cohen, Gerda. 1964. *What's Wrong with Hospitals?* Harmondsworth: Penguin Books.
Council on Tribunals. 1969. *Annual Report 1968*. London: HMSO.
Crossman, Richard. 1977. *The Diaries of a Cabinet Minister. Vol. 3. Secretary of State for Social Services 1968–1970*. London: Hamilton and Cape.
Daniel, Joyce. (Alice Craythorne). 1967. 'No-one smiles here' 37–43. In Robb 1967.
Davie, James. (Frederick Isham). 1967. 'Massive corruption and cruelty' 43–47. In Robb 1967.
DHSS. 1969. *Report of the Committee of Inquiry into Allegations of Ill-treatment of Patients and Other Irregularities at the Ely Hospital. Cardiff*. Cmnd. 3975. London: HMSO.
Dickinson, Tommy. 2015. *'Curing Queers': Mental Nurses and Their Patients, 1935–1974*. Manchester: Manchester University Press.
Goffman, Erving. 1961. *Asylums: Essays on the Social Situation of Mental Patients and Other Inmates*. New York: Anchor Books.
Hilton, Claire. 2014. 'Joint geriatric and old age psychiatric wards in the United Kingdom, 1940s—early 1990s: a historical study'. *International Journal of Geriatric Psychiatry*, 29, 1071–1078.
Hilton, Claire. 2016. 'Developing psychogeriatrics in England: a turning point in the 1960s?' *Contemporary British History*, 30, 40–72.

Mandelbrote, Bertram. 1964. 'Mental illness in hospital and community: development and outcome' 267–290. In *Problems and Progress in Medical Care*, ed. Gordon McLachan. London: Nuffield Provincial Hospitals Trust, OUP.

Martin, Denis. 1962. *Adventure in Psychiatry*. Oxford: Bruno Cassirer.

McCarthy, Helen. 2010. 'Gender inequality' 105–123. In *Unequal Britain*, ed. Pat Thane. London: Continuum.

Ministry of Health. 1966. *Methods of Dealing with Complaints of Patients*. HM (66)15. London: HMSO.

Ministry of Health. 1968. *Findings and Recommendations Following Enquiries into Allegations Concerning the Care of Elderly Patients in Certain Hospitals*. Cmnd. 3687. London: HMSO.

Moodie, Denis. (Michael Osbaldeston). 'Nobody wants to know' 13–18. In Robb 1967.

Oxford English Dictionary. http://www.oed.com, accessed 29 September 2016.

Post, Felix. 1962. *The Significance of Affective Symptoms in Old Age: A Follow Up Study of 100 Patients*. London: OUP.

Prince, John. 1969. 'Statutory inquiry call for patients' complaints'. *Daily Telegraph*, 17 January.

Robb, Barbara. 1967. *Sans Everything: A Case to Answer*. London: Nelson.

Robb, Barbara. 1968. 'Conditions in mental hospitals'. *Times*, 24 June.

Roland, Paul. 1948. 'An exploratory training technique for the re-education of catatonics'. *American Journal of Psychiatry*, 105, 353.

Roth, Martin. 1955. 'The natural history of mental disorders in old age'. *British Journal of Psychiatry*, 101, 281–230.

Royal Commission on Tribunals of Inquiry. 1966. Cmnd. 3121. London: HMSO.

Open Access This chapter is licensed under the terms of the Creative Commons Attribution 4.0 International License (http://creativecommons.org/licenses/by/4.0/), which permits use, sharing, adaptation, distribution and reproduction in any medium or format, as long as you give appropriate credit to the original author(s) and the source, provide a link to the Creative Commons license and indicate if changes were made.

The images or other third party material in this chapter are included in the book's Creative Commons license, unless indicated otherwise in a credit line to the material. If material is not included in the book's Creative Commons license and your intended use is not permitted by statutory regulation or exceeds the permitted use, you will need to obtain permission directly from the copyright holder.

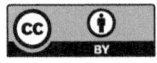

CHAPTER 7

Whitewash and After: 'Most Good Is Done by Stealth'

Early in 1968, disturbing reports about psychiatric hospitals supplemented information presented by AEGIS (Aid for the Elderly in Government Institutions). The media gave generous coverage to: a fire at Shelton Hospital which killed twenty-four patients (Anon. 1968a); appalling overcrowding at Central Hospital, Warwick;[1] a geriatric ward at Powick Hospital, Worcestershire (*World in Action* 1968); and poor care of mentally handicapped children at Harperbury Hospital, Hertfordshire (Shearer 1968). Most reports also highlighted doctors and nurses trying to make improvements. In July 1968, Robinson announced *Findings and Recommendations,* the white paper summarising the outcomes of the *Sans Everything* inquiries (Ministry of Health (MoH) 1968a). Other allegations and investigations about ill-treatment shed light on the *Sans Everything* events and inquiry processes. They help explain why the Ely Inquiry (DHSS 1969), rather than *Sans Everything*, became regarded as pivotal to the reform of the long-stay hospitals (Martin and Walshe 2003, p. 6) although AEGIS paved the way for that to happen.[2]

In October 1968, government reorganisation abolished the Ministry of Health, amalgamating it with the Ministry of Pensions and National Insurance to become the Department of Health and Social Security (DHSS). Robinson stepped down as Minister, and Harold Wilson appointed Richard Crossman as Secretary of State for Social

Services. Crossman appointed Abel-Smith as his chief advisor on health and welfare. Under Crossman, the DHSS acknowledged the importance of improving the psychiatric hospitals. New concepts helped, such as the 'dignity of risk' rather than the 'security of protection', and 'normalisation' which promoted the idea that disabled people should be supported to live as normal a life as possible in the community (Nirje 1969). Following the devaluation of the pound in 1967, the authorities were subject to austerity measures. Economic pressures affected health and welfare services for everybody, but the least-valued members of society— older, mentally ill and mentally handicapped people and others with chronic disorders—were particularly affected. Good intentions for them competed against other demands, such as highly valued acute and high technology medicine and surgery, on a worrying background of increasing real costs of the NHS (OECD 2011).

Improving psychiatric hospitals was tricky, particularly in the context of the long-term goal to close them and to shift services to the community and district general hospitals (DGHs). Plans to close hospitals created new challenges. Work in poorly maintained buildings designated for closure could be grim. Staff whose jobs were threatened had to consider finding alternative employment, which could affect their family life and their home, especially if they lived in tied accommodation.[3] Ensuring improvements in patient care in these circumstances needed support for staff and collaboration between management and clinical leaders to ensure a positive culture change within the hospitals (Carse et al. 1958). Intensive media involvement could produce improvements in the short-term (Shearer 1976, p. 113), but new ways might not be maintained. Severalls Hospital, for example, 'reverted to a situation of poor leadership' when Russell Barton, frustrated by conflict and personality clashes at the hospital and with the Regional Hospital Board (RHB), emigrated to the United States (Gittins 1998, pp. 87–89, 92).

Behind the scenes AEGIS continued to supply information to Abel-Smith,[4] chipped away at the shield defending officialdom and worked to improve hospital provision, assisted by the press. Plans initiated under the Labour government (until 1970), were followed up by the Conservatives (1970–1974). These included establishing a NHS inspectorate, reviewing the complaints system (DHSS 1973), appointing an ombudsman, and creating blueprints for improved services for people with mental handicap and mental illness (DHSS 1971a, 1971b, 1972). Numerous factors influenced health and social care developments, emphasising the risk of ascribing too much, or too little, to any one event, person or organisation, including to AEGIS.

More Psychiatric Hospitals in the News

The stream of press and public interest in the psychiatric hospitals in 1968 contrasted with the situation three years earlier when media reports were rare. Happenings at four hospitals—Shelton, Central, Powick and Harperbury—informed the public of appalling conditions and revealed positive and negative attitudes of the hospital leadership and those higher in the NHS hierarchy. Behind the scenes, Barbara pushed, supported and inspired staff at the hospitals, and the media reporting on them.

On the night of 26 February 1968, a fire on a forty-two-bed ward at Shelton Hospital killed twenty-four women patients (Anon. 1968a). Robinson announced a public statutory inquiry under section 70 of the NHS Act (MoH 1968b).[5] It was the first section 70 inquiry in the history of the NHS that directly concerned patients.[6] Unlike the *Sans Everything* inquiries, it had Council on Tribunals oversight.[7] Various factors contributed to the fire, including hospital bureaucracy, which delayed emergency help because the 'night porter [had] to obtain the authority of one of the hospital fire officers before calling the Fire Service' (Osman 1968).[8] The destroyed ward was locked and minimally staffed,[9] less hazardous than the locked unstaffed wards at Friern[10] and St Lawrence's.[11] Dr JC Barker, a psychiatrist at Shelton, attended the inquiry on several occasions. He told Barbara that staff tried to cover up inadequacies and that 'conflicting evidence is quite horrifying and I am sure is giving this hospital a very bad name'.[12]

Despite the problems, some staff at Shelton, such as David Enoch, did their utmost to make improvements. Among other things, he established an education programme, about which he reflected in 2015:

> I started education days—in Shelton—education for doctors and nurses—in the nurses [home]....There was a big hall for them to have entertainments....I took Thursdays over...and had cases presented, a visiting lecturer, and a debate.
> In the end, of the three other psychiatrists, two of them [asked]:
> 'Could we present a case?'
> 'Of course!' I said, 'I'd love it for you to present a case! Look at the experience you have got.'
> Well, they didn't want to know anything before.[13]

During one of their education days staff highlighted challenges of making improvements:

> Dr Cartwright: wards are overcrowded, the patients are inadequately dressed and there is the very minimum of facilities.... This, in itself tends to make these patients chronic. They are all grouped together and shut up together and there appear to be very few comforts or amenities for them.
> Dr Barker: I quite agree with you.
> Dr Thomas: Try asking for them![14]

In Enoch's opinion, Barbara's high-profile work and *Sans Everything* contributed to initiating this sort of discussion: 'I can't over emphasise its power', difficulties in psychiatric hospitals became 'something that people discussed more'.[15]

A second hospital in 1968 attracted national attention, Central Hospital, Warwick. Similar to Friern, Ely, Storthes Hall and Whittingham, Central had ongoing difficulties that showed no evidence of diminishing with time. Barbara first wrote to medical superintendent Edward Stern in 1966, congratulating him on his 'truly valiant attempt' to improve his hospital.[16] He involved local MPs who made a 'very distressing' three-hour tour of the hospital (Anon. 1966b, 1966c) and asked Robinson to investigate. Robinson agreed that conditions were unacceptable (Anon. 1966d), but little changed. Six months later the press reported deaths of two elderly patients. One drowned in a bath and the other was pushed over, attributed to overcrowding, meal-time chaos and frayed tempers. MPs described the situation as 'desperate'. Stern offered 'to join any delegation' to see Robinson, but Robinson did not reply to his letters (Leamington Spa Reporter, 1967; Robb 1967, pp. 10–11).

In March 1968, days after the Shelton fire, William Price MP told the House of Commons that Central was: 'the most overcrowded mental hospital in Britain. Only by the grace of God have we escaped a major disaster through fire or epidemic'. He described:

> Seventy three men living in a ward made for 38. We saw patients carrying their toothbrushes and other personal belongings in their pockets because there was no room for lockers between their beds. We saw long-term mentally disturbed patients living in adapted corridors and in recreation rooms. We saw a ward where nurses had to move five beds before they could change the clothes on the sixth, and we saw a lot more besides. I am

not by nature squeamish, but the memory of that day will haunt me for the rest of my life.[17]

Shortly after, a patient's family accused two nurses at Central of 'brutality'. A four-hour inquiry reported that the patient 'put up violent resistance' so the staff needed to restrain him, and that although 'no excess force was used', the patient sustained injuries to his face and neck. Particularly vulnerable areas of the body, such as face and neck, should not have been injured in the course of restraint, but no archives have been identified indicating that the committee challenged staff about this. The staff were exonerated. Whether, similar to the *Sans Everything* inquiries, the committee made assumptions that staff actions were justified and patients were in the wrong, is unclear. The family, however, was dissatisfied with the outcome (Anon. 1968i).

A third hospital, Powick in Worcestershire, featured in a *World in Action* television documentary, *Ward F13*. *World in Action* took the then unusual approach of interviewing people directly responsible for social issues and believed that television could change the way people viewed the world (Goddard 2007). With the opening shots of the hospital, the presenter solemnly declared:

> Conditions like these exist in many, but not all, mental hospitals. Most comparable institutions would prefer to stay hidden. Powick didn't evade our enquiries, and the decision was surprising, for the hospital is ashamed of the annexe.

Ward F13 in the Victorian annexe housed seventy-eight women aged fifty-nine to ninety-one, in overcrowded, noisy and undignified conditions. The documentary showed women having their bottoms washed, being dressed or sitting on commodes in the open ward with no privacy. There was visible rough handling, such as when putting a patient onto a bed and locking an uncooperative patient in a chair with a restraining table fixed in front. The nurses appeared hardworking, overstretched and dedicated, doing their best in atrocious circumstances and with no time to spend with patients other than when dealing with their physical needs.

The medical superintendent, Arthur Spencer, took up his post in 1951, succeeding Dr Fenton who retired after forty-three years. Fenton's custodial and ultra-economical approach gave Powick the reputation of being the cheapest asylum in the country. In contrast to Fenton, Spencer developed a therapeutic regime in the admissions section of the hospital, but facilities changed little for elderly people and for patients with chronic mental illness in the four wards of the annexe (Sandison 2001, pp. 31–33). Spencer courageously let the cameras into his hospital. He addressed the circumstances, and the likely responses to them, candidly:

> There are two possible reactions... one is that people will become incensed at some members of the community having to live in these conditions. The other is that people will be so appalled by what they see that they will shut it out of their minds and reject the whole problem as insoluble and something they cannot face up to.

The first reaction was that of AEGIS. The second reflected common patterns of response by NHS leaders, politicians and the committees of inquiry into *Sans Everything*. Spencer's obituary in the *BMJ* (WDS 1979) described his pioneering and modernising approach at Powick, but did not mention *Ward F13*, even though it led to major benefits when the government's Worcester Development Project put Powick at the forefront of developing community psychiatric services nationally (Turner and Roberts 1992). It is conceivable that not mentioning *Ward F13* in Spencer's obituary was because he caused embarrassment and resentment, for colleagues and for the authorities, by saying what needed to be said.

The day after the documentary, Barbara's informal note to 'Vanya', probably Vanya Kewley its researcher, said that some people had a sleepless night after watching it, and it 'was a triumph for everyone concerned with its production'.[18] The style of the note pointed to Barbara's behind-the-scenes contact with the production team. A few days later, the press linked Barbara, the documentary and advice from the Council on Tribunals to proposals for a hospital ombudsman (Roper 1968a; Doyle 1968).

A fourth hospital, Harperbury, under the same RHB as Friern, provided care for children and adults who were 'mentally subnormal'. It was the subject of an article in the *Guardian* by Ann Shearer (1968), a journalist who admired Barbara, Abel-Smith and Barton and for whom AEGIS was 'at the back if not always at the front of my mind'.[19] The *Guardian* took its usual editorial and legal precautions before publishing Shearer's controversial article, which revealed atrocious standards.

The article came about after the *Guardian* received a letter from the aunt of a child living at Harperbury, and Shearer was asked to investigate. The aunt invited Shearer to accompany her to visit her nephew, where she witnessed squalor, including piles of faeces, some on a table. After publication, the staff invited Shearer back: 'they had cleaned the ward, put clothes on those children, and put flowers on the table, and it was the flowers on the table which was the last bloody straw. I was so angry that they would take me for such a fool.'[20] Flowers to admire was an inappropriate, incongruous gesture in a children's ward where toys would have been more fitting.

The RHB was furious about the article and accused Shearer of 'unauthorised entry', which was incorrect, as a patient's relative had invited her. Senior staff at Harperbury rejected Shearer's criticisms, saying that she lacked formal training or experience of working with mentally subnormal people. NHS managers described her as irresponsible, denied the allegations and blamed her for worsening staff morale and recruitment, undermining public confidence, and laying the last straw on the breaking backs of staff (Shearer 1976, p. 110). These defensive responses, eerily similar to those experienced by Barbara and the *Sans Everything* witnesses, give the impression of being automatic rather than stemming from methodical consideration.

Rather than appealing to the Ministry to help put things right, the RHB complained to the Press Council, which investigated and interrogated Shearer. At the inquiry, as she recalled in 2015, Lord Devlin asked her how many piles of excrement she had seen. She found the question so bizarre and irrelevant to the main issue that she angrily replied 'Shit is shit, my lord.'[21] The Press Council upheld the RHB's complaint and criticised the *Guardian* for lack of objectivity and accuracy. Considering the subject important, later in the year the *Guardian* extraordinarily republished the offending article alongside the Press Council's judgement. It did this because the judgement did not specify where the article lacked objectivity or accuracy and it wanted to give readers the opportunity to form their own opinion (Shearer 1976, pp. 109–110). Hackett (1968) was irate about the reprint. He wrote to the *Guardian*: 'I doubt there is another country in the world where the finest nursing service in the world has this kind of ridiculous unnecessary attack made on them by newspapers as the result of a bitter fight for circulation.' Psychiatrist Leopold Field (1968) responded with a letter that NHS managers, when criticised, 'develop an acute attack of paranoia and defend themselves in the most hysterical of terms'. Field rejected Hackett's statement about the 'finest nursing services' as 'impetuous nonsense'. He challenged Hackett's views that hospitals should be immune from press scrutiny and criticised Hackett's 'outrageous statements diametrically opposed to the facts'.

Another television documentary, *Something for Nothing* (BBC 1968), marked the twentieth anniversary of the NHS. It reflected on achievements of the 'technology revolution' and new hospital buildings, but it called the NHS the 'sacred cow of the politicians', and said, 'The NHS today doesn't work.' It criticised the 'British tradition of amateurism' embodied in inefficient Hospital Management Committees (HMCs), and the 'inept, slow, tardy administration' of higher NHS echelons. It discussed the 'burden' of older people and, menacingly sincere, to solve the problem of the number of older people requiring treatment and care, it proposed the option of voluntary euthanasia for those who had 'signed the forms' and were 'of no practical value to society or themselves'. Robinson was livid about the programme, and Crossman was 'disgusted'. Crossman described it as a

> monstrous programme, full of mistakes and also annoyingly... all about euthanasia, where it put people off by its libertarianism, [and] at the end it put people off by guying a hospital committee... it was wrong in every possible way. And we are having an enquiry made.[22]

The government reprimanded the BBC, the consequences of which became apparent after publication of the white paper on *Sans Everything*.

Announcing *Findings and Recommendations*, the White Paper on *Sans Everything*

Robinson wanted to ease the way of the publication of the white paper, *Findings and Recommendations* (MoH 1968a), so he arranged a 'planted' question in the Commons.[23] On 9 July 1968, Labour MP Roy Roebuck asked about progress being made on the inquiries, and when the Minister expected to announce the results. The reply was instant. Robinson announced that the inquiries proved that most of the allegations in *Sans Everything* were 'totally unfounded or grossly exaggerated' and that the committees reported 'very favourably on the standard of care provided'.[24] Robinson concluded his announcement: 'the publication of the White Paper should discourage anyone from making... ill-founded and irresponsible allegations in future.' Roebuck criticised *Sans Everything* for causing distress and wasting public money with 'wild and irresponsible allegations'. MPs responded with relief to Robinson's reassurance, and continued to attack *Sans Everything*. Only Paul Dean, a Conservative MP, probed. He questioned that, if only 'most' were unfounded, then some were founded, and minimum standards needed to be achieved: he asked for an inspectorate. A press release concurred with Robinson's announcement.[25] The Confederation of Health Service Employees (COHSE), which defended its members at the inquiries, rapidly congratulated itself that its 'quiet unwavering year-long stand is vindicated'.[26] Several national newspapers published reports based on the press release, announcing that the white paper vindicated the Ministry (e.g., Jackson 1968; Rawstorne 1968; Wilkinson 1968).

The full text of the white paper became available later in the day. The press made a rapid U-turn after reading it. The *Times* shifted from saying that the hospitals were 'cleared of cruelty' (Roper 1968b) to denouncing the white paper as a 'whitewash' and stating that 'Nurses, distressed by reports of the White Paper, had been ringing AEGIS urging her to continue' (Anon. 1968b). The *Sunday Times* criticised Robinson's complacency, wondered if he had read the white paper and referred to his 'deplorably hostile view' of *Sans Everything* and rejection of criticism from outside the NHS (Young 1968). Rolph wrote about journalists' embarrassment when they realised the inconsistency between the press release and the full white paper: they 'could see how they had been misled. I don't remember hearing pressmen so angry' (Rolph 1968).

In the *Observer*, the National Association for Mental Health (NAMH) and Spastics Society criticised Robinson for his handling of the inquiries (Staff reporter 1968). Helen Hodgson (1968) in the *Guardian* condemned the inquiry methods and regarded Robinson as 'deluded' if he thought the allegations were 'authoritatively discredited'. The Patients Association (PA), backed by the NAMH and the National Council for Civil Liberties[27] wrote directly to Harold Wilson, asking him to establish an independent inquiry into conditions for older people in psychiatric hospitals (Anon. 1968h).[28] Wilson redirected their appeal to the Ministry,[29] which was ineffective, unsurprising considering that ministerial apathy about older people's care was the rationale for their request.

The medical profession did not know which way to step. One report commended the inquiry committees: 'unsentimental, impartial and intelligent men and women authorised to investigate the total situation at each hospital and guided by Queen's Counsel' (Anon. 1968f). The same report noted that 'throughout the country the psychiatric services in general and particularly the psychogeriatric services, are in an appalling mess'. The *Lancet* described Robinson as well intentioned but said that the inquiries should have been under the Council on Tribunals to ensure they were done 'in way that the man on the Clapham omnibus would regard as impartial' (Anon. 1968g). A *BMJ* editorial highlighted the 'deplorable hospital facilities with which valiant staffs are trying up and down the country to provide satisfactory care and treatment of their patients' and that 'the sordid conditions in which many are condemned to live out their days in hospital are a disgrace to the nation' (Anon. 1968j). One letter in the *BMJ* told doctors not to be complacent: they were part of the cause (Mathers 1968). The British Medical Association (BMA) recognised that it 'would have to put continual pressure on the Government, on the local authorities, and on Regional Hospital Boards (RHBs) if the necessary urgent financial assistance was to be obtained' to tackle the problems (Greenberg 1968).

Crossman understood Barbara's fury about Robinson, 'that what he was doing was to smother perfectly legitimate criticism of what was going on'.[30] He criticised Robinson's announcement as

> obviously untrue. In fact the reports didn't by any means deny all the allegations and if he had had the common sense to say they deny all the most important, the gravest and most serious allegations, well there are of course a number of criticisms about geriatric hospitals. If he had emphasised the criticisms and welcomed them and said that of course they were not fully met and he was going to meet them, that was right. But he didn't. He gave a sense of complacency and complete defending which he does as a bit of a bureaucratic minister.[31]

An editorial in *New Society*, attributed to Townsend (Cochrane 1990, p. 117), also described Robinson's statements in the Commons as 'untrue', and criticised him for disbanding a group of professors and doctors that he set up in 1966 to plan hospital geriatric services (Anon. 1968e). Applebey of NAMH reportedly said that she 'nearly dropped' when she heard Robinson's announcement (Anon. 1968c; Rolph 1968). Rolph (1968) declared that he almost did likewise and criticised the committees of inquiry, especially at Friern, which, by failing to interview the *Sans Everything* witnesses, drew conclusions based on 'blind and inaccurate guesses about the information of which it stupidly deprived itself'. The *Daily Mail* summarised the government's response: 'Whitehall washes whitest' (Anon. 1968d).

Barbara did not shrug off the humiliation and discrediting but became more cautious, sometimes wrongly interpreting criticisms as malicious, to the extent of risking losing allies and supporters.[32] Brian and the AEGIS friends supported Barbara emotionally as much as they could during very stressful periods of the campaign.[33] Harvey wrote to Rolph about his 'characteristically splendid article' in the *New Statesman*: 'How glad I am that you have given Barbara some of the enormous credit she deserves. I wish it could be known how you have helped with the kind of expert advice that I was unable to give, and the non-stop backing.... Much love, Audrey.'[34] Davie wrote to Barbara:

> I have just finished reading the latest fiction entitled *Findings and Recommendations*....Overriding my own feelings of disquiet and anger is my sympathy for you over the treatment accorded you in this nauseous little blue book. But one must admit that, in its way, this book is a masterpiece—of the art of distortion by omission and the application of overwhelming bias. In short, fiction of a nasty kind featuring 'Goodies' and 'Baddies' with the Hospitals cast in the former role... and our goodselves in the latter.[35]

Barbara worked with Desmond Wilcox, editor of BBC2's *Man Alive* current affairs series, to create a programme about *Sans Everything* to coincide with publication of the white paper.[36] Barbara's cast included Barton, Cross, Daniel and the Cowley Road witnesses. Part of the programme was filmed in advance, including scenes of patients and staff at Severalls. Barbara contacted her solicitor before the screening, concerned that some of the recorded interviews did not follow the agreed plan. For example, the interview with Daniel went over old ground of the allegations and did not include new material—namely, the hostile atmosphere of the inquiry and that she received threatening phone calls.[37] The *Man Alive* team invited trade union representatives, members of RHBs and Robinson, although Barbara was not informed that Robinson was involved until the day. In part, that might have been because Wilcox had trouble persuading him to appear. Wilcox's telegram to Robinson on 12 July revealed the latter's ambivalence and the Ministry's pressure on RHB chairmen to conform. Wilcox wrote:

> I sincerely regret your decision not to appear in next Tuesdays Man Alive.... I think your confidence that the BBC will still be able to make a balanced programme is not being helped by your own Ministry advising

those chairmen of Regional Hospital Boards invited by us to appear that it is not in the Ministry's interests that they should do so.... May I now solicit your cooperation in allowing representatives of Regional Hospital Boards to appear in the discussion. It must be considered a matter of public concern if fair balance is prevented because of pressure of this sort.[38]

The live discussion was a shambles, including three interviewees introduced incorrectly and a crash interrupting the proceedings. Similar to *24 Hours* the previous year, the programme allocated Barbara and her supporters little time compared to her opposition, and Robinson had the last word:

> I think this White Paper speaks for itself, to anyone who reads it with an unprejudiced eye.... Basically, the crucial element in this book were the stories of deliberate, calculated cruelty. This is what made the book sell;... The credibility of the book, I think, has been destroyed. I wouldn't, Mr Wilcox, expect the authors of the book to apologise for the damage, the harm they have caused. This cannot have helped the recruitment of nurses. This cannot have helped the morale of the nursing profession.... But by and large, this task [of looking after elderly and mentally ill people] is discharged, in my view, extraordinarily well, by a dedicated body of nurses, who certainly do not deserve the generalised smear that this book conveyed on them.[39]

Neither 'a generalised smear' nor 'deliberate cruelty' formed part of Barbara's allegations (e.g., Robb 1967, pp. xiii–xvi; Rolph 1968). Despite the evidence, including within the white paper, there was no leeway in Robinson's argument that NHS practices were right and Barbara and AEGIS were wrong.

Crossman was delighted with the programme, which he watched with Abel-Smith, without realising that Abel-Smith contributed to *Sans Everything* and was a force behind AEGIS.[40] Barbara was enraged by the programme, particularly because Wilcox had assured her it would be impartial. She wrote to Wilcox outlining the distribution of air time in the discussion: Robinson had eight minutes, the 'opposition' to *Sans Everything* had seventeen, while she with her team had eight. She wrote that the programme 'was very far from typical of the impeccable behaviour I have learned to expect from the BBC.' Wilcox replied only that 'we made the best programme possible under the circumstances.'[41] 'The circumstances', Crossman explained, was due to the government reprimanding the BBC about *Something for Nothing*. Wilcox was 'under control from on top to give fair play to Kenneth Robinson and fair play to the Hospital system'.[42] The BBC showed its subservience to the government, at the expense of *Sans Everything*. The public did not know about the political furore behind the bias, but some complained to the BBC about the programme. One wrote that it lacked cohesion, 'none of the statements which were flung into the pool were taken up or followed through', Robinson was allowed 'to evade a straight answer to a plain question' and 'Mrs Robb was allowed practically no time to say anything'.[43] Another viewer wrote to Barbara that she was 'appalled by the lack of manners on Mr Robinson's part, and the small opportunity given to you to speak'.[44] Harvey was 'quite ill with anger at the *Man Alive* thing'.[45]

THE AFTERMATH

In the immediate aftermath of the white paper, the Ministry asked AEGIS not to complain further about the inquiry processes until it had put into action various vital reforms, including an inspectorate and an ombudsman. Barbara later reflected: 'it was with misgivings that we agreed to protest no more until the health ombudsman was appointed. Little did we guess that meant a five year wait.'[46] However, other changes emerged. Some, such as the Health Services and Public Health Act (1968), appeared politically tokenistic. Sections of this Act relevant to older people built on earlier legislation that permitted local authorities to provide domestic help and fund 'recreation or meals for old people'.[47] The new Act gave permissive powers to local authorities 'to make arrangements' for promoting their welfare. However, given that it coincided with publication of the Seebohm Report (DHSS 1968), which originated in concerns about probation and children's social services (Lowe 1999, p. 268) and prioritised local authorities' commitment to families, the sections of the Act about older people were unlikely to be implemented in the short-term.

Despite the authorities' lethargy, constructive responses emerged elsewhere, including from individual politicians and the medical profession. Eric Moonman MP asked Barbara to speak at Labour Party events, including in a lecture series that also featured the Archbishop of Canterbury. Moonman wrote to thank Barbara: 'You were splendid.'[48] Some psychiatric hospitals were more proactive in paying attention to the needs of older people. Goodmayes Hospital advertised for a consultant psychiatrist to work specifically with them, and Tom Arie commenced work there in

January 1969.[49] Enoch wrote to Barbara informing her about his geriatrician–psychiatrist planning group on psychogeriatric services.[50] It comprised enthusiastic pioneers in the field, including psychogeriatricians Brice Pitt and Klaus Bergmann. Their pamphlet linked to Whitehead's (1965) scheme at Severalls and emphasised the importance of 'care of the aged in the community, for clinical, economic, social and humanitarian reasons' (Enoch and Howells 1971, p. 17). It encouraged the British Geriatrics Society (BGS) and Royal College of Psychiatrists (RCPsych) to establish a joint working party on older people, which produced recommendations for clinical practice endorsed by both organisations, feeding into other developments at the RCPsych.[51]

Changes occurred in several domains of nursing practice and organisation. For example, the organiser of a King's Fund Hospital Centre project, which explored nurses' attitudes to patients and produced guidance for nurses who wanted to start discussion groups with colleagues about this,[52] informed Barbara that her work inspired it.[53] Also in 1968, demonstrations took place at Westminster about nurses' pay and conditions (Eade 1968). Demands included a living wage so nurses were not dependent on tied accommodation. That would give them greater professional independence as they would not fear losing their job and home if they spoke out. A photograph in the *Daily Telegraph* of protesting nurses on their way to the Commons suggested a link with recent events: one nurse held a copy of *Sans Everything* (Anon. 1968k). Peter Nolan (1998 p. 135) commented that when nurses realised that recourse to outside agencies could be more effective in redressing the wrongs of an institution than invoking the authority of senior nurses, 'the tradition of secrecy within the mental hospitals was broken'. The NAMH newsletter also noted that more doors were open in psychiatric hospitals, affecting patient care and indicating less concealment: 'If this trend continues, Mrs Robb's book will have had a considerable secondary effect—one of which is all to the good.'[54]

THE ELY HOSPITAL INQUIRY

Martin (1984 p. 5) wrote that after *Sans Everything* 'By a strange coincidence another inquiry was set up at the same time.' It was hardly coincidence: the Ely allegations emerged directly from Roxan's (1967) announcement about *Sans Everything* in the *News of the World*. In another analysis of NHS and social care scandals, Butler and Drakeford

(2005, p. 113) commented: 'Ely marked the start...of an avalanche of scandal in mental health.' However, several of these scandals surfaced after publication of *Sans Everything* and before Ely became public knowledge. The sequence of events, particularly concerning Ely, is worth exploring because it sheds light on AEGIS and on the *Sans Everything* inquiries, their flaws and outcomes.

Ely was in Wales, where the UK government was in an unfavourable spotlight following the Aberfan disaster (Report 1967). Geoffrey Howe (a Conservative politician, later Lord Howe) 'one of the cleverest Conservative lawyers',[55] represented the colliery managers' unions at the inquiry. Howe and Abel-Smith knew each other since their student days at Cambridge, and on Abel-Smith's recommendation, the Welsh Hospital Board (WHB) appointed Howe to chair the Ely Inquiry (Sheard 2014, pp. 47, 236–237). Howe, following his experiences at Aberfan and unlike the *Sans Everything* chairmen, was acutely and personally aware that public authorities could turn a blind eye to unsatisfactory and dangerous practices (Hillman and Clarke 1988, p. 86).

Allegations at Ely resembled those in the *Sans Everything* hospitals. The Ely Inquiry committee had the same terms of reference as its *Sans Everything* predecessors (MoH 1968a, p. 21; DHSS 1969, pp. 2–3), although under Howe's chairmanship, the planning and conduct of the inquiry differed from them. Howe challenged the Ministry's instructions if he disagreed with them. For example, when the Ministry advised him not to publicly announce a private inquiry,[56] he argued for the benefits of *privacy* during an inquiry, as opposed to *secrecy* about it.[57] Thus for Ely, the inquiry included an appeal for witnesses, compatible with Council on Tribunals guidance (Howe 1999, p. 303).[58] Howe also broke with the Lord Chancellor's advice to 'keep this kind of inquiry narrow' and intended to investigate up to Ministry level if necessary (Crossman 1977, p. 426).[59] Howe requested documentation about NHS services and complaints procedures,[60] unlike Lowe at Friern, who the Council on Tribunals criticised for being unaware of protocols.[61]

Michael Pantelides, the informant, made many allegations about Ely, including staff teasing, assaulting, hitting and inappropriately secluding patients, pilfering food, trying to fit the wrong dentures into a patient's mouth, and inflicting pain when clumsily cutting toenails (DHSS 1969, pp. 122–124). The Ely committee cautiously evaluated Pantelides' integrity: despite being unreliable and mistaken at times, 'he seldom, if ever, identified smoke in the absence of fire' (p. 9). His allegations thus deserved serious attention. The committee's analysis of Pantelides' integrity resembled the Springfield Inquiry's opinion of Davie.[62]

The Ely committee upheld many of the complaints. Nursing care was 'old fashioned, unduly rough and [of] undesirably low standards' (DHSS 1969, p. 24). Staff who complained were victimised. The HMC was ineffective as a management body. Overcrowding (Fig. 7.1), understaffing, and deficits at all levels of administration were largely responsible for failings (pp. 127–133). Recommendations from Howe's committee affected all aspects of hospital function. They included: employing more domestic staff so nurses could nurse; adequate time for nursing handovers between shifts; in-service training; creating better links with the surrounding community and with voluntary organisations; and publishing an information booklet for patients and their families (p. 115). The committee recommended instigating disciplinary proceedings against one charge

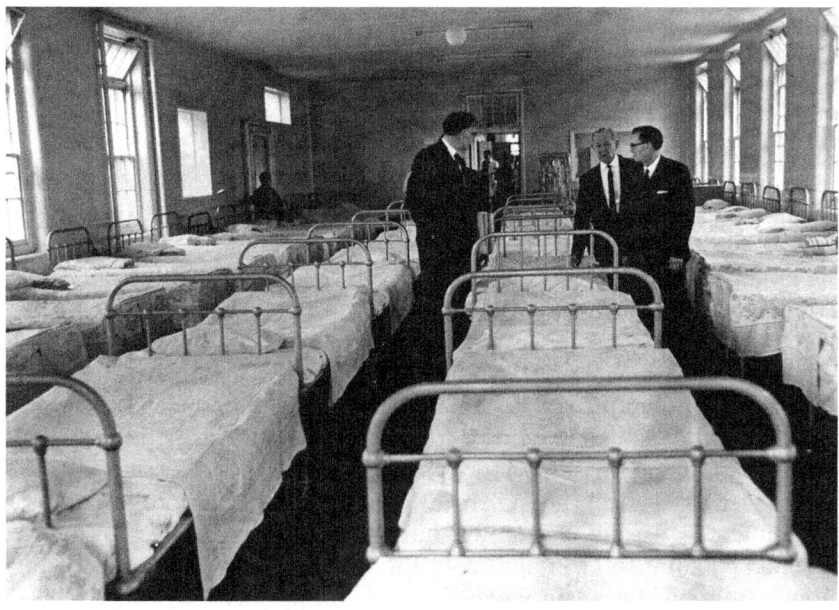

Fig. 7.1 Officials inspect a men's ward at Ely Hospital, 1969.
Source: South Wales Echo, April 1969. Reproduced with permission from Media Wales.

nurse who 'contrived complaints' against other staff (pp. 55, 132), supporting the impression that dishonesty and victimisation of staff occurred in psychiatric hospitals. The committee also criticised the WHB, which needed to make greater efforts to achieve improvements (p. 132). In addition to local recommendations, Howe proposed wider ranging remedies. Notably, a better system of investigating complaints, a body to consider 'complaints and disciplinary matters which had not been satisfactorily handled in some other way' and a system of independent inspection (p. 133) aligned closely with proposals in *Sans Everything* (Abel-Smith 1967, pp. 128–135).

Howe commented that it was a matter of speculation how long the situation at Ely would have persisted without Pantelides' report to the *News of the World* (DHSS 1969, p. 123). Howe's investigation lacked the logical fallacies of the *Sans Everything* inquiries, such as deference to seniority and discrediting witnesses because of their status and presumed personalities, rather than what they had to say. Malpractice was malpractice even if condoned by senior staff or due to overwork, understaffing or stress. Howe acknowledged the difficulties of the subject matter, especially categorising cruelty, as did the Springfield committee, and was 'conscious of obscurity about the burden of proof to be applied and constantly aware of the risk of coming to unjust conclusions' (p. 120). On several occasions the report described events as 'probable' (pp. 122–124), but steered towards 'probably true', whereas the *Sans Everything* committees in similar circumstances verged towards 'probably false'.

The DHSS was embarrassed by the content of Howe's report, especially when it came to light that the Ministry had filed deplorable reports about Ely three years earlier (Crossman 1977, p. 411).[63] The WHB described Howe's report as 'a devastating indictment not only of the hospital staff but of pretty well all concerned with it', and informed the DHSS that 'it is not suitable for publication', on grounds that it was too long—83,000 words—and repetitious, 'particularly in its treatment of the specific allegations'.[64] As with the *Sans Everything* inquiries, the DHSS requested an abridged version for publication. Howe undertook this, rather than delegate it to the WHB. By stylistic change, he reduced the length to 76,000 words, the 'eleven twelfths' ('11/12') version.[65] 'Under pressure' he also produced a 20,000-word summary, in which he referred to editorial interference, indicated that it did not do justice to the case (Hillman and Clarke 1988, p. 91) and noted that the DHSS and WHB sought to conceal damaging information.[66] The summary would whet the appetites of journalists and lead to demands for publication of the full version. Howe would not bow to embedded attitudes determined to avoid negative publicity: he did not just *ask* for the full report to be published, as Polson did for St Lawrence's,[67] but he *fought* for it.[68] Abel-Smith ensured that the full report and the 11/12 version got onto Crossman's desk (Howe 1994, p. 42). Crossman regarded the report as 'explosive' and feared that if he did not publish at least the 11/12 version, he would 'be at the mercy' of Howe who 'would be entitled to go on the tele and talk about the report which had been supressed'.[69] Crossman also knew that Barbara had regular contact with Abel-Smith so would probably know what was happening to the Ely Report, and he regarded her relationship with the press as a 'terrible danger' to the government (Crossman 1977, p. 727).[70] Crossman also had unpleasant recollections of his own family's care, which could have made him more sensitive to the issues. In particular, his mother died in a poorly run nursing home: 'Heavens its (*sic*) disgusting. I could almost smell the stale smell again, and think how odious it is, and it stirred all the feelings in me.'[71]

Critical of Robinson for his management of *Sans Everything*, Crossman, a shrewd politician, did not want to receive similar, potentially career-damaging, criticism by having his image maligned by the press (Cochrane 1990, p. 121). Crossman made his plan: 'The report completely vindicated the *News of the World* story and I might as well make the best of it by outright publication. But I could only publish and survive politically if in the course of my statement I announced necessary changes in policy.'[72] Before the announcement he briefed the RHBs, and the press, and promised an exclusive interview to the *News of the World*. He briefed Howe, who was delighted with the 11/12 publication plan. Howe modestly and honourably refused to join Crossman on television, because he wanted to remain as the independent chairman of the inquiry, rather than introduce party politics.[73]

Crossman announced the Ely Report in the Commons in March 1969, eight months after Robinson announced *Findings and Recommendations*. The announcement, content, response and consequences were startlingly different. Crossman wrote in his diary: 'I felt a great gulp in my throat when I started because I think I really do care about this, I do feel righteous and indignant about it, and I launched it out and read it and within 30 seconds I knew I had gripped the House.'[74] Crossman announced that most of the specific incidents of ill-treatment took place and victimisation of well-intentioned staff who made complaints was 'odious and alarming'. The report, he said, 'should be used at once as a basis for remedial action', creating an inspectorate, protecting staff from victimisation, and improving long-stay provision for mentally handicapped people. Remedial action could prevent the report shaking staff morale. Crossman sent copies of the report to RHB chairmen, announcing his intention that it 'shall be made a springboard for action rather than a setback for morale in the hospital service.'[75]

Unlike Robinson, Crossman did not blame individuals but expressed a sense of collective responsibility, as nursing leaders, doctors and journalists had done earlier, and hinted at a revision of spending:

> We all bear responsibility for leaving it there, and unless we think of these things without blaming others we shall not get them put right. Public opinion has to face it, that if we are spending vast sums, as we are, on making wonderful new hospitals for acute illness and acute surgery, we must bear in mind the hundreds and thousands of people in these other places.

The House supported Crossman's proposals. Tom Driberg MP asked if the new inspectorate would make an early visit to South Ockendon 'from which there have been some very disturbing reports'.[76] The press latched onto the plans for an inspectorate and the concerns about South Ockendon (Roper 1969; Anon. 1969b).

Baroness Beatrice Serota (Minister of State for Health and an acquaintance of Barbara's in Hampstead) read an identical statement in the Lords. Lord Amulree referred to the government's courage in publishing the report. Baroness Summerskill made the obvious deduction that if intimidation of staff who wish to raise alerts happened elsewhere, ill-treatment would be unknown to the authorities. Lord Segal, a medically qualified peer, commented on a sense of relief at the publication of the report: 'These conditions have been known to exist for quite a long time... and have given rise to an enormous amount of uneasiness.'[77] The Lords accepted the Ely Report, in contrast to their rejection of Strabolgi's allegations in 1965.[78] Strabolgi's revelations then were too shocking to believe: as Spencer said during the documentary about Powick, people can react by shutting appalling situations out of their minds and rejecting them (*World in Action* 1968). Since 1965, engineered by Barbara, the media had drip-fed the politicians, professionals and public about abuse in hospitals, sensitising their outlook and expectations. The Ely announcement was within the bounds of government and public credibility and provoked constructive responses.

Publication of the Ely Report was a team effort. Barbara was a threat to the Labour government. Howe was highly respected, determined and had a fierce sense of justice. His biographers, Judy Hillman and Peter Clarke (1988, p. 91), regarded achieving publication of the 11/12 version as Howe's 'toughest and most formative challenge' against the 'Whitehall mandarins'. Abel-Smith, dedicated to the cause, had a foot in the AEGIS camp, knew Howe and was respected at the DHSS. Crossman reframed the deficits of the hospitals as a problem for society that could be dealt with, rather than blaming the patients and informants and portraying the situation as inevitable and insurmountable. Anthony Howard (1979, p. 11), editor of Crossman's diaries, described his action to publish the 11/12 report, contrary to official advice, as 'perhaps the bravest political action' of his career.

Ely's centrality to the process of reforming the psychiatric hospitals was due largely to its allegations being upheld, in contrast to similar allegations in *Sans Everything* being overturned. Webster's view (1998, p. 80) that 'the Ely Hospital scandal...suddenly precipitated long-stay hospitals to the head of the policy agenda' is an oversimplification. AEGIS played vital roles in triggering the allegations, channelling Ely into the limelight and setting the policy agenda. Barbara breached the wall of NHS bureaucratic paternalism, secrecy and the myth of universal high standards of NHS care, Howe undermined the foundations, and Crossman took up the cudgel and began to demolish what remained. Barbara congratulated Crossman on his announcement and initiating remedies to improve the hospitals and complaints mechanisms. She recognised that Crossman sought to prevent his predecessor losing face at the same time as he called public attention to some particularly grisly aspects of the NHS. She wrote that the Ely Report 'marked the end of the ostrich era. Doubtless the old bird still lingers, its bad habits dyed in the feather; but its days are numbered' (Robb 1969). The Ely Report vindicated Barbara, but there was no official acknowledgement about the way *Sans Everything* was swept under the carpet. Barbara did not seek an apology and placed clearing her name as unimportant relative to succeeding with her campaign (Robb 1970). She shifted from working outside government circles to being an inside lobbying advisor to the DHSS (Cochrane 1990, p. 140).[79]

After Ely, Crossman took particular interest in the subnormality hospitals (Crossman 1977, pp. 607, 664, 726).[80] This partly detracted from AEGIS's original concerns. The imperative to prevent stripping and other indignities encountered by older people moved away from centre stage. However, Barbara's demands for an inspectorate, ombudsman and improved complaints procedures shifted into the formal policy arena when Crossman set up the Post-Ely Working Party (PEP). Crossman or Serota chaired the PEP. Members included Howe, Townsend, and senior doctors, nurses and local authority representatives.[81] Abel-Smith, AEGIS, the PA and NAMH fed into it.[82] It set the foundations for *Better Services for the Mentally Handicapped* (DHSS 1971a), a strategy to provide community services as an alternative to hospital accommodation.[83] Some critics, however, such as Townsend, regarded these proposals as little better than the Royal Commission (1957), and the local authorities, charged with much of the work, were unenthusiastic (Sheard 2014, p. 315). The PEP also used information gleaned from Barbara's correspondence with the Council on Tribunals[84] and discussed a broad range of challenges, including how to handle complaints from staff.[85]

Crossman demonstrated his intention to take the issues seriously by openly visiting long-stay hospitals, thus encouraging the press to report on them. He described Chelmsley Hospital, Birmingham, as 'Bleak, and oh their lavatory architecture, ghastly buildings, and ghastlily overcrowded; I have never seen overcrowding like it, beds absolutely jammed together.'[86] Coleshill Hospital nearby, was more modern but had seventy-two beds in a ward designed for thirty-six, with only three toilets (Squire 1969; Anon. 1969d). Birmingham RHB, a remaining 'ostrich', was horrified by the publicity caused by these visits and blamed Crossman's discoveries on press leaks.[87] To prevent recurrences, the RHB clamped down on its members who now had to seek permission to publicise matters that had not been finalised by the Board. The RHB chairman rationalised his decision as a way to control *when*, rather than *if*, information was passed to the public (Adeney 1969), but his actions gave the impression that the RHB preferred to keep problems secret. Crossman negotiated with and cajoled hospital authorities in Birmingham. He reflected in his diary:

> My crusade, and I'm going to win this now, there is no doubt about it, in the Birmingham area they couldn't go on, they are going to concede, they are going to do some building...we didn't come to conclusions, but I pressed on rations, I pressed on personal possessions, I pressed on dealing with overcrowding.[88]

Publicity probably assisted Crossman to pledge more funding to long-stay hospitals, backed by public opinion. In 1970, he reallocated £4 million to them,[89] hardly enough, but it was a start (Crossman 1977, p. 726).[90]

More Inquiries

Other allegations of abuse, including at Whittingham, Farleigh and South Ockendon hospitals preceded publication of the Ely Report, although the public inquiries to investigate them commenced after it. As with Ely, Barbara's work influenced the course of these inquiries and the implementation of recommendations. In particular, *Sans Everything* triggered the nurses' allegations at Whittingham (see Chapter 5 pp. 162–164), AEGIS helped develop NHS guidance from recommendations made in the Farleigh Report (Anon. 1971b; 1971c; DHSS 1971c, Appx.5),[91] and behind-the-scenes, Barbara ensured that events at South Ockendon received appropriate attention (Anon. 1974a).

The inquiry at Farleigh demonstrated unhelpful senior staff behaviours and victimisation of complainants. In 1968 Greta Saunders, a new nurse, alleged ill-treatment of patients. From the timing, it is conceivable that *Sans Everything* influenced her disclosure. The hospital's chief nurse did not investigate because he 'thought her an emotional young woman'. He sacked her but offered to reinstate her if she withdrew her claims (DHSS 1971c, p. 22), hardly an ethical way to confront alleged deficits of care. Greta Saunders informed the RHB of her concerns, but still nothing was done. Her husband, Kenneth Saunders, then a student nurse at the hospital, was suspended soon after, for alleged 'insubordination, using bad language, and failing to obey instructions' (Fishlock 1969). When a senior doctor and the hospital secretary questioned him about his behaviours, details about the allegations of ill-treatment emerged, and the hospital secretary informed the police. Subsequently, three nurses received prison sentences, each between two and three years, for offences of ill treatment contrary to the Mental Health Act (DHSS 1971c, p. 3). Notably, one of the nurses convicted was allowed to continue working when Mrs Saunders was dismissed (Robinson 1970; DHSS 1971c, p. 22). The committee of inquiry explained: 'The nursing staff fell into two incompatible groups. The one, tough minded, experienced and in control. The other younger, new to the hospital and at the bottom of the nursing hierarchy. The first group was implicitly trusted, the second disregarded' (DHSS 1971c, p. 20). This contributed to Abel-Smith's opinion that complaints against Mr Saunders were probably 'framed' by senior staff.[92]

The criminal trial delayed the Farleigh Inquiry. The committee of inquiry was alarmed by staff 'stating, or restating, their views that no ill treatment of patients had ever taken place at Farleigh. This was a most unhelpful and unfortunate attitude to adopt in the face of many findings of guilt by a jury' (DHSS 1971c, p. 24). Alongside the contradictory evidence given at Shelton and Howe's findings of 'contrived complaints' at Ely, this highlighted the lengths to which staff could go to justify their work patterns and attempt to protect their reputations (p. 19) and pointed towards a probable oversight by the *Sans Everything* inquiry committees. The report added another, worrying, dimension: Farleigh was small with 270 patients (p. 3), indicating that abuse did not occur only in large hospitals. Like Ely, the Farleigh Report recommended national policy changes to ensure better standards of care and complaint management (p. 23; Roper 1972).

Staff also raised concerns at South Ockendon Hospital. In December 1968, Barbara received several pages, posted to her anonymously, that appeared to be from the official record of Beech Villa from the night of 16/17 June 1968. They recorded severe injuries to Michael Pardue, a twenty-three-year-old 'subnormal' patient. The nursing report did not mention disturbances on the ward that night, nor identify the cause of the injuries but noted that all patients 'appear well and comfortable'. The hospital reported the injuries to the police and an internal inquiry resulted in the dismissal of one nurse. However, the conflicting statements in the night report suggested a coverup by night staff and unquestioning acceptance of the report by day staff. The hospital would not allow any public scrutiny of the incident: for them, the matter was closed. Barbara and her AEGIS advisors agreed that if the original reports were genuine, then the internal inquiries into the circumstances of Pardue's injuries were inadequate.[93] Thus began another hospital scandal that continued to occupy Barbara until 1974. That an anonymous member of staff sent the original report to Barbara testified to her reputation of being able to handle staff concerns sensitively. Her independent position reaffirmed the need for an autonomous ombudsman who staff could approach directly.

Other baffling disasters on the same ward included the death of patient Robert Robinson. David Burles, another patient, was accused of his manslaughter, and at trial was found 'unfit to plead' (Anon. 1969c). This verdict designated him a criminal with an order for long-term detention in a hospital, and implied that no other perpetrator need be sought. That contrasted with a verdict of 'not guilty', which would have meant that the search for the perpetrator continued (Whitehead 1971). The difference between the two verdicts was poorly understood, and Barbara Castle MP had to explain it to Keith Joseph.[94] The 'unfit to plead' outcome alarmed Barbara Robb, who, through Abel-Smith, approached Howe. Howe took the case to appeal, which quashed the verdict, and found Burles 'not-guilty' (Anon. 1972). By implication, the perpetrator was still at large, but the authorities did nothing further to find him.

In 1970, Barbara sent her own dossier of evidence to the Director of Public Prosecutions, who passed it to Joseph. He did not respond, so Abel-Smith contacted Howe, (by then a MP): 'Barbara Robb has collected together a great file of facts and is having considerable difficulty in getting them properly investigated. I was wondering whether you could help.'[95] Howe called Joseph's attention to Barbara's 'friendship with the press, and the fact that, if the press were gagged, there would be publicity about it. Joseph said he would look into the matter.'[96] The South Ockendon Inquiry began in 1972.

Six years after the alarm was raised at South Ockendon, Barbara Castle (Secretary of State for Social Services, 1974–1976; Labour government under Harold Wilson), published the inquiry report (DHSS 1974a). Announcing it in the Commons, she paid tribute to Barbara Robb 'who made such strenuous and successful attempts to ensure that the events which had occurred were not swept under the carpet' (Anon. 1974a). The day after the announcement, the *Times* carried seven separate reports on South Ockendon, including one on the front page, emphasising the need to provide better facilities for mentally handicapped people and better management of violence in hospitals (Anon. 1974b). South Ockendon added another worrying dimension: it was a new hospital, and recently had £1 million spent on it.[97] Thus new buildings, like small hospitals, were not immune from abusive practice.

Following South Ockendon, and linked to recommendations from the Farleigh Report, Barbara collaborated with the Royal College of Nursing (RCN), NAMH, RCPsych and others to develop the first NHS guidance on managing violence in hospitals.[98] The initial draft focussed on staff education about causes of violence, observing warning signs, seeking help, documenting events, and ensuring that nurses maintain correct professional relationships with patients. AEGIS's critique added more person-centred ideas, including the importance of team working, preventing violence, providing a 'therapeutic milieu' for patients, and pointing to the need to specify techniques included under the term 'restraint'.[99] Creating the guidance was frustratingly slow. The final document was published around the time of Barbara's death (DHSS 1976).

'THE ANSWERS' PROPOSED IN *SANS EVERYTHING*: OUTCOMES

The main 'answers' given in *Sans Everything*, to improve the situation of older people in psychiatric hospitals, comprised creating comprehensive psychogeriatric services; establishing a NHS inspectorate, an ombudsman and complaints procedures; and providing housing and raising revenue through Project 70. They met with various levels of success by the early 1970s.

At Friern, change was slow. In 1969, four years after Barbara visited Amy Gibbs, Crossman visited Friern. He described its 'deplorable atmosphere' compared, for example, to Littlemore Hospital under Mandelbrote's leadership. Friern had the same hospital secretary and HMC chairman as in 1965 and still lagged behind expected standards of good practice.[100] Soon after Crossman visited, Peggy Jay, a Labour 'grande dame' from Hampstead (Harrington 2008), became chairman of the HMC.[101] Barbara was impressed with Jay.[102] By 1971 she had recruited 180 domestic staff so that nurses could nurse rather than do domestic chores, and she had overseen the renovation of six wards. Nevertheless, there was still much to do. A *Daily Mail* reporter, Douglas Thompson, worked as a nursing assistant at Friern and reported on his experience. Unlike earlier Ministry and RHB condemnation of journalists such as Shearer at Harperbury, Crossman accepted the *Mail*'s approach: 'naturally the hospital staff are furious with the *Daily Mail* for smuggling a reporter into Friern.... But I fear this is the kind of trick which must be used in order to shake the public out of its apathy' (Crossman 1971).

In 1972, the General Nursing Council (GNC) noted patchy improvement at Friern compared to its visit in 1967. There were more nurses of all grades, a greater emphasis on rehabilitation, and better staff morale, including on older people's wards. A third-year nursing student contrasted his experiences on one ward, two years apart. In 1970, 'it was considered a "heavy" ward with the majority of psychogeriatric and infirm patients confined to bed, frequently incontinent and a considerable number suffering from pressure sores.' In 1972, 'the same patients are all up, none have pressure sores, and incontinence is kept to a minimum by a habit training programme', a well-tried effective proactive intervention. Contrary to Robinson's and the RHB's fears that bad publicity created low morale, in line with Crossman's views, when deficits were addressed and the authorities supported change, morale and staffing improved.

On a national level, Crossman implemented his plan for a hospitals' inspectorate, the Hospital Advisory Service (HAS), soon after the Ely Report. Opinions varied on the need for it, including among the medical profession. The BMA Joint Consultants' Committee (JCC) canvased responses from the Medical Royal Colleges, indicating diverse opinions, including strong opposition. The Pathologists said that the HAS had little relevance to them and would not be very useful, and that 'resources hitherto directed to other purposes of the NHS would be taken up in correcting revealed deficiencies in mental and geriatric hospitals.'[103] The Royal College of Physicians of Edinburgh regarded it as 'sinister' and that 'advice' might become 'instruction'.[104] Representative bodies of psychiatrists supported it, proposing that it should be established in all hospitals in line with other policies that mental illness should be provided for in the same way as physical illness.[105] The chairman of the JCC, Sir John Richardson, a physician at a prestigious teaching hospital, disagreed. He stated that a NHS-wide plan was unsupportable: 'The psychiatric hospitals are a special case.'[106]

The *Daily Telegraph* commissioned an article from Barbara (Robb 1969).[107] She was enthusiastic about the HAS, which would be Crossman's 'eyes and ears',[108] but she also had reservations. Her concerns included that, if set up by the DHSS, the HAS might not be sufficiently independent: it might function better as part of a NHS ombudsman service. Ways to protect nurses and overcome their fear of victimisation were particularly important if the HAS were to feed back fully to individual hospitals. It would need to see all parts of the hospitals, not just those that the HMCs wanted it to see. Barbara was also sceptical about the director of the HAS, Dr Alex Baker. Before being appointed Senior Principle Medical Officer at the Ministry in 1967, he was 'medical administrator' at Banstead Hospital which was implicated in *Sans Everything*. In 1990, he recalled his time at the Ministry and the instruction given to him that his 'first duty was to protect the Minister, i.e. to make sure that any advice, or anything the Minister said, was in keeping with accepted policies and would not lead to criticism in Parliament' (Baker 1993, p. 200). He would need to break with that instruction to establish an independent inspectorate.

Crossman, anxious about Barbara's influence through the media, sought to placate her. He and Serota invited her to meet Baker over lunch at the House of Lords. The meeting was initially tense. Barbara noted: 'poor Dr Baker was as outraged at having to discuss his problems with me as I was to say anything to him.' Nevertheless, they discovered common ground, discussion was lively, and revealed much about the challenges faced by the HAS and within the DHSS, including an extreme lack of lateral thinking among the department's civil servants. Baker described: 'everyone was digging his own little hole, straight down, and getting embedded deeper and deeper in it', and Barbara added, 'and what is more they're not even digging it with spades. They are using tiny little trowels.'[109] Crossman, offered an alternative unflattering description of his department: they were 'pen pushers' and 'the only thing which corresponds to them I should think in British History is the old Colonial Office which used to run the Empire from inside the Ministry'.[110] The DHSS might no longer be an ostrich with its head in the sand (Robb 1969), but lateral thinking and effective communication were alarmingly weak. Barbara left the meeting and, 'As we shook hands Mr Crossman said, "So we've met—at last!" We had—and for me it had been fun.' [111]

The HAS visited many hospitals with long-stay wards in England and Wales, and found good and bad practice. Standards of communication varied, at all levels in the hospital, from senior management to day-to-day care of patients. In many large psychiatric hospitals, staffing levels were the same on wards for younger active psychiatric patients requiring less nursing care as on those for frail and dependent older people, who often had nursing needs more in line with patients in geriatric wards of general hospitals that were better staffed (DHSS and Welsh Office 1971, pp. 2, 25). Baker's first round of visits targeted known trouble spots. The HAS annual reports anonymised hospitals but described situations similar to those at Powick, where elderly patients:

> sleep, eat, excrete, live and die in one large room. As would be expected, under such conditions, the wards will be quite sordid with foul smells, and all kinds of personal activities and distress publicly exposed. Sometimes the nurses concerned seem to become so hardened to the sight, sounds and smells of this type of accommodation that they seem unable to realise the impact on first visitors, and indeed on new admissions. Doctors therefore may continue to admit to these hospitals and maintain this type of degrading situation (NHS 1972, p. 26).

Thus problems were particularly evident to newcomers. Baker was determined to listen to them because valuing them would help reduce victimisation. The HAS made constructive suggestions, such as encouraging community psychogeriatric nurses to treat patients in their own homes (NHS 1974, p. 31).

Many staff found the HAS visits helpful in understanding and solving problems,[112] others did not:

> we had been hospital advised. They arrived in the middle of a strike... they said, well, we'll try to make it as gentle as possible. So we had our week. They found 25 things wrong which we knew about, and as my new hospital management said, 23 of them had financial implications. How do we set about that? And they said, well, let's start on the other two. [113]

If managers ignored the HAS reports, they were open to criticism from the RHBs and DHSS,[114] although at least one RHB also ignored HAS reports, irritated that the HAS could recommend changes without providing money to implement them.[115] Overall, the credibility and official status of the HAS raised awareness of service inadequacies and led to changes within the hospitals. However, the magnitude of the problems, including the need to improve the wards and modify staff practices within a conforming rigid hospital culture, precluded rapid transformation. Particularly important, the HAS ensured that the responsible authorities officially endorsed frank discussion about NHS quality of care.

The HAS impacted on two other *Sans Everything* 'answers': Project 70 and comprehensive psychogeriatric services. The HAS described 'Dumping Syndrome', the tendency to place 'rejects' from the community in the psychiatric hospitals (HAS 1971, pp. 20–21). This reignited Project 70 ideas, to create housing estates on the sites of psychiatric hospitals, advocated by AEGIS since 1966 and rejected by Robinson (Anon. 1966a).[116] Independent from AEGIS and Project 70, Lord Hayter (1972), in a letter to the *Times*, drew public attention to the possibility of building on hospital land, and MIND (the campaigning name adopted by NAMH in 1972 (Mind 2016)) took up the theme in 1975.[117] Project 70 was ahead of its time. Building homes on psychiatric hospital land and refurbishing hospital buildings for domestic housing became common in the 1990s. By then, in a consumer-led housing market keener to purchase than to rent, the original financial model of Project 70 was not implemented. After Friern closed in 1993, like many similar hospitals, the estate was sold to a housing developer.

The HAS influenced the development of psychogeriatric services, in conjunction with new enthusiastic psychogeriatricians who had forged links with the DHSS. The blueprint *Services for Mental Illness Related to Old Age* (DHSS 1972) provided psychogeriatricians with clear objectives and a baseline for negotiating future provision (Hilton 2008, p. 304). As earlier, recommendations were permissive and lacked dedicated funding, but they provided a timely mandate for clinicians beginning to develop, lead and improve services (Arie 1973). A nucleus of enthusiastic psychogeriatricians began to meet, including Bergmann and Pitt (previously in Enoch's study group), and Arie and Whitehead, all at least indirectly influenced by AEGIS. The group grew and in 1973 became the RCPsych Special Interest Group for the Psychiatry of Old Age (GPOA).[118] The GPOA (in 2017, a RCPsych Faculty) aimed to promote good practice by sharing experiences, developing services, training staff, encouraging research, exerting pressure on government and other bodies, and commenting on all matters relating to the mental health of older people.[119] In many ways it adopted and broadened AEGIS's initial ideals of dedicated and proactive mental health services for older people.[120] However, Barbara was less prominent publicly, and the GPOA overlooked its AEGIS inheritance.

Despite more professional and government interest, change was slow, as in other 'low-tech' specialties that overlapped with social needs. In 1971, the *Times* reported that the amount of home help provided by most authorities 'was derisory', and that the 'geriatric service must become the top medical priority' because delays would only add to longer-term costs (Anon. 1971d). Age Concern (now Age UK) and MIND carried out a survey of provision for older people in psychiatric hospitals (MIND 1973). They identified important deficits, including inadequate assessment facilities, 'wards of nearly 50 deteriorated and incontinent patients in the care of four nurses' and staff discouraging visitors. The DHSS had set no timetable for transferring older people from psychiatric hospitals (p. 7), an obstacle to longer-term planning. DHSS-led mental health meetings tended to consider older people's services peripheral to their main business (Cawley 1973, p. 4) and postponed discussions about them (DHSS 1974b, p. 12). MIND questioned the DHSS's commitment to psychogeriatric services (MIND 1973). Prioritising older people would be hard to achieve, despite the need and enthusiastic clinical leadership, because financial constraints, competing NHS and social care priorities, stereotypes about older people and low expectations about their health, militated against it. Nevertheless, dedicated psychogeriatric services expanded, from about six in 1966 to 120 in 1980 and then across the entire NHS (Arie and Jolley 1999, p. 262). Experience in the HAS whetted Baker's own appetite to work in psychogeriatrics, and when he stepped down after four years as HAS director, he opted to specialise in the field (Baker 1993, p. 204).

As well as contributing to establishing the specialty of psychogeriatrics, AEGIS made many broader contributions to the NHS, including towards creating the office of ombudsman (MoH 1968c; DHSS 1970). The Council on Tribunals advised on robust procedures for this role, prompted by Barbara's complaints to them.[121] Nurses welcomed the proposals (Anon. 1969a). Similar to establishing the HAS, opinions differed in the medical profession, which was overall conservative when considering changes that it perceived would affect its autonomy. The BMA opposed an ombudsman to whom patients could complain directly, on the grounds that it would destroy the 'trust, respect and mutual rapport' that characterised the doctor–patient relationship (Anon. 1970a). Whitehead (1970) took an alternative view, criticising the 'usual biased, illogical, and egocentric claims...that hospital staff are better at investigating themselves than anyone else'. The *Lancet* (Anon. 1970b) endorsed Whitehead's view: 'For once, cannot the profession shake itself free from its occupational obscurantism?'. Joseph announced plans for the 'Health Service Commissioner' in Parliament in January 1972,[122] with intentions to formalise the role in the NHS Reorganisation Act. During early readings of the reorganisation bill, Barbara and Strabolgi campaigned for, and achieved, amendments to ensure that staff who complained on behalf of a patient were allowed to go straight to the ombudsman, thus bypassing the internal hospital hierarchy and helping overcome concerns about reprisals.[123]

AEGIS's proposals for improving NHS complaints mechanisms (Abel-Smith 1967) received prompt initial attention, but conclusive outcomes were tardy. DHSS research in 1969 corroborated evidence about victimisation of staff and patients who made complaints, and that NHS investigations often left complainants dissatisfied and without knowing how to take the problem to a higher authority. The DHSS report incorporated evidence from voluntary bodies 'not confined to the less reasonable organisations', which it did not name.[124]

The DHSS and Welsh Office (1973) appointed the Davies Committee in 1971 to review complaints procedures, the first comprehensive review in the history of the NHS. The Committee included Applebey and Shearer, social scientists and health service professionals (p. iv). It acknowledged the role of the scandals, particularly at Ely, Farleigh and Whittingham, which 'by themselves would have amply justified our appointment' (p. 3). It took evidence broadly, including from most HMCs, AEGIS, the Council on Tribunals, the BMA, and from 1,000 other organisations and individual members of the public, indicating a high level of concern (pp. 112–113). It produced a twenty-six-page code that covered all aspects of complaint management, including guidance for chairmen of inquiries and recommendations to protect staff who feared victimisation. The code endorsed many of AEGIS's suggestions (e.g., pp. 125, 158). Doctors disliked the recommendations but patients' groups, including the PA, supported them. Implementation was slow, related to the relative lack of power of patients' groups compared with professionals (Mold 2012, p. 2034). Only in 1985, after a House of Commons Select Committee, did the Hospital Complaint (Procedure) Act make it compulsory for hospitals to establish procedures for handling complaints (Mulcahy 2003, p. 41).

BARBARA, OPPONENTS AND ALLIES

Many people influenced the course of the AEGIS campaign. Within the higher ranks of NHS management, three stand out: Robinson, Hackett and Crossman. Their personal influence was huge, but at times it is difficult to fathom out the reasons for their course of action. Robinson and Hackett shared an unchallengeable belief in the adequacy of NHS long-stay provision. Their attitudes matched those of other establishment figures, such as chairmen of the *Sans Everything* inquiry committees. In contrast, Crossman's perspective was closer to that of AEGIS and was associated with steps to improve provision.

Robinson did not publish a memoir and there are no substantial biographies. His entry in the *Oxford Dictionary of National Biography* praised his achievement of remaining popular with the government and the medical profession and contributing significantly to developing the NHS, such as by negotiating the general practitioners' (GP) charter (Jeger 2004). A medical journal (Anon. 1965), based on an interview with an anonymous 'member of the Government', described him in glowing terms: 'He wants to provide the sick with the most humane and effective means of getting better' and 'he is roused to high indignation by injustice, unnecessary suffering, exploitation of the weak...but indignation does not drive him to personal quarrels or enmities.' Obituaries may be biased, tending to praise the deceased, but in the absence of other biographical sources, Robinson's requires consideration. The obituary in the *Independent* (Dalyell 1996) praised Robinson unconditionally for his firm adherence to socialist principles, profound understanding, good judgement and expert knowledge. It cited surgeon Sir Roy Calne, who described Robinson as 'one of the few Ministers of Health that the medical profession have liked', because of his 'transparent compassion and his understanding of the profession.'

Praise for Robinson from GPs and surgeons did not concur with psychiatrists' and social scientists' experience of him. Enoch, for example, described him as 'hardworking, but defensive', rather less impressive than some of his predecessors.[125] In 1969, Townsend criticised him for discrediting *Sans Everything* because, by doing so, he deferred the possibility of major reform of the psychiatric hospitals.[126] Townsend also commented that he failed to promote better mental health services for which he argued previously (Robinson 1958), and that he ignored the authoritative work of experts, including Russell Barton, Martin Roth, Norman Exton-Smith and Doreen Norton, about the mental and physical health of older people (Anon. 1968e).

Abel-Smith and Rolph tried to fathom out the reasons for Robinson's hostility to the situation on the long-stay wards and to Barbara, AEGIS and *Sans Everything*.[127] Rolph (1968) thought that his complacency was 'a mask for anger', but could not work out the cause for that. Crossman claimed to have identified a cause that stemmed back to Barbara's student days: Robinson's wife, Elizabeth, was an alumna of Chelsea College of Art, contemporary with Barbara, Brian and Strabolgi (Cochrane 1990, p. 397),[128] and at some point a personal disagreement arose. Barbara and Crossman discussed this when they met in April 1970, a dialogue that Barbara rapidly committed to paper:

BR: What can I tell the press?
RC: Tell them that I will not investigate the White Paper but will investigate the hospitals. The White Paper arises out of a family quarrel.
BR: What are you saying?
RC: Well, it's linked with a family quarrel.
BR: What family are you talking about?
RC: You and the Robinsons.
BR: I beg your pardon, Sir. I am not related to or connected in any way with the Robinsons.
RC: They're old friends of yours.
BR: I have known Elizabeth Robinson for a long time. I have nothing whatever against her. I have only met Kenneth twice....

BR: Am I to tell the press that you regard the White Paper as part of a family quarrel between the Robinsons and the Robbs?
RC: No, you are *not* to tell the press. If you were warm-hearted you wouldn't be bothering about the White Paper. You'd be concerned only about investigating the hospitals.
BR: Can't you ask one of our mutual friends about the state of my heart?
RC: I've discussed you with Bea Serota. When things go wrong and we're very depressed, she and I often cheer ourselves up by asking one another what you would say about the problem.[129]

The dialogue revealed as much about Barbara and Crossman as about Robinson. It demonstrated her wittiness, her uninhibited confidence to contest people in authority and her immediate response to 'tell the press'. It also indicated Crossman's characteristic frankness, and a mixture of impertinence, humour and respect when he described Barbara's effect on Serota and himself. Crossman described the same meeting in his diary. He said that *Sans Everything*

> was her pound of flesh to destroy Kenneth Robinson. I said it is a pity to have a personal squabble, (this is the only time she got really angry) because of course it is true she and Elizabeth Robinson were bosom friends together until Kenneth Robinson failed to give Mrs Robb's husband the key appointment he thought was his due, whereupon she turned against the Robinsons. At least that is what Brian Abel-Smith tells me and I can well believe it.[130]

The likelihood of Robinson having a post to offer Brian, an artist, seems remote. In an internal memo at the DHSS, Abel-Smith referred to the importance of his confidential discussions with Barbara,[131] but whether he broke a confidence or if Abel-Smith was in fact Crossman's source of information or if there was any foundation to the rumour is unknown.

Despite a reputation for his interest in psychiatric hospitals,[132] Robinson was complacent about the older people in them. Crossman tried to justify Robinson's approach, speculating that he took little action on their behalf because he expected that the 'new hospitals would have a fair proportion of geriatric and psychiatric beds',[133] which would solve the difficulties. New facilities in most places, however, were beyond the horizon. Crossman (1977, p. 727)[134] did not criticise Robinson in public but wrote in his diary: 'he mishandled her [Barbara] and instead of treating *Sans Everything* sensibly Kenneth set up committees of investigation into her charges and then published a white paper as a non-controversial document to answer her, which it didn't. This left a very dirty impression.' Robinson seemed oblivious to public opinion and he misjudged Barbara's tenacity and strength of character, even in the face of public humiliation.[135] Crossman (1977, p. 134)[136] stated: 'I feel he has done nothing whatsoever to silence Mrs Robb because the bare picture [that psychiatric hospitals are adequate] is not terribly convincing.'

In an oral history interview in 1991, Robinson clung to the conviction that his stance towards *Sans Everything* was correct, and still sounded exasperated by Barbara:

> I thought at the time and I still think, that it was very much exaggerated and emotionally weighted. She was a very strange and almost hysterical woman... maybe I resisted it too strongly, but this was a terrible slander on the mental nursing profession.... It conveyed the impression that they were a whole lot of sadistic people who were only concerned to make life hell for the patients. Maybe I over reacted, I don't know.[137]

Robinson did not like Barbara, but whether an element of personal animosity fuelled a conflict about *Sans Everything* is unconfirmed. If Robinson behaved in the manner Crossman described, it was unprofessional.

Robinson and Hackett mishandled 'Diary of a Nobody' and *Sans Everything*, fuelling Barbara's campaign. Both men were authoritarian and patronising. Hackett's self-righteousness in the media, his hand-in-glove working relationship with Robinson (Hackett 1965b), his probable underhandedness with staff at Friern and his complicity with Friern's shortcomings, did not enhance the well-being of patients, despite his claim to 'guard and protect' them (Hackett 1965a). Hackett and the RHB ignored criticism rather than using it to seek ways and resources to achieve improvements, a pattern mirrored by the Friern HMC. He was heavy-handed with staff who might spoil his, or his RHB's, reputation. Hackett appeared unaware that belittling complainants, rejecting genuine concerns and accusing critics of ignorance and exaggeration, inhibited improvements and antagonised the public, some of whom saw through his methods (Field 1968). Others disliked his leadership style, including the distinguished advisory body, the South-East Economic Planning Council. Hackett was appointed its chairman while his brother-in-law George Brown was in a related role of Secretary of State for Economic

Affairs. On the Planning Council he 'upset a fair proportion of the leading academics, lay planners and men from industry... by a curiously unendearing brusqueness in the chair and a proneness to cut off respected experts in mid-exposition' (Anon. 1967).

Hackett was knighted for services to the RHB and to the Planning Council (Anon. 1970c, 1970d). Undoubtedly some positive events happened in the region under his leadership, such as building and opening Northwick Park Hospital. However, one wonders how much his knighthood related to who he knew rather than what he did and how much he sought recognition for himself rather than benefit for those he represented, particularly the most vulnerable and stigmatised people in the psychiatric hospitals. Crossman described Hackett as 'gloomy' and a 'bore'.[138] In Shearer's words, Hackett was 'an idle jobsworth'.[139]

Robinson and Hackett contrasted with Crossman in their responses to Barbara and to the issues that concerned AEGIS. However, like them, Crossman also knew how to manipulate the system, revealed by his nicknames 'Tricky Dicky' (Cochrane 1990, p. 120) and 'Double Crossman' (Rolph 1987, p. 183). Abel-Smith (1990, p. 259) later reflected:

> I've always been slightly puzzled... and never really satisfied myself as to why it was that Richard Crossman made this such a personal crusade.... it was definitely as much a personal crusade to try and get things right as it was for Barbara Robb to draw attention to what was wrong. Most people don't realise the extent to which the change was initiated by Crossman, but he started a movement which, once the Department had got on to it, took on its own momentum. This was what a great minister can do. Long after he had died, the ripple effects of the whole thing were still going on. I don't usually go for the 'great man' thesis in history, but he will be remembered, or ought to be remembered, as a rather unlikely person to have done something like this.

Crossman was more perceptive about Barbara's determination and public influence than Robinson. Crossman described her as collecting 'ammunition for an attack on us',[140] and that

> She is a dangerous woman because people go to her, people write to her, the most terrible stories about the hospitals are collected by her. She is always ready with some great scandal to break, and there are, God knows, enough scandals to break.[141]

On one occasion, on her way to meet Crossman at the Commons, an usher escorted her to his office. Barbara remarked to the usher that the Commons was a labyrinth, to which the usher replied: 'and at the end of the labyrinth you meet the Minotaur.' Barbara relayed the comment to Crossman during their meeting.[142] Rolph (1987, p. 182) commented that Barbara's sense of humour was 'effervescent and mischievous... without ever giving offence'. Crossman said about Barbara: 'I happen rather to like her.... it's better for us to have her investigations useful and her on relatively friendly terms with me.' He described her as 'a curious little thing, terribly neat, precise, cold, venomous, with a certain serpentine charm'.[143]

Crossman's approach to NHS complaints contrasted with Robinson's. Crossman gambled with his reputation by publishing the Ely Report, and survived, by committing himself to, and implementing, policy changes. When Crossman became a back-bencher in 1970, he returned to journalism, editing the *New Statesman*. He commissioned a series of articles, 'Snakepits of the seventies', which declared in large print on the cover of the *New Statesman* that in overcrowded 'asylums' patients were still 'stripped of self-respect along with their personal property and clothes' (Anon. 1971a). That was probably the nearest Crossman came to criticising Robinson in public for rejecting *Sans Everything*. At the end of the snakepits series, Donald Gould and Ann Shearer (1971) wrote: 'To the medical profession's shame, it was a politician, Richard Crossman, who made us take notice of the ugly state of the mental health scene.' In view of his short period as Secretary of State (twenty months) it is likely that his impact would have been far less without Barbara's groundwork, expertise and influence.

Comment

Many people including Townsend, journalists and psychiatrists, and organisations such as AEGIS and the PA, were not deceived by the 'sacred cow' image of the NHS as propagated by Robinson, Hackett and others in authority. Fear of adverse publicity about the NHS, and reproach by the Ministry to those, including the BBC, who spoke out, supported the notion that the NHS sought to protect its workforce from criticism, over and above the needs of patients. Robinson doubted that such a 'conspiracy against the patients' existed.[144] However, some in NHS positions of authority indicated little respect for the 'man on the Clapham omnibus', whether as patient or as healthy member of the public, corroborating Cohen's *What's Wrong with Hospitals?* (1964) and the PA's and AEGIS's experiences. This attitude jarred with changing public perceptions in the 1960s, such as about personal autonomy, paternalism, and public ownership of the NHS.

Various factors contributed to the authorities ignoring or concealing bad practice, including believing that the problems were insurmountable, hoping they would go away (MoH 1961, p. 98) or, more positively, that developments already under way, such as the *Hospital Plan,* would overcome them (MoH 1962, 1963). The Ministry believed that criticism of the NHS would lower morale and adversely affect staff retention and recruitment, but evidence suggests the contrary. The Ministry did not perceive that openness about deficits could inspire hope, raise morale, lead to improvements for patients and make mental health service employment more attractive. Fear of the effects of negative publicity was associated with defensiveness, deception and coverups in various NHS settings, from individual hospitals to the Ministry, including Robinson's announcement of *Findings and Recommendations* in the Commons.

Sans Everything and subsequent inquiries revealed unhelpful patterns of NHS administration, such as seniors denying allegations of malpractice, rejecting criticism from those without formal qualifications and victimising whistle-blowers. Barbara, Abel-Smith, Baker, Crossman and Howe, discouraged, and probably lessened, these methods during the period covered in this chapter, such as by improving complaints guidance, creating the ombudsman and by the HAS encouraging staff to speak out. Nevertheless, ongoing vigilance remains necessary to prevent defensive responses creeping back (e.g., NHS 2016).

In 1969, the NAMH reflected that recent events marked a turning point in the history of the psychiatric hospitals:

> When the history of the treatment and care of the mentally ill and subnormal in England in the twentieth century comes to be written, there will be a chapter devoted to the last 12 months....

> Everyone concerned may want to forget the *causes célèbres*—Sans Everything, Shelton, Ely, Farleigh—the public because it is distasteful, the government because it cries out for a massive reallocation of funds and the hospital service because it damages their image—but we believe that the time has come when everybody should be urged to remember, to think and to discuss a subject which inexorably will become a major medical, political and social problem in the 'seventies' (NAMH 1969, pp. 5, 7).

Barbara heavily influenced many aspects of this, publicly or behind the scenes, from supporting and encouraging individual nurses and doctors, to face-to-face meetings with the Secretary of State. *Sans Everything* inspired clinicians, such as psychiatrists Arie, Enoch and Whitehead, and nurse Peter Carter, later Chief Executive of the RCN, for whom 'it made a life-long impression'.[145] The Ely Report took the policy proposals raised in *Sans Everything* beyond the walls of the mental illness and 'subnormality' hospitals into the broader NHS, including creating a health service ombudsman and better complaints processes. However, the effectiveness of top-down policies and guidance was, and is, variable, as with the stripping guidance in 1965 and complaints memorandum in 1966; committed clinicians who adopt a bottom-up approach dedicated to ensuring improvements in the care of patients and morale of staff (Arie 1971) are likely to increase the chances of policy success. Thus by inspiring individuals and influencing policy, Barbara, despite the odds stacked against her, achieved her goals. As Enoch reflected in 2015: 'Her effect was far more than Robinson's in the end.'[146] In Abel-Smith's words (1990): 'For one woman who had really very little background in the mental hospital area… to suddenly do so much in such a short period—and tragically, to die so soon—is a remarkable story.'

Notes

1. Hence the title of this chapter: 'Most good is done by stealth': Quentin Blake, interview by author, January 2016, citing Brian Robb.
2. 'Central Hospital, Warwick', *Hansard* HC Deb 4 March 1968, vol 760 cc.189–200.
3. DHSS/Royal College of Psychiatrists meeting, RCPsych Council minutes, 8 September 1972 (RCPsych Archives).
4. See Abel-Smith memoranda (University of Warwick Modern Records Centre, UWMRC).
5. 'Shelton Hospital, Shrewsbury (Inquiry)', *Hansard* HC Deb 19 March 1968, vol 761 cc.216–217.
6. MoH, 'Formal Inquiries under S 70 NHS Act 1946', 1967, MH159/213 (The National Archives, TNA).
7. Letter, FDK Williams to Council on Tribunals, 4 August 1967, MH159/213 (TNA).
8. 'Shelton Hospital, Shrewsbury (Fire)', *Hansard* HC Deb 16 December 1968, vol 775 cc.268–270W.
9. 'Shelton Hospital (Fire)', *Hansard* HC Deb 26 February 1968, vol 759 cc.945–947.

10. Blofeld Report, 11–13 (London Metropolitan Archives, LMA).
11. St Lawrence's transcript, 15 September 1967, 44, MH159/226 (TNA).
12. Letter, JC Barker to Robb, 10 July 1968, AEGIS/2/3 (AEGIS archives, London School of Economics).
13. David Enoch, interview by author, 2015.
14. JC Barker, Mabel Miller, 'The problem of the chronic psychiatric patients', Shelton Hospital, postgraduate education programme, 14 December 1967, 24–25, AEGIS/2/3.
15. David Enoch, interview by author, 2015.
16. Letter, Robb to Edward Stern, August 1966, AEGIS/1/18/3.
17. 'Central Hospital, Warwick', *Hansard* HC Deb 4 March 1968 vol 760 cc.189–200.
18. Robb, note to 'Vanya', 21 May 1968, AEGIS/1/6.
19. Letter, Shearer to Robb, 24 October 1967, AEGIS/1/6; Ann Shearer, interview by author, 2015.
20. Ann Shearer, interview by author, 2015.
21. Ann Shearer, interview by author, 2015.
22. Crossman Diaries, July 1968, 64 and 152/68/SW (UWMRC).
23. Memo, Robinson, 29 June 1968, MH159/216 (TNA).
24. '*Sans Everything* (Reports of Inquiries)', *Hansard* HC Deb 9 July 1968 vol 768 cc.213–216.
25. MoH press service, 'Enquiries into allegations made in the book *Sans Everything*: Findings published in White Paper', 9 July 1968, AEGIS/B/3.
26. COHSE flyer, AEGIS/A/2.
27. Also AEGIS, National Corporation for the Care of Old People, and National Old People's Welfare Committee.
28. Letter, Helen Hodgson to Harold Wilson, 2 August 1968, AEGIS/1/7.
29. Letter, Hodgson to Robb, 9 September 1968, AEGIS/1/7.
30. Crossman Diaries, May 1970, 168/JH/70/26 (UWMRC).
31. Crossman Diaries, 16 July 1968, 151/68/SW (UWMRC).
32. Correspondence and discussion, Robb and Applebey; Townsend, NAMH Annual Conference, 20 February, 1969, manuscript of speech, and letters, AEGIS/2/8, AEGIS/B/4.
33. Note, Barbara and Brian Robb, 8 November 1967, AEGIS/2/10; Letter, Shearer to Robb, 24 October 1967, AEGIS/1/6.
34. Letter, Harvey to Rolph, 19 July 1968, AEGIS/B/3.
35. Letter, Davie to Robb, 28 July 1968, AEGIS/2/7/A.
36. Plan for *Man Alive* programme, February 1968, AEGIS/B/3.
37. Letter, Robb to solicitor, 1 July 1968, AEGIS/2/7/A.
38. Telegram, Wilcox to Robinson, 12 July 1968, MH159/220 (TNA).
39. BBC2, *Man Alive*, 16 July 1968, transcript, 18, AEGIS/2/7/A.
40. Crossman Diaries, 16 July 1968, 150/68/SW (UWMRC).

41. Letters, Wilcox and Robb, 18 and 22 July 1968, AEGIS/2/7/A.
42. Crossman Diaries, 16 July 1968, 151/68/SW (UWMRC).
43. Letter, viewer in Kent (signature illegible) to Wilcox, 17 July 1968, AEGIS/2/7/A.
44. Letter, Mrs Gwatkin to Robb, 25 July 1968, AEGIS/1/17/5.
45. Letter, Harvey to Rolph, 19 July 1968, AEGIS/B/3.
46. Robb, 'Record of a campaign', vol 8, 10, AEGIS/1/8.
47. NHS Act 1946 and National Assistance Act 1948.
48. Labour Party, Blackpool, 'A new, urgent approach to mental health', 2 October 1968; Eric Moonman, guest lecture series list; Letter, Moonman to Robb, AEGIS/1/10/A.
49. Tom Arie, discussions, 2004.
50. Letter, Enoch to Robb, 1 October 1968, AEGIS/1/10/A.
51. BGS/RCPsych, minutes, 22 June and 11 July 1972; BGS/RCPsych, 'Joint report', 1973 (Tom Arie's archives).
52. Boorer, David. Craig, Janet and Kirkpatrick, Bill. 1971.'Nurses attitudes to their patients', King's Fund Hospital Centre, AEGIS/6/1.
53. Letter, DJ Dean (Deputy Head of Nursing, Napsbury) to Robb, 15 October 1968, AEGIS/1/5.
54. Robb, 'Progress report' 1967–8, AEGIS/6/13.
55. Crossman Diaries, 10 March 1969, 129/69/SW (UWMRC).
56. Letters, Howe to WHB, 18 September 1967; Memo, Croft to Franklyn Williams, 17 October 1968, MH96/2198 (TNA).
57. Letters, Howe to Robinson, 22 October 1968; Robinson to Howe, 6 November 1968, MH96/2198 (TNA).
58. The *Sans Everything* inquiry at Banstead publicised its investigation in a similar way (MoH 1968a, pp. 3–9).
59. 24 March 1970.
60. Letter, Howe to WHB, 18 September 1967, MH96/2198; Letter, Baroness Burton to Crossman, 26 March 1969, MH159/217 (TNA).
61. Letter, Burton to Crossman, 26 March 1969, MH159/217 (TNA).
62. Springfield Report part 1, 2, MH159/233 (TNA).
63. 12 March 1969.
64. Memo, WHB to Mr Merifield, MoH, 9 September 1968, MH159/221 (TNA).
65. Crossman Diaries, 10 March 1969, 129/69/SW (UWMRC).
66. Note, Croft, January 1969, MH159/222 (TNA).
67. Memo, Hales to Hewitt, 15 February 1968, MH159/225 (TNA).
68. Memo, Croft to Hedley, 4 February 1969, MH159/218 (TNA).
69. Crossman Diaries, 10 March 1969, 127 and 129/69/SW (UWMRC).
70. 27 November 1969.
71. Crossman Diaries, 16 July 1968, 152/68/SW (UWMRC).

72. Crossman Diaries, 10 March 1969, 127/69/SW (UWMRC).
73. Crossman Diaries, March 1969, 160 and 177/69/SW (UWMRC).
74. Crossman Diaries, 27 March 1969, 183/69/SW (UWMRC).
75. Letter, Crossman to RHB chairmen, 27 March 1969, MH159/219 (TNA).
76. 'Ely Hospital, Cardiff', *Hansard* HC Deb 27 March 1969, vol 780 cc.1808–1820.
77. 'Ely Hospital, Cardiff: Inquiry findings', *Hansard* HL Deb 27 March 1969, vol 300 cc.1384–1393.
78. 'Community Care', *Hansard* HL Deb 7 July 1965, vol 267 cc.1332–1410.
79. Howe attributed ongoing respect for the Ely Report to 'the fact that it was the first inquiry of its kind from which—albeit *conducted* in private—the veil of secrecy was decisively removed' (Howe 1999, p. 302). Howe's firmness, according to a fellow barrister, also 'stiffened the position of chairmen of all subsequent inquiries' (Hillman and Clarke 1988, p. 92).
80. 6 August 1969; 3–4 October 1969; 12 November 1970.
81. 'Hospitals Scrutiny (Working Party)', *Hansard* HC Deb 24 April 1969, vol 782 cc.123–124W.
82. NAMH, 'An inspectorate for hospitals?' Annexe to PEP(69)21, MH159/219 (TNA).
83. Note, KDK Williams, 'Post Ely Policy Working Party', April 1969, MH159/219 (TNA).
84. Letters for consideration by the PEP committee on complaints, MH159/236 (TNA).
85. PEP, Working group on complaints procedures: first meeting 5 May 1969, minutes, MH159/236 (TNA).
86. Crossman Diaries, 6 August 1969, CD 23/69 (UWMRC).
87. Crossman Diaries, 6 August 1969, CD 24/69 (UWMRC).
88. Crossman Diaries, 6 August 1969, CD 24/69 (UWMRC).
89. Post-Ely Working Party, 'Re-allocation of resources in favour of long-stay hospitals', c.1970, MH150/450 (TNA).
90. 12 November 1969.
91. 'South Ockendon Hospital (Report)', *Hansard* HC Deb 15 April 1974, vol 873 col 1293–1303.
92. Memo, Abel-Smith to Mr Mottershead, 'Report of Working group on complaints procedures', 6 August 1969, 154/3/DH/46/13 (UWMRC).
93. Robb, 'Record of a campaign', vol 9, Introduction and pp. 10–11, AEGIS1/9/1.
94. 'South Ockendon Mental Hospital', *Hansard* HC Deb 11 April 1972, vol 834 cc.1024–1026.
95. Letter, Abel-Smith to Howe, 22 December 1970, AEGIS/1/9/2.
96. Robb, 'Record of a campaign', vol 9, 29–30, 32, AEGIS/1/9/2.
97. Crossman Diaries, 11 April 1969, CD1082 (UWMRC).

98. RCN/RCPsych, 'The care of the violent patient', 1972, AEGIS/B/7.
99. DHSS, 1974. Draft 'Management of violent or potentially violent hospital patients', 2, 3. AEGIS/2/5/A.
100. Crossman Diaries, February 1969, 54/69/SW (UWMRC).
101. New Southgate HMC, minutes, 24 July 1969, 7585 (LMA).
102. Robb, letter (typescript) to *Hampstead and Highgate Express*, 27 January 1970, AEGIS/1/10/A.
103. Letter, James Howie to Gray-Turner, 1 May 1969, E/2/367/1 (BMA).
104. Letter, Christopher Clayson to Gray-Turner, 7 May 1969, E/2/367/1 (BMA).
105. Letters, WAS Falls to Richard Crossman, 16 May 1969; Francis Pilkington to Dr Wilson, BMA, 2 June 1969, E/2/367/1 (BMA).
106. Letter, Sir John Richardson to Gray-Turner, 19 June 1969, E/2/367/1 (BMA).
107. Colin Welch, senior *Daily Telegraph* reporter, Aegis/B/2.
108. Crossman Diaries, March 1969, 158/69/SW (UWMRC).
109. Report of meeting at House of Lords, 12 November 1969, AEGIS/6/16.
110. Crossman Diaries, 10 March 1969, 133/69/SW (UWMRC).
111. Report of meeting at House of Lords, 12 November 1969, AEGIS/6/16.
112. Letter, Alex Baker to Gray-Turner, BMA, 24 June 1970, E/2/367/2 (BMA).
113. Anon. psychiatrist, interview, 2016.
114. South West Thames Regional Health Authority, 'Report of Committee of Enquiry, St Augustine's Hospital, Chartham, Canterbury', 1976, 4 (RCPsych Archives).
115. Normansfield Inquiry, transcript, 17 January 1978, 7, 10, H29/NF/F/6/117 (LMA).
116. Letter, Joseph to Robb, 28 June 1972, AEGIS/2/5/A; Report, Rolph to Robb, about meeting with Robinson, February 1967, AEGIS/1/18/3.
117. MIND, Campaign for the Mentally Handicapped and Spastics Society, 'Hospital land—a resource for the future?' July 1975, AEGIS/1/10/F.
118. GPOA, minutes 9 February 1973, 2 (RCPsych Archives).
119. GPOA, 'Draft Memorandum on the readiness of the group for the Psychiatry of Old Age now to become a section of the Royal College of Psychiatrists', c. October 1977 (RCPsych Archives).
120. Robb, 'Aims of AEGIS', AEGIS/7/2.
121. 'Comments by Mrs Bell on the Minister's reply of 30th July 1968', Annex B, BL2/862 (TNA).
122. 'Health Service Commissioner', *Hansard* HC Deb 22 February 1972, vol 831 cc.1104–1114.
123. NHS Reorganisation Act 1973, 35 clauses 2 and 4: Robb, '*Sans Everything* and the health ombudsman', c.1974, AEGIS/1/8.

124. DHSS, 'Procedure for investigating complaints and proposals for a Health Commissioner', Annexe 2, March 1969, MH159/218 (TNA).
125. David Enoch, interview by author, 2015.
126. Townsend, Peter. 1969. NAMH Annual Conference, 20 February, and correspondence, Rolph, Robb and Townsend, April 1969, AEGIS/B/4.
127. AEGIS meeting, 16 March 1967, 34, AEGIS/1/20.
128. Kenneth Robinson, interviewed by Margot Jeffreys, 1991 (British Library Sound Archive, BLSA).
129. Robb, 'Report of a discussion in Mr Crossman's office at the Commons, 30 April 1970', AEGIS/2/12/2.
130. Crossman Diaries, May 1970, 168/JH/70–27 (UWMRC).
131. Memo, Abel-Smith to Mr Farrant, 'South Ockendon Hospital', July 1969, DH/45/56 (UWMRC).
132. See Chapter 2, p. 78.
133. Crossman Diaries, March 1969, 132/69/SW (UWMRC).
134. 12 November 1969.
135. Crossman Diaries, 16 July 1968, 151/68/SW (UWMRC).
136. 14 July 1968.
137. Kenneth Robinson, interviewed by Margot Jeffreys, 1991 (BLSA).
138. Crossman Diaries, 6 February 1969, 195/69/SW (UWMRC).
139. Ann Shearer, interview by author, 2015.
140. Crossman Diaries, 12 November 1969, JH/69–40 (UWMRC).
141. Crossman Diaries, 16 March 1970, 166/70/SW 116–7 (UWMRC).
142. Robb, 'Report of a discussion in Mr Crossman's office at the Commons, 30 April 1970', AEGIS/2/12/2.
143. Crossman Diaries, May 1970, 168/JH/70–26 and 27 (UWMRC).
144. 'Care of the elderly', Hansard HC Deb 11 July 1967, vol 750 cc.431–554.
145. Peter Carter, discussion, October 2016.
146. David Enoch, interview by author, 2015.

Bibliography

Abel-Smith, Brian. 1967. 'Administrative solution: a hospital commissioner?' 128–135. In Robb 1967.

Abel-Smith, Brian. 1990. Interviewed by Hugh Freeman. *BJPsych Bulletin*, 14, 257–261.

Adeney, Martin. 1969. 'Clampdown on hospital press leaks'. *Guardian*, 25 September.

Anon. 1965. 'What manner of man is he? Kenneth Robinson—romantic radical or physician manqué?' *British Hospital Journal and Social Service Review*, 13 August, 1531–1532.

Anon. 1966a. 'Project 70'. *Nursing Times*, 10 June.
Anon. 1966b 'Disgusting, disgraceful, degrading'. *Sunday Mirror*, 14 August.
Anon. 1966c. 'MPs call for inquiry into hospital overcrowding'. *Times*, 17 August.
Anon. 1966d. 'Team to study hospital'. *Times*, 30 September.
Anon. 1967. 'Steamrolling chairman'. *Times*, 2 November.
Anon. 1968a. 'Shelton hospital fire toll rises to 24'. *Times*, 28 February.
Anon. 1968b. 'Hospitals report a "whitewash"'. *Times*, 11 July.
Anon. 1968c. 'Minister under fire on "cruel hospitals" probe'. *Observer*, 14 July.
Anon. 1968d. 'Whitehall washes whitest'. *Daily Mail*, 15 July.
Anon. 1968e. 'Haste, ignorance and inhumanity'. *New Society*, 18 July.
Anon. 1968f. 'An official indictment'. *Medical Tribune*, 18 July.
Anon. 1968g. 'Not good enough'. *Lancet*, ii, 202–203.
Anon. 1968h. 'New inquiry sought on hospitals: aged patients'. *Daily Telegraph*, 3 August.
Anon. 1968i. 'Male nurses are exonerated'. *Times*, 17 August.
Anon. 1968j. 'Old people in hospital'. *BMJ*, iii, 135.
Anon. 1968k. 'Tug of war at nurses' Commons protest'. *Daily Telegraph*, 14 December.
Anon. 1969a. 'Editorial'. *Nursing Mirror*, 24 January.
Anon. 1969b. 'Constant watch on conditions in long-stay hospitals'. *Times*, 28 March.
Anon. 1969c. 'Patient unfit to plead'. *Times*, 26 April.
Anon. 1969d. 'Crossman sees the worst—and pledges better'. *Guardian*, 7 August.
Anon. 1969e. 'Hospital overcrowding shocks Crossman'. *Daily Telegraph*, 7 Augustt.
Anon. 1970a. 'Special report of Council'. *BMJ*, ii, supplement, 28.
Anon. 1970b. 'Complaints in hospitals'. *Lancet*, i, 759.
Anon. 1970c. 'Birthday honours'. *Times*, 15 June.
Anon. 1970d. *Hampstead and Highgate Express*, 19 June.
Anon. 1971a. 'Snakepits of the seventies.' *New Statesman*, 19 February.
Anon. 1971b. 'Shut away'. *BMJ*, ii, 119.
Anon. 1971c. 'Nurses at Farleigh Hospital'. *BMJ*, ii, 180.
Anon. 1971d. 'Patients need total care, doctors told.' *Times*, 26 November.
Anon. 1972. 'Burles was not guilty'. *Grays and Thurrock Express*, 19 April.
Anon. 1974a. 'Disturbing report on a hospital: health authorities to be asked to review standards of care'. *Times*, 16 May.
Anon. 1974b. 'Pledge by Mrs Castle after hospital report'. *Times*, 16 May.
Arie, Tom. 1971. 'Morale and the planning of psychogeriatric services'. *BMJ*, iii, 166–170.
Arie, Tom. 1973. 'Psychogeriatrics'. *Age and Ageing*, 2, 195–197.

Arie, Tom and Jolley, David. 1999. 'Psychogeriatrics' 260–265. In *A Century of Psychiatry*, ed. Hugh Freeman. London: Mosby-Wolfe.

Baker, Alex. 1993. Interviewed by Hugh Freeman [1990], edited transcript, 192–206. In *Talking About Psychiatry*, ed. Greg Wilkinson. London: Gaskell.

BBC1. 1968. *Something for Nothing: A Birthday Celebration*, 27 June, http://www.bbc.co.uk, accessed 24 December 2015.

Butler, Ian and Drakeford, Mark. 2005. *Scandal, Social Policy and Social Welfare*. Bristol: Policy Press.

Carse, Joshua, Panton, Nydia and Watt, Alexander. 1958. 'A district mental health service: the Worthing experiment'. *Lancet*, i, 39–41.

Cawley, Robert. 1973. 'Planning for the future'. *News and Notes* (of the RCPsych) May, 1–5.

Cochrane, David. 1990. 'The AEGIS campaign to improve standards of care in mental hospitals: A case study of the process of social policy change'. PhD thesis, University of London. http://etheses.lse.ac.uk, accessed 17 September 2016.

Cohen, Gerda. 1964. *What's Wrong with Hospitals?* Harmondsworth: Penguin Books.

Crossman, Richard. 1971. 'London diary'. *New Statesman*, 22 October.

Crossman, Richard. 1977. '*The Diaries of a Cabinet Minister*'. In Vol. 3. *Secretary of State for Social Services 1968–1970*. London: Hamilton and Cape.

Dalyell, Tam. 1996. 'Obituary: Sir Kenneth Robinson'. *Independent*, 21 February.

DHSS. 1968. *Committee on Local Authority and Allied Personal Social Services*. Cmnd. 3703 (Seebohm Report). London: HMSO.

DHSS. 1969. *Report of the Committee of Inquiry* into *Allegations of Ill-Treatment of Patients and Other Irregularities at the Ely Hospital, Cardiff*. Cmnd. 3975. London: HMSO.

DHSS. 1970. *The Future Structure of the National Health Service in England*. London: HMSO.

DHSS. 1971a. *Better Services for the Mentally Handicapped*. London: HMSO.

DHSS. 1971b. *Hospital Services for the Mentally Ill*. HM (71)97. London: HMSO.

DHSS. 1971c. *Report of the Farleigh Hospital Committee of Inquiry*. Cmnd. 4557. London: HMSO.

DHSS. 1972. *Services for Mental Illness Related to Old Age*. HM (72)71. London: HMSO.

DHSS. 1973. *Report of the Committee on Hospital Complaint Procedures*. (Chair: Sir Michael Davies). London: HMSO.

DHSS. 1974a. *Report of the Committee of Inquiry into South Ockendon Hospital*. HC. 124. London: HMSO.

DHSS. 1974b. *Providing a Comprehensive District Psychiatric Service for the Adult Mentally Ill*. London: HMSO.

DHSS. 1976. *The Management of Violent or Potentially Violent Hospital Patients.* HC (76)11. London: HMSO.

DHSS and Welsh Office. 1971. *NHS Hospital Advisory Service, Annual Report for 1969–70.* London: HMSO.

Doyle, Christine. 1968. 'Ombudsman plan for hospitals wins support'. *Observer*, 26 May.

Eade, Christine. 1968. 'Nurses march with banners to No 10'. *Guardian*, 16 August.

Enoch, M David and Howells, John. 1971. *Organisation of Psychogeriatrics.* Ipswich: SCP.

Field, Leopold. 1968. 'Harperbury: paranoia and hysteria in the National Health Service'. *Guardian*, 20 December.

Fishlock, Trevor. 1969. 'Patients were beaten up, coroner told.'. *Times*, 12 August.

Freeman, Sue. 1968. 'A problem that can't be whitewashed'. *Daily Express*, 8 August.

Gittins, Diana. 1998. *Madness in Its Place: Narratives of Severalls Hospital 1913–1997.* London: Routledge.

Goddard, Peter, Corner, John and Richardson, Kay. 2007. *Public Issue Television: World in Action 1963–98.* Manchester: Manchester University Press.

Gould, Donald and Shearer, Ann. 1971. 'Snakepits: a summing up: knock down those walls'. *New Statesman*, 9 July.

Greenberg, RC. 1968. Cited in 'Annual Representative Meeting (Geriatric Hospital Beds)' *BMJ*, Suppl, 6 July, iii, 13.

Hackett, Maurice. 1965a. 'Old people in mental hospitals'. *Times*, 18 November.

Hackett, Maurice. 1965b. 'Mental hospitals'. *Times*, 1 December.

Hackett, Maurice. 1968. 'Ill informed, ill considered, and unkind'. *Guardian*, 14 December.

Harrington, Illtyd. 2008. 'Peggy Jay'. *Guardian*, 22 January.

Hayter. 1972. 'Surplus hospital land'. *Times*, 14 August.

Hillman, Judy and Clarke, Peter. 1988. *Geoffrey Howe: A Quiet Revolutionary.* London: Weidenfeld and Nicolson.

Hilton, Claire. 2008. 'The provision of mental health services for people over 65 years of age in England 1970–78'. *History of Psychiatry*, 19, 297–320.

Hodgson, Helen. 1968. 'Patients sans everything'. *Guardian*, 15 July.

Howard, Anthony. 1979. *Selections from the Diaries of a Cabinet Minister.* California: Hamilton.

Howe, Geoffrey. 1994. *Conflict of Loyalty.* London: Macmillan.

Howe, Geoffrey. 1999. 'The management of public inquiries'. *Political Quarterly*, 70, 295–304.

Jackson, John. 1968. '*Sans Everything* hospitals cleared'. *Sun*, 10 July.

Jeger, Lena. 2004. 'Robinson, Sir Kenneth (1911–1996)'. *Oxford Dictionary of National Biography.* http://www.oxforddnb.com, accessed 15 February 2016.

Leamington Spa Reporter. 1967. 'Call for action over crowded hospitals'. *Times*, 18 March.
Lowe, Rodney. 1999. *The Welfare State in Britain Since 1945*. Houndmills: Macmillan Press.
Martin, John (and Evans, Debbie). 1984. *Hospitals in Trouble*. Oxford: Blackwell.
Martin, John and Walshe, Kieran. 2003. *Inquiries: Learning from Failure in the NHS?*. London: Nuffield Trust.
Mathers, James. 1968. 'Old people in hospital.' *BMJ*, iii, 374.
Mind, 'Achievements'. www.mind.org.uk, accessed 11 March 2016.
MIND. 1973. *Psychogeriatric Services—The Questions Answered*. London: MIND.
Ministry of Health. 1961. *Report for the Year 1960. Part II: On the State of the Public Health*. Cmnd. 1550. London: HMSO, 1961.
Ministry of Health. 1962. *A Hospital Plan for England and Wales*. Cmnd. 1604. London: HMSO.
Ministry of Health. 1963. *Health and Welfare: The Development of Community Care: Plans for the Health and Welfare Services of the Local Authorities in England and Wales*. Cmnd. 1973. London: HMSO.
Ministry of Health. 1966. *Methods of Dealing with Complaints of atients*. HM (66) 15. London: HMSO.
Ministry of Health. 1968a. *Findings and Recommendations following Enquiries into Allegations Concerning the Care of Elderly Patients in Certain Hospitals*. Cmnd. 3687. London: HMSO.
Ministry of Health. 1968b. *Report of a Committee of Inquiry into the Circumstances Leading to a Fire at Shelton Hospital on the Night of 25th to 26th February 1968, and to the Deaths of 24 Patients*. London: HMSO.
Ministry of Health. 1968c. *The Administrative Structure of the Medical and Related Services in England and Wales*. London: HMSO.
Mold, Alex. 2012. 'Patients' rights and the National Health Service in Britain, 1960s–1980s'. *American Journal of Public Health*, 102, 2030–2038.
Mulcahy, Linda. 2003. *Disputing Doctors: The Socio-Legal Dynamics of Complaints About Medical Care*. Berkshire: Open University Press.
NAMH. 1969. *Annual Report. 1968–1969*. London: NAMH.
NHS. 1972. *Annual Report of the Hospital Advisory Service to the Secretary of State for Social Services and the Secretary of State for Wales for the Year 1971*. London: HMSO.
NHS. 1974. *Annual Report of the Hospital Advisory Service to the Secretary of State for Social Services and Secretary of State for Wales for the Year 1974*. London: HMSO.
NHS Improvement and NHS England. 2016. *Freedom to Speak up: Raising Concerns (Whistleblowing) Policy for the NHS*. https://improvement.nhs.uk, accessed 8 October 2016.

Nirje, Bengt. 1969. "The normalisation principle and its human management implications' 19–23. In *Changing Patterns in Residential Services for the Mentally Retarded*, eds. R. Kugel and W. Wolfensberger. Washington, DC: President's Committee on Mental Retardation.

Nolan, Peter. 1998. *A History of Mental Health Nursing*. Cheltenham: Stanley Thornes.

OECD (Organisation for Economic Co-operation and Development). 2011. 'Health expenditure as a share of GDP, 1960–2009, selected OECD countries'. http://dx.doi.org/10.1787/888932523215, accessed 1 February 2016.

Osman, Arthur. 1968. 'Vital lapse in hospital fire warning'. *Times*, 17 December.

Rawstorne, Philip. 1968. 'Inquiry clears hospitals of cruelty to old'. *Guardian*, 10 July.

Robb, Barbara. 1967. *Sans Everything: A Case to Answer*. London: Nelson.

Robb, Barbara. 1969. 'Detecting those sins of the health service'. *Daily Telegraph*, 18 June.

Robb, Barbara. 1970. 'Sans Everything'. *Daily Telegraph*, 12 April.

Robinson. Anne. 1969. 'Nurse goes after whipping'. *Sunday Times*, 26 January.

Robinson, Anne. 1970.'Whitewash in the old folks' wards'. *Sunday Times*, 5 April.

Robinson, Kenneth. 1958. *Policy for Mental Health*. London: Fabian Society.

Rolph, Cecil. 1987. *Further Particulars*. Oxford: OUP.

Rolph, C.H. 1968. 'Whiter-than-white paper'. *New Statesman*, 19 July.

Roper, John. 1968a. 'Call for hospital ombudsman'. *Times*, 27 May.

Roper, John. 1968b. 'Hospitals cleared of cruelty'. *Times*, 10 July.

Roper, John. 1969. 'Nurse XY's complaints of ill-treatment and irregularities at a hospital upheld by committee of inquiry'. *Times*, 28 March.

Roper, John. 1972 'Health service ombudsman'. *Times*, 22 January.

Roxan, David. 1967. '"Old folk beaten in hospital" allegation'. *News of the World*, 25 June.

Royal Commission on the Law Relating to Mental Illness and Mental Deficiency 1954–1957. Cmnd. 169. 1957. London: HMSO.

Sandison, Ronald. 2001. *A Century of Psychiatry, Psychotherapy and Group Analysis*. London: Jessica Kingsley.

Seebohm Report. See DHSS 1968.

Sheard, Sally. 2014. *The Passionate Economist*. Bristol: Policy Press.

Shearer, Ann. 1968. 'Dirty children in a locked room: A mental hospital on a bad day'. *Guardian*, 28 March.

Shearer, Ann. 1976. 'The news media' 109–118. In *Changing Patterns of Residential Services for the Mentally Retarded*, eds. Robert Kugel and Ann Shearer. Washington, DC: President's Committee on Mental Retardation.

Squire, Kingsley. 1969. '"Worst ward I've ever seen": hospital shocks minister'. *Daily Express*, 7 August.

Staff Reporter, 1968. 'Minister under fire on "cruel hospitals" probe'. *Observer*, 14 July.
Turner, R. and Roberts, G. 1992. 'The Worcester Development Project'. *British Journal of Psychiatry*, 160, 103–107.
WDS. 1979. 'AM Spencer'. *BMJ*, ii, 1718.
Webster, Charles. 1998. *The National Health Service: A Political History*. Oxford: OUP.
Welsh Office. 1967. *Report of the Tribunal Appointed to Inquire into the Disaster at Aberfan on October 21st 1966*. HL 316, HC 553. 1967. London: HMSO.
Whitehead, Anthony. 1965. 'A comprehensive psychogeriatric service'. *Lancet*, ii, 583–586.
Whitehead, Tony. 1970. 'Hospital Commissioner'. *Lancet*, i, 774.
Whitehead, Tony. 1971. 'Fitness to plead and fitness to be a victim'. *Lancet*, i, 234.
Wilkinson, James. 1968. 'Hospital old folk are not treated badly'. *Daily Express*, 10 July.
World in Action. 1968. *Ward F13*, Granada Television, 21 May. https://www.youtube.com, accessed 2 October 2016.
Young, Hugo. 1968. 'Nothing to be smug about in the plight of the aged sick'. *Sunday Times*, 14 July.

Open Access This chapter is licensed under the terms of the Creative Commons Attribution 4.0 International License (http://creativecommons.org/licenses/by/4.0/), which permits use, sharing, adaptation, distribution and reproduction in any medium or format, as long as you give appropriate credit to the original author(s) and the source, provide a link to the Creative Commons license and indicate if changes were made.

The images or other third party material in this chapter are included in the book's Creative Commons license, unless indicated otherwise in a credit line to the material. If material is not included in the book's Creative Commons license and your intended use is not permitted by statutory regulation or exceeds the permitted use, you will need to obtain permission directly from the copyright holder.

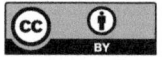

CHAPTER 8

Then and Now: Concluding Remarks

In the 1960s, health and social care authorities generally ignored research indicating that accurate psychiatric diagnosis and proper treatment, in hospital and in the community, could improve the well-being of older people and reduce the need for long-term institutional care. The research findings contradicted time-honoured teaching and widespread assumptions about decline rather than recovery in old age. Most of the medical profession lacked interest, the public rarely demanded improvements, and the government, which had other priorities and feared an insurmountable 'burden' of more older people living longer, did not allocate resources to meet needs. These factors contributed to poor-quality care and overcrowding in the psychiatric hospital back wards. The AEGIS (Aid for the Elderly in Government Institutions) campaign, led by Barbara Robb, brought the situation to the fore.

These concluding remarks draw together aspects of the AEGIS campaign and Barbara's work. They also touch on the significant role of women in the campaign, the last years of Barbara's life, and AEGIS's legacy for twenty-first century health and social care policy and practice.

The AEGIS Campaign

The AEGIS campaign developed in response to Barbara's and Strabolgi's anguish about the care Amy Gibbs received in Friern Hospital and dissatisfaction with official responses to their complaints. The Ministry could have dealt with many of their criticisms about standards of care early on, when it received the 'Diary of a Nobody' or after Barbara's meeting with Tooth, but a bureaucratic, defensive and self-justifying culture militated against this. The NHS administrative hierarchy was secretive, hostile to criticism, and sometimes deceitful, exemplified by the Friern Hospital Management Committee disregarding independent research about the adequacy of hospital staffing, the Regional Hospital Board (RHB) ignoring the Blofeld Report, and Kenneth Robinson announcing that *Findings and Recommendations* concluded 'very favourably' about standards of care provided.

During the AEGIS campaign, patterns emerged of disrespectful ill-treatment towards older, chronically mentally ill and 'subnormal' people in long-stay hospital wards. Practices that patients, visitors and new staff perceived as cruel included slapping, teasing, rough handling, undignified bathing, lack of privacy and deprivation of personal possessions. Overcrowding and understaffing were associated with time saving, sometimes harsh, methods, which nurses perceived as legitimate. Unkind practices were also founded on out-of-date knowledge, and negative attitudes towards patients. Staff rarely intended harm.

Patterns also emerged about the author-witnesses and other whistleblowers. Most were new to the hospital, idealistic about the well-being of their patients, and lacked formal health service–related professional qualifications. Some who were new to nursing in middle age probably worked below their potential in terms of their personal and intellectual ability. The authorities did not address the issues that they raised and harassment by colleagues led some to resign.

Similar to the attitudes within the NHS, the *Sans Everything* committees of inquiry were hostile towards the author-witnesses, discrediting their evidence as false, unreliable or exaggerated. They based their perceptions on the witnesses' status and presumed character, rather than impartially evaluating the material presented to them. They grounded their decisions on standards set by the senior staff who they were judging, rather than on independent sources about clinical practice. Some ignored, or were unaware of, recent recommendations about NHS complaint management, and they lacked professional experience of investigating statutory bodies who neglected their responsibilities to the detriment of the public. Overall, their evaluation of the evidence was flawed. Their conclusions revealed their stereotypical assumptions about nurses, older people, mental illness and the excellence of the NHS. The Council on

Tribunals and the events at Ely, Whittingham, Farleigh and South Ockendon highlighted many shortcomings of the *Sans Everything* inquiries, casting doubt on the conclusions drawn from them.

In the complex field of health service policy development, AEGIS was only part of the process, albeit a significant one. AEGIS contributed by identifying issues and suggesting answers, stirring up public and professional support, pressurising the government and persisting until it took action. Helped by the media and idealistic social-rights investigative journalists and editors, Barbara's frankness jolted the conscience of people who already knew about inadequacies on the back wards but had failed to take action and those to whom the revelations were new. Robinson and Hackett regarded the press as primarily aiming to improve the circulation of their newspapers, and Barbara as wanting to sell copies of *Sans Everything*. They disregarded the sincerity of AEGIS and its supporters, and ignored the sense of justice that motivated them. It is a credit to the media that they sustained their interest. This helped overcome the normal human tendency to disengage with unappealing and distressing subjects and helped maintain public, professional and political awareness at levels that could produce constructive debate about policy change.

Through its psychiatric advisors, Barton, Whitehead and Enoch, AEGIS fed into the process of developing proactive, non-custodial, comprehensive psychogeriatric services and the Royal College of Psychiatrists' Group for the Psychiatry of Old Age (GPOA). Psychogeriatricians introduced best clinical practice and continued to lobby NHS authorities to resource proactive and effective community and hospital mental health services for older people. AEGIS also advocated for improvements in long-stay NHS hospitals more broadly, and thus contributed to establishing the Hospital Advisory Service, a NHS ombudsman and more effective complaints procedures. These encouraged the NHS to improve services, and promoted strategies to deal with criticism, including transparent and balanced investigations that could result in corrective action if necessary. AEGIS helped develop guidance to manage violence in hospitals and stimulated nurses to examine their practices and terms of employment. It also helped inspire voluntary organisations, such as the National Association for Mental Health (NAMH), to adopt less apologetic and more assertive campaigning roles.

In contrast to the dissonant relationship between Barbara and Robinson, Barbara and Crossman saw eye-to-eye about the need to make improvements. Crossman, assisted particularly by Abel-Smith,

Baker and Howe, contributed to AEGIS achieving its objectives. Following up on Crossman's plans, Keith Joseph (1972, p. v) acknowledged that NHS acute physical illness hospitals previously had 'legitimate priority', but stated that the Department of Health and Social Security (DHSS) now intended to improve health services for people with chronic disorders. How far and how fast these proposals materialised, to provide effective services which met needs, merits further study.

AEGIS operated relentlessly from 1965 until 1974, and then modestly until Barbara's death two years later. AEGIS existed only because of Barbara, but she did not function in isolation. She did not try to create a large organisation, and there is no evidence that she or AEGIS trained a successor to take over her role. AEGIS remained small, elite and financially and organisationally independent. Independence ensured that Barbara could be forthright and publicly outspoken, more than academics, nurses, doctors, lawyers and politicians who might jeopardise their reputation and future livelihood by doing so. When Barbara Castle invited Barbara Robb to join the Central Health Services Council, an advisory body to the DHSS, Barbara Robb and the AEGIS advisors agreed that: 'AEGIS functions best as a totally independent body, and has the best hope of being of service to the Secretaries of State and to the public by continuing in that capacity.'[1]

Reflections on Barbara

Jung, White, Robinson and Crossman could not quite fathom Barbara out. Jung wrote 'She decidedly leaves you guessing'; White did not know quite how to 'deal with' her;[2] and Robinson and Crossman both described her as 'strange'.[3] Journalist Anne Robinson said that politicians 'really didn't know the beast they were battling with. They totally underestimated her'.[4] To a degree, she was the 'misunderstood genius' of Jung's 'intuitive introvert' personality type (Jung (1923) 1971, pp. 401-402). She was able to engage with people in all social classes and to treat them as partners in her campaign. Her psychotherapy skills helped them express their concerns and ideas, to which she paid the utmost attention.[5] People who worked with Barbara, such as the author-witnesses, were intensely loyal to her. Barbara also had her faith, which was central to her life and work,[6] and Brian (Fig. 8.1) supported her emotionally and helped practically with cooking and domestic tasks, enabling her to lead AEGIS (Allen 1967).

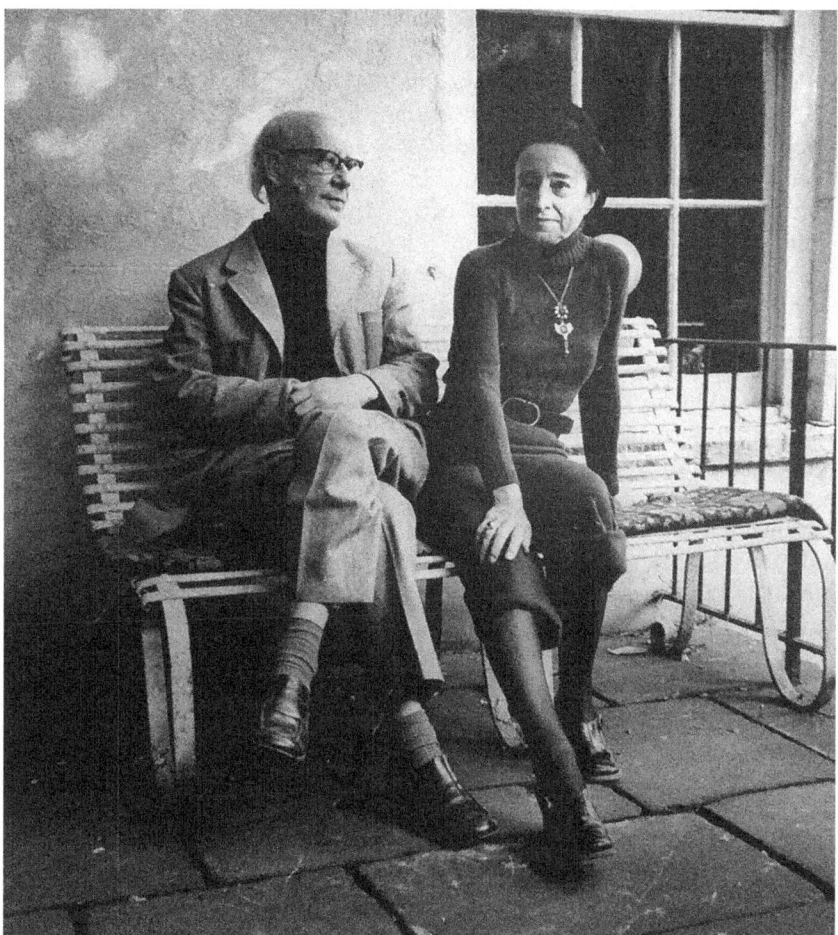

Fig. 8.1 Barbara and Brian Robb, c.1972. Reproduced courtesy of Elizabeth Ellison-Anne.

Harvey (1976) attributed Barbara's ability to command, and to work as an equal in elite ranks of society without feeling intimidated, to her upper-class background. She fought politically, went to the top and inspired individuals and organisations. She would not be thwarted by officialdom. Barbara's determination, self-confidence, skills and sense of justice antagonised the authorities who described her as a 'bloody nuisance' (Rolph 1987, p. 182). Barbara described her campaign style (Anon. 1976): 'I'm better suited to Walls of Jericho than to Trojan Horse tactics.' The *Sunday Times* described her extraordinary drive and her punishing schedule, twelve hours a day, six days a week, including acting as counsellor to 'hundreds of distressed nurses'[7] and responding personally to a constant stream of correspondence. AEGIS's address list comprised 1,600 names by 1973.[8]

Anne Allen (1967) compared Barbara to notable forebears, such as Lord Shaftsbury and Florence Nightingale: 'When everyone else accepted, as facts of life, women working down mines, parents having the right to beat their children, or soldiers dying for lack of good nursing, one person condemned—and won.' Unlike her forebears, public, political and personal factors contributed to Barbara being largely forgotten, despite the role she played in overcoming abusive practices and shaping health policy. Public and political factors included Robinson discrediting *Sans Everything*, the Ely Inquiry overshadowing it and Barbara being eclipsed by people more formally prominent, and career-wise determined to be so, within government and political circles. Personal factors included Barbara pursuing her campaign rather than personal recognition, her move to behind-the-scenes lobbying after 1970 and her and Brian's untimely deaths. Rolph discussed with Barbara her intention to write a book about AEGIS and *Sans Everything*, but there was no time to do so during her campaign,[9] and her death, while still in the middle of her work, precluded it. Some people recognised Barbara's achievements in her lifetime. Strabolgi, in 1969, suggested 'an award of some kind' for her, and discussed this with Brian. Brian replied to Strabolgi that Barbara had refused two similar proposals and that she would not accept this one because 'the attainment of her objectives is so incomplete.'[10] Barbara Castle wrote to her in 1974: 'Dear Barbara,... You can feel proud at the outcome of all your efforts. Yours, Barbara.'[11] For all Barbara Robb's objectives to be moving towards fulfilment by the time she died was remarkable.

WOMEN AND THE AEGIS CAMPAIGN

In the 1960s, the women's movement tended to focus on young women. Campaigning related mainly to employment, welfare rights, pay, taxation and women's control of childbearing (McCarthy 2010, pp. 109-110). It overlooked the needs of the oldest and most dependent women. It would require more research to be conclusive about whether sexism contributed to the neglect of older people on back wards, who were mainly women with no financial means, and underprovision of alternative community social support for them.

Among women of working age, relatively few walked the paths of power in government, in the health service or in journalism. Many who were idealistic, and had the means and the time, worked voluntarily for the betterment of society. Thus, in some ways, Barbara worked within the framework expected of her class and generation. Looking after people was considered women's work, and this probably reflected the forty or so women who contributed significantly to the AEGIS narrative. Some worked as volunteers, and others were paid, but the content of their jobs, either of their own choice or offered to them by employers, exemplified the traditional female caring role relocated to the public arena. Examples are Helen Hodgson, Mary Applebey, Ann Blofeld and Yvonne Cross. In the days when female journalists on national newspapers were rare, male editors would allocate them the health and welfare stories, in line with social expectations about their gender, a tacit sexism. At the *Guardian*, if 'they needed somebody to cover a bed-pan story... where did their eyes go, you can do that Ann,' recollected Shearer.[12] Thus three female journalists on national newspapers—Anne Allen, Anne Robinson and Ann Shearer—reported on psychiatric hospitals. Similar to Barbara and the *Sans Everything* witnesses (male and female), they experienced hostility, personal criticism and attempts by NHS authorities to intimidate them in the course of their reporting about *Sans Everything*, Harperbury and South Ockendon.[13]

Barbara's appearance was startling, as the men-folk discussed with emotional overtones and in ways that could have affected their working relationships with her. Jung described Barbara as 'an eyeful and beyond!' and White called her 'quite a corker'.[14] Rolph described in his memoir asking Crossman whether Barbara impressed him: 'Impressed?' Crossman responded, 'Have you seen the hats she wears?' In Rolph's opinion (1987, p. 183): 'Even if it were possible to forget Barbara, it would not be possible to forget those extraordinary, carefully chosen, and obviously expensive hats, with which she seemed to transmute every occasion into a kind of one-woman Ascot.' Women also commented on Barbara's appearance and manner, but in ways that were more factual and related to her role. Anne Robinson described her appearance: 'immaculately dressed with the makeup and the hair.... with quite long black skirts, and a rather good cashmere roll neck sweater.... She was charming, and exotic in a way.'[15] Harvey (1976) commented that Barbara 'must have been the most elegant of hospital researchers, the most tender and the sharpest eyed'. Despite being 'tender', Barbara openly admitted that she could 'cut up rough' especially if she thought officials were obstructing her (Robb 1967, p. 83).

More overt than sex discrimination in the course of the AEGIS campaign, was arrogance from those in authority, bordering on bullying, related to designated status within the NHS hierarchy. Men and women who challenged higher tiers of staff in the hospitals, RHBs or the Ministry, were disparaged almost automatically. Although this was particularly common for staff without formal qualifications, seniority did not protect a critic. The authorities ostracised Barton, for example, despite being a male medical superintendent. Being a peer did not protect Strabolgi from Robinson reprimanding him for his speech in 1965, and a senior Home Office civil servant ominously challenged Rolph about his involvement with AEGIS without further explanation: 'Why are you signing letters for AEGIS?... you've no idea the trouble there is going to be about that business.'[16]

AFTER AUGUST 1974

Barbara's page-to-a-day desk diary suddenly stopped in August 1974. A note sent to the telephone-diversion answering service that she usually used when on holiday read: 'Please explain that AEGIS is temporarily closed down but hopes to re-open in October, organised on a rather different basis.'[17] Her diary began to fill again at the beginning of November, but never regained its sense of busy-ness.

In the last few months of her life, Barbara began to sort her archive (Cochrane 1990, p. 26). At the end of her life Brian cared for her at home, with the help of a nurse (a black woman who was also an opera singer) and Henrietta Charlton, her niece and god-daughter.[18] Barbara died on 21 June 1976, age sixty-four. A service took place at St Mary's Catholic Church, Hampstead. Barbara was cremated and her ashes were deposited in the Anne family cemetery at Burghwallis where a modest stone commemorates her. Her epitaph reads: 'Fearless champion of the cause of old people in hospitals.' An obituary appeared in the *Hampstead and Highgate Express* (Anon. 1976) and Harvey (1976) wrote one in the *Times*. She attributed Barbara's success to 'a mind free from academic restraints, to a gift for witty and trenchant expression, to upper class nerve, Yorkshire doggedness, an inbuilt Catholic faith, and above all, a near perfect marriage to Brian.'

Brian wrote, illustrated and published two children's stories, *My Grandmother's Djinn* (1976) and *The Last of the Centaurs* (1979). Both are allegories about Barbara's work to rectify unethical situations. *My Grandmother's Djinn* is an adventure about the rescue of a single 'victim', a djinn or genie in a bottle, by 'Ursula' (Barbara) assisted by the narrator (Brian) and a small band of helpers. They faced challenges and obstacles demanding determination, kindness, insight and ingenuity, ultimately rescuing hundreds more djinns from imprisonment in bottles. The symbolism is clear: Barbara's work to rescue one person, Amy Gibbs, achieved much wider and lasting outcomes (Fig. 8.2). Illustrations of Ursula show her with two long dark plaits, as Barbara wore her hair in childhood (Figs. 8.3 and 8.4). In *The Last of the Centaurs* (1979) Barbara is represented by Ursula and Achilles, a centaur. Achilles, disguised as a horse, won the Epsom Derby in an escapade to support Ursula's impoverished uncle who had lost his job due to a boss who would not listen. Brian, as narrator, wrote:

> It aroused in her mind a sequence of ideas that was eventually to carry the day. The first inklings of these came when one morning I saw her retire, with a bundle of newspapers, some paint and some paste, up into the attic. But I quite failed to guess their significance, and merely thought how odd it seemed for her to fritter away her time...
>
> Later I was to feel ashamed to have so much misjudged her...
> She had always been something of a loner...
> For though the victory was due entirely to Achilles... I received an undeserved measure of praise, and must confess that I enjoyed my share of the glory.

Brian was devastated after Barbara died and then had to cope with his own disabling neurological disorder.[19] Quentin Blake, who visited him in the institution where he was cared for, recalled that even when confused, his conversation was more interesting than most other people's most of the time.[20] Brian died in 1979. His name shares Barbara's memorial stone at Burghwallis, with the epitaph 'A painter of distinction'.

Relevance to Current Practice

Since the 1960s, many positive changes have taken place in health and social care provision for mentally and physically unwell older people. Proactive treatment and rehabilitation services exist across the NHS.

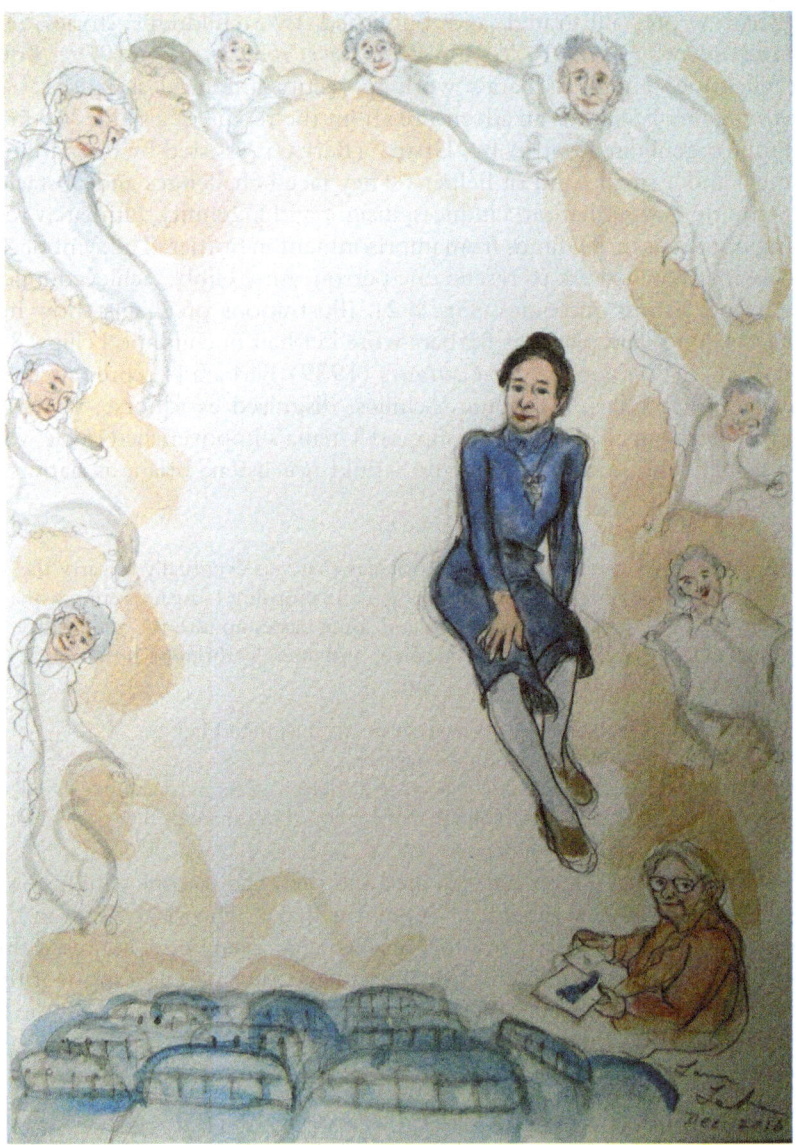

Fig. 8.2 'Older women, djinns and beds' by Laura Lehman, 2016, inspired by *Ward F13*, photographs of Barbara and Amy, and Brian Robb's illustrations. Ursula first rescued her grandmother's djinn and Barbara first rescued Amy. Both ultimately achieved much wider and lasting outcomes, freeing many more from overcrowded, custodial and undignified conditions.

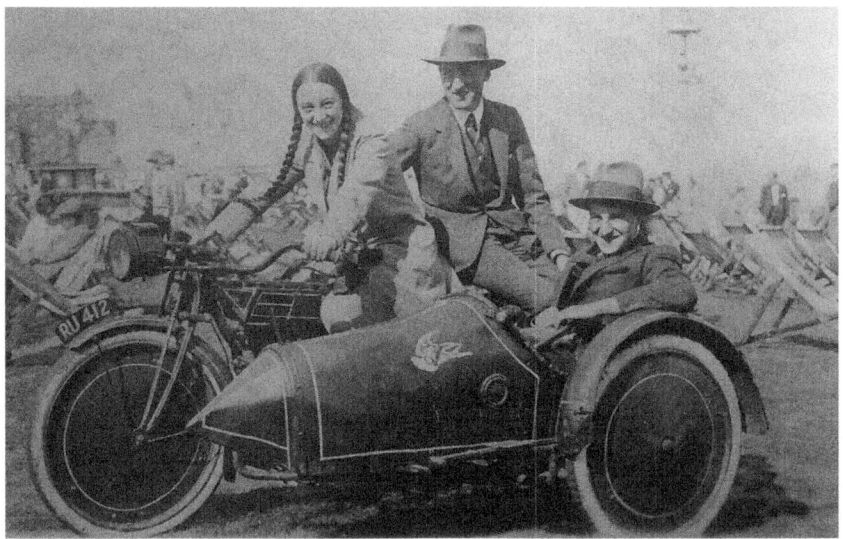

Fig. 8.3 Barbara in the driving seat: at the seaside with her father George and brother Michael, 1928. Reproduced courtesy of Elizabeth Ellison-Anne.

People who might have been resident in psychiatric hospital back wards in the 1960s today live either in their own homes, despite disability and frailty, or in a myriad of mainly privately run care homes. Standards of care still vary, from very bad to very good, whether in care homes, general hospitals or the person's own home. In Bergmann's view (2009, p. 62), 'if one wants to sum up the difference between the old psychiatric hospital scandals and nowadays it's sweeping it under one big carpet or hundreds of small rugs'. In terms of providing adequate NHS resources to create and run services, mental illness lags behind physical illness (Hilton 2016) and psychiatric services for older people lag behind those for younger people (Hilton 2012a, 2012b). Mental health provision for older people today aims to be evidence based, rehabilitative, dignified and humane, as AEGIS sought to achieve. The GPOA, now a Faculty, and its members throughout the NHS and beyond, collaborate with government bodies, local authorities, care homes, voluntary organisations and other health service disciplines, aiming to achieve high standards.

Angie Ash's (2014) study of scandals of care since 2010 found alarming similarities to *Sans Everything*, including ageist attitudes, underresourced

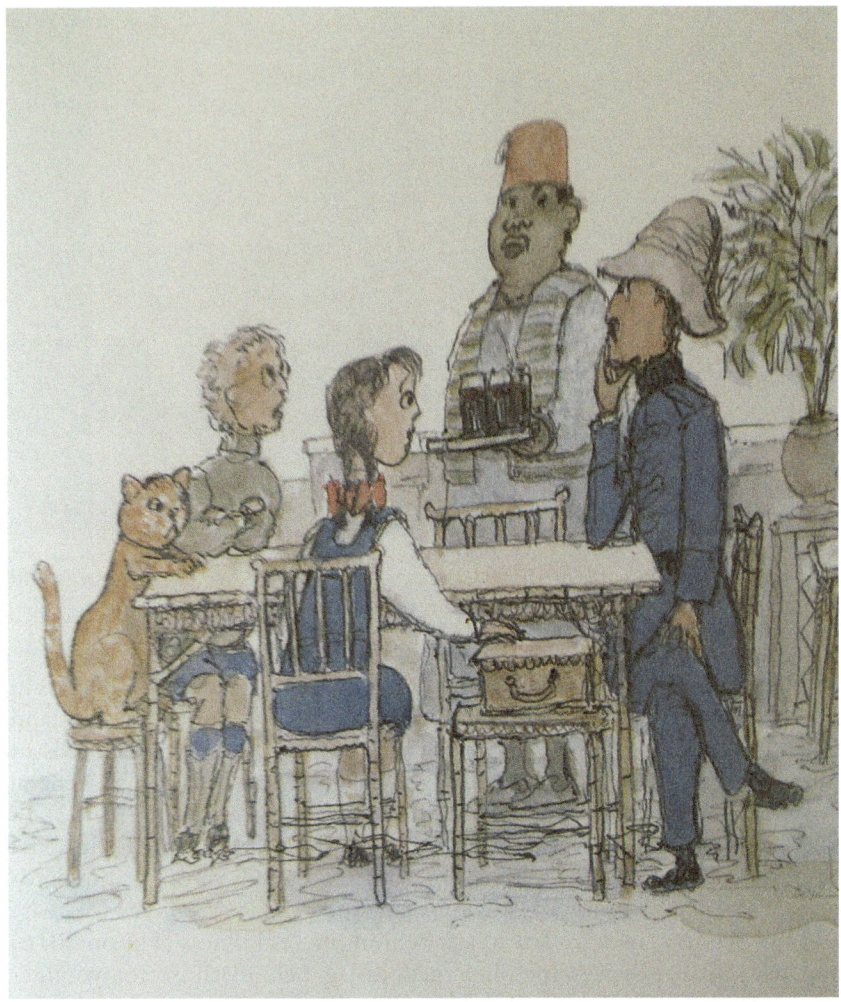

Fig. 8.4 'Ursula', with long plaits, by Brian Robb. Originally published in *My Grandmother's Djinn* (London: André Deutsch, 1976). Copyright: Carlton Books Ltd holds the rights for the *book* but was unable to ascertain if it holds the rights to the *images*. Presumed orphan work.

and target-driven services, and organisational cultures of blame and scapegoating. Harsh treatment of whistle-blowers recurs, as does institutional secrecy about bad practice. Examples of these occurred at a hospital in Carlisle (1996–2000), a sequence of events uncomfortably reminiscent of the 1960s. An internal report identified low standards of care, including tying elderly patients to commodes, forcing them to eat while restrained, and staff washing their genitals with a flannel later used to clean their face. The report was concealed from the hospital's senior management. Student nurses who helped expose the abuse were disciplined and pilloried by staff, while some accused staff 'received a lot of support from colleagues', similar to the events at Farleigh Hospital. In Carlisle, the subsequent inquiry found 'degrading—even cruel—practices', vindicating the students (Herbert and Laurance 2000). The National NHS Staff Survey (2015) included three questions concerning 'unsafe' clinical practice: would staff know how to report concerns (86 percent answered yes), feel secure in raising them (70 percent 'agree' or 'strongly agree') and be confident that their organisation would address them (56 percent 'agree' or 'strongly agree')? Similar to the questions the *Nursing Mirror* asked its readership in 1967, the responses indicate that difficulties still exist for staff who observe, or who are expected to carry out, practices that disturb them. Victimisation of activists who criticise the NHS in the course of seeking improvement still happens. Local people accused Julie Bailey, a patient's relative who led the Stafford Hospital campaign 'Cure the NHS' (2007–2013), of lying and wanting to close the hospital rather than improve it, even after a public inquiry revealed gross failings (Anon. 2013, 2014). Similar to findings by AEGIS, the Parliamentary and Health Service Ombudsman (2015) reported that patients over sixty-five often did not know how to raise concerns or were too scared to complain about their care, fearing negative consequences. Chris Smyth (2015) reported in the *Times* that 'The NHS gets away with complacency because people are so grateful for their care.' In Barbara's time, undercover newspaper journalists worked in hospitals and exposed callous and harsh treatment. In 2014, covert television journalists revealed similar inhumanities (Panorama 2014).

Barton (1967, p. ix) stated that complaints and criticisms 'may cause management... to embark on over cautious supervising'. Tighter monitoring and control is often employed in an attempt to raise standards, but it has drawbacks. In 1960s psychiatric hospitals rigid hierarchical management and strict obedience to seniors had damaging effects. Similar problems occur today when NHS staff are expected to conform to strict clinical protocols or 'care pathways'. Many pathways were created idealistically, but rigid interpretation means that they can become associated with unthinking, mechanistic practice that can detract from individual, person-centred care, demotivate staff and stifle creativity. Top-down monitoring means that it is difficult for staff to deviate from pathways deemed to be correct, even if they do not fit with an individual's care needs (Department of Health 2013). Thus some hospital and care home regimes are uncomfortably close to the mechanistic and task-driven care on the back wards in the 1960s, with accompanying risks of objectifying and dehumanising the person requiring care.

Other difficulties identified by AEGIS related to overcrowding and understaffing, problems that reemerge in modified forms. Today the NHS has fewer beds, associated with rapid throughput, with some patients being discharged before they are sufficiently well. This is less visible than excessive numbers of beds on a ward but is nevertheless a pernicious form of overcrowding, in time rather than in space. In particular, managers take pride in rapid patient throughput and may assume incorrectly that discharge indicates adequate and effective treatment in a shorter time, and therefore a lower financial cost. If staffing levels have not increased in line with the demands caused by shorter admissions, staff under pressure may work too fast for the patient's comfort, with insufficient time to give patients explanations for the care or treatment they require. Staff may inadvertently tolerate rough handling, undignified and untherapeutic care, and cause patients unnecessary distress. A report from the public services trades union UNISON (2015, p. 7) commented on dangerously low ward staffing levels associated with management inaction, and it highlighted complacency about achieving satisfactory standards. UNISON stated: '62% of respondents who had had a nursing "red-flag" [unsafe staffing level] event occur on their ward said that the ward was not immediately allocated additional staff.' Not only was the 'red-flag' unremedied, but managers' unresponsiveness linked to the risk of future underreporting of difficulties because staff lacked confidence that the process would achieve the desired outcome. This risks inadequacies being accepted as normal, irremediable or 'the best under the circumstances', linking to low standards, as happened in the psychiatric hospitals.

Today, most care homes are small, modern and well equipped, and facilities suggest that residents receive dignified care. As the scandals of Farleigh and South Ockendon demonstrated, the size and the modernity of the buildings did not relate to the standards within them. The physical environment in 2017 is usually good, but as Barton commented, there is the risk that superficial inspections assume that an obviously pleasant environment equates with good care. Recent investigations into small, modern homes have identified uncaring and dangerous practices, such as slapping residents, ignoring their calls for help and unsafe management of medication, hydration and nutrition (e.g., West Sussex 2014). On inspection days—in 2016 by the Care Quality Commission—staff are carefully briefed in advance and all is well prepared, as Barbara described at Friern and Davie at Storthes Hall. The pros and cons of announced and unannounced inspections merit further historical consideration to inform contemporary debate.

NHS hospitals today provide only short-term in-patient treatment and usually have active departments of geriatric medicine and 'mental health services for older people', (formerly psychogeriatrics). However, standards of care can still drop, as demonstrated by the Mid Staffordshire Inquiry (2013). Patients of all ages were affected at Stafford Hospital, but the report specifically mentioned older people, including that basic standards of care were not met: 'No patient should be expected to tolerate the neglect and assault on their dignity that some were exposed to' (p. 1370). It recommended: 'Much of what needs to be done does not require additional financial resources, but changes in attitudes, culture, values and behaviour' (p. 1499). Recommendations since the 1960s for tackling inadequate care have been broadly similar: increasing staff levels, more training, improving supervision and inspection processes, and aiming to change institutional culture. These are important, and much has improved, although there is less evidence that fundamental attitudes have changed. In Martin's view (1984, p. 246), 'The bedrock on which the quality of care depends consists of staff and the ethics which motivate and guide them.' Tasks may be taught successfully through traditional practical training, but it is less easy to teach ethics, compassion or kindness in that way or to ensure that staff can effectively manage their emotional responses when stressed or when looking after behaviourally challenging patients. For staff to become more aware of their behaviours and responses, which they may regard uncomfortably as failings, requires thought, tact and reflection, not just knowledge of what ought to be done. This is important, especially for staff working with dependent, frail older people, confused due to delirium or dementia, who may unknowingly be irritating, repetitive, aggressive, ungrateful, demanding or physically unpleasant. If the older person's behaviours are interpreted as deliberate, staff are more likely to adopt punitive or demeaning ways of managing them, such as at Storthes Hall by the nurse who said he was treating rather than punishing a patient or at St Lawrence's when floor-cleaning soap was used to wash patients. Hands-on staff need the ability to recognise, and confidence to discuss, their negative and positive feelings towards patients. Senior staff need to listen and support. In conjunction with top-down approaches, more bottom-up opportunities for hands-on staff, in the form of discussion about ethics, morals, attitudinal and emotional aspects of workplace challenges, might help prevent unacceptable practices and recurrence of scandal.

It was apparent in *Sans Everything* that people new to the hospital and with minimal formal training often had the greatest insights into the humanity and quality of the care provided. Students may be particularly innovative, creative and idealistic, not yet having been conditioned to the views that their profession is *meant* to hold. The 'new eyes' effect is underutilised in the NHS. New staff are the least likely to be asked their views about standards of practice. It might be valuable if their feedback could be sought, preferably face to face, and if necessary by a member of staff in a different department, taking into account ongoing insecurities about criticising the authorities.

Barbara's work significantly influenced change for the better in hospital practice and NHS policy in the 1960s and 1970s, but inadequate care in the twenty-first century still requires rectifying. Recurrence of scandal does not invalidate the importance of her work, or that of other social reformers. Fry did not solve all the problems in prisons, nor Nightingale all those of nursing. Wilberforce and Shaftsbury would still have work to do today, such as dealing with modern slavery and people trafficking, exploited migrant workers, minimum wages and zero hours contracts. The nature of the difficulties in all these contexts centres round the imbalance of power between those in authority and others who are more vulnerable, for mental, physical, social, political or other reasons, thus risking exploitation, neglect or abuse. To a degree that had not been achieved previously, all the pioneers broke the chain of officialdom that overlooked or ignored inhumane practices. None of the pioneers provided all the answers, but each made crucial, pivotal contributions, consequently relieving much suffering and raising public awareness, with the potential to inform future eventualities.

Barbara's grandfather Ernest told her as a child, 'when you see somebody needing help—help him', do not be a bystander to human suffering. Barbara illuminated the happenings on the back wards and broke through a conspiracy of silence about them. Her sense of justice, and her determination—*Sans Varier*—to make improvements, enthused many people during her lifetime, including doctors, nurses, journalists, academics, politicians and the author-witnesses. Her personal story is inspiring and lessons from her campaign remain pertinent. Fifty years since *Sans Everything* and forty years since Barbara died, it is rightful to recognise her place in history.

Notes

1. Letter, Robb to Hedley, 30 April 1974, AEGIS/1/10/D (AEGIS archive, London School of Economics).
2. Letters, Jung and White, 21 September and 7 October 1951 (in Lammers and Cunningham 2007).
3. Kenneth Robinson, interviewed by Margot Jeffreys, 1991 (British Library Sound Archive); Crossman Diaries, 16 March 1970, 166/70/SW 116-117 (University of Warwick Modern Records Centre, UWMRC).
4. Anne Robinson, interview by author, 2015.
5. Tape recorded meetings, 11 May and 6 July 1971, AEGIS/4/27.
6. Mamie Charlton, letter, 2015.
7. *Sunday Times*, labelled 12 November 1972 (no title on archived cutting) AEGIS/9/1.
8. List of names and addresses, 1966–1973, AEGIS/9/13 and AEGIS/2/3.
9. Letter, Bill (Rolph) to Robb, 1 April 1968, AEGIS/B/3.
10. Letter, Brian Robb to Strabolgi, 29 October 1969, AEGIS1/10/A.
11. Letter, Castle to Robb, May 1974, AEGIS/1/10/E.
12. Ann Shearer, interview by author, 2015.
13. Anne Robinson, interview by author, 2015.
14. Letters, Jung and White, 21 September and 7 October 1951 (in Lammers and Cunningham 2007).
15. Anne Robinson, interview by author, 2015.
16. Note by Robb, checked and approved by Rolph, 21 March 1974, AEGIS/1/10/D.
17. Letter, Robb to Answering Ltd, 30 July 1974, AEGIS/9/3.
18. Letter, Mamie Charlton to author, 2015; Note, Henrietta (Hinny) Varley to author, 2016.
19. Elizabeth Ellison-Anne, discussion, 2016.
20. Quentin Blake, interview by author, 2016.

Bibliography

Allen, Anne. 1967. 'One woman who refused to pass by..'. *Sunday Mirror*, 9 July.
Anon. 1976. 'The patients' campaigner'. *Hampstead and Highgate Express*, 25 June.
Anon. 2013. 'Stafford Hospital campaigner Julie Bailey to leave "hostile" town'. *BBC News*, 6 June.
Anon. 2014. 'Julie Bailey: NHS campaigner suffers online abuse'. *BBC News*, 2 January.
Ash, Angie. 2014. *Safeguarding Older People from Abuse: Critical Contexts to Policy and Practice*. Bristol: Policy Press.
Barton, Russell. 1967. 'Foreword' ix–xi. In Robb 1967.
Bergmann, Klaus. 2009. In *The Development of Old Age Psychiatry in Britain 1960–1989*, (Guthrie Trust Witness Seminar 2008) ed. Claire Hilton. University of Glasgow. http://www.gla.ac.uk, accessed 18 September 2016.
Cochrane, David. 1990. 'The AEGIS campaign to improve standards of care in mental hospitals: A case study of the process of social policy change'. PhD thesis, University of London. http://etheses.lse.ac.uk, accessed 17 September 2016.
Department of Health. 2013. *More Care, Less Pathway: A Review of the Liverpool Care Pathway*. https://www.gov.uk, accessed 14 April 2016.
Hackett, Maurice. 1968. 'Ill informed, ill considered, and unkind'. *Guardian*, 14 December.
Harvey, Audrey. 1976. 'Mrs Barbara Robb', *Times*, 28 June.
Herbert, Ian and Laurance, Jeremy. 2000. 'Trainee nurses blew the whistle on abuse of elderly patients', *Independent*, 15 November.
Hilton, Claire. 2012a. 'Sans teeth, sans eyes, sans taste, sans everything: resourcing mental health services for older people, a long term view'. *Journal of the Royal Society of Medicine*, 105, 146–150.
Hilton, Claire. 2012b. 'No scope for complacency: observations on the guidance from the Royal College of Psychiatrists on the Equality Act and achieving non-discriminatory, age-appropriate services', *BJPsych Bulletin*, 36, 441–443.
Hilton, Claire. 2016. 'Parity of esteem for mental and physical health care in the United Kingdom: a hundred years war?' *Journal of the Royal Society of Medicine*, 109, 133–137.
Joseph, Keith. 'Foreword' v–vii. In DHSS 1972. *National Health Service Reorganisation. England*. Cmnd. 5055. London: HMSO.
Jung, Carl. (1923) 1971. *Psychological Types*. (translation: H Godwyn Baynes, revised by RFC Hull). New York: Pantheon Books.
Lammers, Ann and Cunningham, Adrian, eds. 2007. *The Jung-White Letters*. London: Routledge.
Martin, John (and Evans, Debbie). 1984. *Hospitals in Trouble*. Oxford: Blackwell.

McCarthy, Helen. 2010. 'Gender equality' 105–123. In *Unequal Britain*, ed. Pat Thane, London: Continuum.
Mid Staffordshire NHS Foundation Trust. 2013. *Mid Staffordshire NHS Foundation Trust Public Inquiry* HC. 947 (Francis Report) London: TSO.
National NHS Staff Survey Co-ordination Centre. 2015. NHS Staff Survey. http://www.nhsstaffsurveys.com, accessed 16 March 2016.
Panorama. 2014. *Behind Closed Doors: Elderly Care Exposed*, BBC1, 30 April.
Parliamentary and Health Service Ombudsman. 2015. *Breaking Down the Barriers*. http://www.ombudsman.org.uk, accessed 10 October 2016.
Robb, Barbara. 1967. *Sans Everything: A Case to Answer*. London: Nelson.
Robb, Brian. 1976. *My Grandmother's Djinn*. London: André Deutsch.
Robb, Brian. 1979. *The Last of the Centaurs*. London: André Deutsch.
Rolph, Cecil. 1987. *Further Particulars*. Oxford: OUP.
Smyth, Chris. 2015. 'Grateful patients unwilling to expose NHS failings'. *Times*, 21 December.
UNISON. 2015. *UNISON's Staffing Level Survey 2015: Red Alert: Unsafe Staffing Levels Rising*. London: Unison.
West Sussex Adult Safeguarding Board. 2014. *Orchid View Serious Case Review*. http://www.westsussex.gov.uk, accessed 17 September 2016.

Open Access This chapter is licensed under the terms of the Creative Commons Attribution 4.0 International License (http://creativecommons.org/licenses/by/4.0/), which permits use, sharing, adaptation, distribution and reproduction in any medium or format, as long as you give appropriate credit to the original author(s) and the source, provide a link to the Creative Commons license and indicate if changes were made.

The images or other third party material in this chapter are included in the book's Creative Commons license, unless indicated otherwise in a credit line to the material. If material is not included in the book's Creative Commons license and your intended use is not permitted by statutory regulation or exceeds the permitted use, you will need to obtain permission directly from the copyright holder.

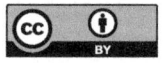

INDEX

A
Abel-Smith, Brian, 3, 8, 81, 84, 99–100, 102, 109–110, 124, 132, 159–160, 222
  chief advisor at DHSS, 202
  and Crossman, 202, 212, 218, 220, 233, 235, 253
  and Harvey, 69, 86
  and Howe, 215, 217–218, 220, 224
  reflection on Barbara Robb, 238
  and Robinson, 108, 232–233
  See also London School of Economics
Aberfan disaster, 148, 160, 165, 215
AEGIS, *see* Aid for the Elderly in Government Institutions
Ageism, 11–12, 261
Age UK
  Age Concern, 14n8, 229
  Help the Aged, 10, 14n8
  National Old People's Welfare Committee, 10
Aid for the Elderly in Government Institutions (AEGIS)
  aims, 11, 97–98, 108–113, 126, 261
  archive, 12, 58, 61, 64, 114

charitable status, 129–130
correspondence, 256
and Ely Inquiry, 162, 201, 214–215, 220
expert advisors, 122–126, 132, 223, 253
finances, 65, 129
independence, 254
letter to *Times*, November 1965, 100–102
libel concerns, 130
and media (radio and television), 151–153, 201, 206
origin and meaning of name, 97
outcomes, 251–254
and press, 9, 98, 99, 144–148, 164, 193, 232
See also Robb, Barbara; *Sans Everything*; Project 70
Aix, Dr., 71
Allen, Anne, 257
Allsop, Kenneth, 151–152, 159–160
Altschul, Annie, 23
Amulree, Lord, 78, 219
Amy, *see* Gibbs, Amy
Anne, Edith Charlton, 61
Anne, Ernest Charlton, 59, 60, 267

272 INDEX

Anne, Ernestine 'Missie', 61, 75, 130, 153
Anne (Charlton), Frederick John, 12, 61, 62
Anne, Michael, 61
Anne, Robert, 61, 62
Antipsychiatry, 27, 46
Applebey, Mary, 83, 127, 146, 148, 153, 210, 230, 257
  See also National Association for Mental Health
Arie, Tom, 86, 158, 213–214, 229, 238
Association of Hospital Management Committees, 84
Asylums, 5, 13, 19–20, 29, 104, 105, 122, 123, 205, 236
  See also Colney Hatch; Prestwich

B
'Baby Peter', 4
Bailey, Julie, 7, 263
Baker, Alex, 226–228, 237
  lunch with Barbara Robb, 226–227
  psychogeriatrician, 230
Barbara, see Robb, Barbara
Barton, Russell, 20, 33, 34, 43, 85, 123–126, 202, 211, 232, 253, 258
  Belsen, 128–129, 163
  institutional neurosis, 22
  See also Severalls
BBC, see British Broadcasting Corporation
'Bed blocking', 32, 35
  See also General hospitals
Benson, Sheila, 81
Bergmann, Klaus, 86, 214, 229, 261
Bethlem-Maudsley Hospital, 31, 40
Bevan, Aneurin, 34, 36, 46, 84, 147
Beveridge, William, 34

Biss, Jean, 116, 120, 154, 190
Blake, Quentin, 86, 259
Blessed, Garry, 86, 154
Blofeld, Ann, 102–103, 106, 257
Blofeld Inquiry, 102–107, 179
  and Hackett, 106–107, 157, 179
  and Regional Board, 157, 252
BMA, see British Medical Association
Board of Control, 5, 20, 21, 35, 37, 113
British Broadcasting Corporation (BBC), 9, 145
  Man Alive, 211–213
  Panorama, 4
  Something for Nothing, 208, 213
  Ten O'clock, 143, 151
  24 Hours, 143, 151–153, 159–160, 165
British Geriatrics Society, 214
British Medical Association (BMA), 210
  on NHS inspectorate, 226
  on older people, 35
  on ombudsman, 230
Burghwallis, 58, 59, 62, 63, 258, 259
Buss, Eric, 69, 71, 72, 86

C
Campbell, Malcolm, 39, 41, 43, 45, 47n2, 177
Castle, Barbara, 224, 254, 256
Cathy Come Home, 9
Central Health Services Council, 254
Central Hospital, Warwick, 201, 204–205
Charlton, Barbara, 59
Charlton, Frederick John, *see* Anne
Charlton, William, 61, 100
Chelsea School of Art, 61, 62, 86, 232

Child Poverty Action Group
    (CPAG), 8, 9, 99
Claybury Hospital, 20, 26, 40, 121,
    146, 164
Climbié, Victoria, 4
Cloake, Miss, 71, 73, 75,
    84, 175
Cochrane, David, 5, 7, 12
Cohen, Gerda, 10, 34,
    58, 178
COHSE, *see* Confederation of Health
    Service Employees
Colney Hatch Asylum, 19–20
    Fire, 104–105
    See also Friern Hospital
Commissioner, *see* Ombudsman
Complainants, 106
    doctors, 5, 25, 45
    nurses, 25, 117–119, 120, 123,
        145, 146, 152, 153, 178, 195,
        216, 222, 223
    patients, 10, 70, 145, 188,
        230–231
    psychology student, 178
    relatives, 44–45, 79, 80, 101,
        110, 111–112, 119, 152,
        178, 251
Complaints
    back wards, 80
    contrived/distorted, 176, 217, 223
    Davies Committee, 230–231
    guidance and procedures, 106,
        108–112, 150–151, 160, 181,
        192, 215, 217, 221, 223, 225,
        230, 253
    handling by DHSS, 218, 220, 230,
        236
    handling by HMC, 44–45, 84, 119,
        163
    handling by Ministry, 80, 83, 100,
        106, 109, 110, 149–151, 153,
        154–156, 161–162
    handling by RHBs, 109, 111, 112,
        131, 150, 160, 163
    lack of, 9, 119
    measure of quality, 162
    See also Inquiries; named inquiries;
        RHBs; Robinson, Kenneth;
        Ombudsman; Council on
        Tribunals
Confederation of Health Service
    Employees (COHSE), 147–148,
    150, 209
Consumers' Association, 8
Cosin, Lionel, 32, 34, 121
Cossett Hospital, *see* Friern Hospital
*Cost of the National Health Service,
    Report of the Committee of
    Enquiry* (Guillebaud Report),
    37, 46
Council on Tribunals, 149, 156, 174,
    203, 206, 221, 230, 231
    correspondence with Barbara
        Robb, 192–193
    criticism of inquiry
        processes, 191–193, 210, 215
    reprimand Kenneth Robinson, 192
Cowley Road Hospital, 116, 121, 190
    allegations, 121
    See also Cosin; Porter; Skrine
CPAG, *see* Child Poverty Action
    Group
Craythorne, Adeline, *see* Daniel, Joyce
Crichton Royal Hospital, 33, 41, 76
Crofts, Dorothy, 116, 121,
    174, 176
Cross, Yvonne, 146, 152–153, 257
Crossman, Richard, 3, 9, 201,
    212, 235
    and Abel-Smith, 202, 212,
        218, 235
    editor of *New Statesman*, 236
Ely Report, 217–220
    hospital funding, 222

Crossman, Richard (*cont.*)
  meetings with Barbara
    Robb, 226–227, 232–233, 236
  opinions on; Graham Bryce, 156;
    Hackett, 235; Robb,
    Barbara, 57, 131, 145, 210,
    225–226, 232–234, 235, 236,
    254, 257; Robinson,
    Kenneth, 208, 210, 232–234,
    236
  Post-Ely Working Party, 221
  visit to Chelmsley and
    Coleshill, 221–222
  visit to Friern, 106, 225

D

Daily Mail, 144
  Friern, 210, 225
  Harperbury, 111
  survey, 82, 83–84
Daniel, Joyce, 115–117, 151,
    181–186, 190, 211
  threats to her, 186
  See also St Lawrence's
Davie, James, 116, 118–119, 151,
    187–189, 190, 216
  comments on *Sans Everything* white
    paper, 211
  See also Storthes Hall Inquiry;
    Springfield Inquiry
Department of Health and Social
    Security (DHSS), 201–202, 217,
    220, 226, 228, 229, 230
  lack of lateral thinking, 227
Depressive illness
  ('depression'), 31–32, 34, 38, 61,
    76–77
  failure to identify, 31–32, 34, 184
DHSS, *see* Department of Health and
    Social Security
'Diary', *see* 'Diary of a Nobody'

'Diary of a Nobody', 57, 58, 69–77,
    103, 153, 174, 234
  decision to publish, 107
  response by Ministry of
    Health, 80–84
  sent to Kenneth Robinson, 79–80,
    101
Dickens, Mrs, 44–45, 112, 178, 188
Dumping older people, 29, 30, 32, 40,
    159, 228

E

ECT, *see* electroconvulsive therapy
Elderly people, *see* Older people
Electroconvulsive therapy (ECT), 31,
    77–78
Ely Hospital, Cardiff
  HMC, 161, 162
  scandalous report, c.1965, 162, 165
Ely Inquiry, 3, 6, 201, 214–220, 222,
    223, 230
  allegations, 161
  contrived complaints, 217, 223
  outcomes, 201, 220–221, 226, 237,
    238, 253
  See also Howe; Pantelides; Post-Ely
    Working Party
Enoch, M David, 30, 123, 124, 126,
    154, 164, 203–204, 214, 229,
    232, 238, 253
  See also Shelton Hospital
Enquiries, *see* Inquiries
Ethics, 61, 69, 126, 128–129, 146,
    192, 222, 265, 266

F

Fabian Society, 102
Faculty for the Psychiatry of Old Age
    (RCPsych), 229, 261
Farleigh Hospital, 222–223, 237, 263,
    264

criminal trial, 223
  outcome, 224, 230
  Saunders, Greta, 222
  Saunders, Kenneth, 222
Fenton, Louisa, *see* Skrine, Susan
Findings and Recommendations, *see*
  Sans Everything white paper
France, Arnold, 7, 127, 154
Francis Report, *see* Mid Staffordshire
  Inquiry
Franks, Mabel, 143, 190
Friern Hospital, 1, 7, 19–20, 39–45,
  69–73, 102–106
  Crossman's visit,
    106, 225
  GNC inspections, 40–42, 225
  Halliwick, 27, 104, 164
  HMC, 39–44, 46, 106, 107, 111,
    179, 180, 225, 252
  medical superintendent, *see* Sutton,
    Isaac
  report on nurse staffing, 42–43, 179
  RHB, 43–47, 81, 83, 102–106,
    111, 131, 179–180, 206,
    234, 252
  ward E3, 41, 69, 72, 104
  See also Blofeld Inquiry; Colney
    Hatch; Friern (*Sans Everything*)
    Inquiry; Gibbs, Amy
Friern (*Sans Everything*) Inquiry
  committee, 156, 157, 174
  criticism of RHB, 106,
    179–180
  legal representation for
    witnesses, 174–175, 192
  locked wards at night, 182
  recommendations, 179
  standards used to judge
    practice, 176–178
Fry, Elizabeth, 1, 8,
  131, 266

G
General hospitals, 2, 32, 34, 38, 120,
  159, 202
  See also 'Bed blocking'
General Nursing Council
  (GNC), 39–42, 225
General practice/practitioner
  (GP), 29, 30–31, 32, 34, 78,
  231, 232
Geriatrician, 2, 32, 37, 85, 173
  See also Amulree; Cosin
Geriatric medicine, 12, 28, 32, 33, 87,
  100, 121, 158, 159, 173, 191,
  194, 265
Gibbs, Amy, 66–68, 104, 259, 260
  at Friern, 1, 41, 69–73, 75–78,
    81–83, 175, 176, 177
  mental health, 63, 67, 68–69, 70,
    76–78
  at St Peter's, 72–76, 153
Giddie, Dr., 72
GNC, *see* General Nursing Council
Goffman, Erving, 22, 27, 127–128
Goodmayes Hospital, 213
GP, *see* General practice
GPOA, *see* Group for the Psychiatry of
  Old Age
Graham Bryce, Isabel, 156, 174
Group for the Psychiatry of Old Age
  (GPOA, RCPsych), 3, 229, 253,
  261
Guillebaud Report, *see Cost of the
  National Health Service*

H
HAC, *see* Hampstead Artists Council
Hacker, Rose, 43
Hackett, Maurice, 101–102, 106–107,
  131, 156–157, 165, 207, 231,
  234–235, 253

Hackett, Maurice (*cont.*)
  and Friern Inquiry, 174, 179–180, 234
  television interview, 159–160
  See also Robinson, Kenneth
Halliwick Hospital, *see* Friern
Hampstead Artists Council (HAC), 68, 69, 86
Hampstead, London, 62, 67, 77, 110, 130, 219, 225, 258
Harperbury Hospital
  Daily Mail, 111
  Guardian, 206–207, 225, 257
Harvey, Audrey, 69, 73, 83, 86, 98, 100, 102, 122, 211, 213
HAS, *see* Hospital Advisory Service
Help the Aged, *see* Age UK
Heneage, Laura, *see* Biss, Jean
Hesleyside Hall, 63
Hewitt, Bill, *see* Rolph, CH
HMC, *see* Hospital Management Committee
Hodgson, Helen, 10, 112, 209, 257
Hospital Advisory Service (HAS), 226–228, 230, 237, 253
  See also Baker, Alex
Hospital Management Committee (HMC)
  appointment of, 20
  inspection visits, 21, 84, 86, 162
  role, 21
  See also named hospitals
Hospitals' inspectorate
  proposals for, 82, 112–113, 146
  See also Board of Control, Hospital Advisory Service
House of Commons, 34, 36, 114, 123, 145, 155, 204, 207, 214, 224, 236
  announcement of Ely Report, 218–219
  announcement of *Sans Everything* white paper, 208–209, 210, 237
  'inspired', 'planted' questions, 82, 150–151, 162, 208
  mental health, 79
  older people, 78
  stripping, 82, 107
House of Lords
  announcement of Ely Report, 219
  lunch organised by Beatrice Serota, 226–227
  Strabolgi's speech, 58, 81–82, 84, 98, 123, 219
Howe, Geoffrey, 223
  Aberfan, 215
  Ely Inquiry, 215–218, 220, 221
  South Ockendon, 224

I

Inquiries, 3, 5–7, 173–195
  established by RHBs, 143
  independent, 101, 103, 110, 148–150, 160
  NHS Act section, 70, 149, 150, 163, 165, 192, 203
  oversight of statutory inquiries, 149, 156, 192, 203 (*see also* Council on Tribunals)
  private, 83, 101, 102–106, 143, 149, 154–155, 215
  processes, 149–150, 215
  secrecy, 154–155, 215
  See also Complaints; named inquiries
Institute of Hospital Administrators, 110
Institutional neurosis, *see* Barton, Russell
Investigative journalism, 9, 164, 253
Isham, Frederick, *see* Davie, James

J

Jay, Peggy, 225
Jones, Kathleen, 5, 25–26
Joseph, Keith, 163–164, 224, 230, 254
Journalists, 9, 144, 257
  access to RHB meetings, 145
  anger, after white paper press release, 209
  'collective guilt', 147
  support for AEGIS, 129, 147
  undercover, 111, 225, 263 (*see also* Rolph, CH; Shearer, Ann)
Jung, Carl, 63–66, 86, 254, 257

K

King Edward's Hospital Fund, *see* King's Fund
King's Fund, 42, 153, 214
Kirkpatrick, WJA 'Bill', 7, 25, 123, 126

L

Last Refuge, The, 99
  See also Townsend, Peter
Littlemore Hospital, 20, 225
Loach, Ken, 9
Local Authorities, 12, 27, 29, 84, 99, 113, 179, 191, 210, 213, 221
Lomax, Montagu, 5, 122, 147
London School of Economics (LSE), 3, 8
  AEGIS archive, 12
Lovat, Miss, 71
Lowe, Douglas, 174–175, 179–180
  criticism by Council on Tribunals, 192, 215
Loyalty to colleagues, *see* National Health Service

LSE, *see* London School of Economics
Lubbock, Eric, 107, 123–124
Lunacy Commission, 20

M

Macmillan, Duncan, 85
Manchester RHB, report *Care of the Aged*, 159, 164
Mandelbrote, Bertram, 20, 26, 225
Martin, Denis, 20
Martin, John, 6–7, 214, 265
Mental handicap
  Better Services for the Mentally Handicapped 1971, 221
  See also Mentally subnormal
Mental Health Act 1959 (MHA), 13, 21, 22, 37, 78, 113
  section, 126, 150
Mental health services for older people (psychogeriatrics), 85–86, 214, 225, 228–229, 230, 253, 265
  Services for Mental Illness Related to Old Age 1972, 229
  See also Group/Faculty for the Psychiatry of Old Age
Mental hospitals, *see* Psychiatric hospitals; named hospitals
Mental subnormality hospitals
  Chelmsley, 221
  Coleshill, 221
  Harperbury, 111, 201, 206–207, 225
  See also Ely Hospital; Ely Inquiry
Mental Treatment Act 1930, 5, 13
MHA, *see* Mental Health Act 1959
Michelmore, Cliff, 151–152
Mid Staffordshire Inquiry, 4, 6–7, 265
MIND, *see see* National Association for Mental Health
Ministry of Health, 80, 102, 118, 127, 145, 162, 201, 211–212, 217

Ministry of Health (*cont.*)
  appointment of HMCs, 20
  financial considerations, 46
  guidance, 21, 38, 109–112, 131–132
  handling of complaints, *see* Complaints
  preparations for inquiries, 143, 147, 148–151, 154–157, 160, 173–174, 215
  response to 'Diary of a Nobody', 80–84
  See also France, Arnold; Tooth, Geoffrey; *Sans Everything* white paper
Missie, *see* Anne, Ernestine
Moodie, Dennis, 116, 120, 129, 151, 174, 177, 190
Moody, Roger, 115, 116, 121, 174
Morale of hospital staff, 79, 104, 123, 179, 207, 212, 219, 225–226, 237, 238

N
NAMH, *see* National Association for Mental Health
National Association for Mental Health (NAMH, MIND), 11, 20, 38, 78, 83, 87, 98, 103, 146, 153–154, 209, 214, 221, 224, 228, 237–238, 253
  survey of provision for older people, 229
National Council for Civil Liberties, 147, 209
National Health Service (NHS)
  'best', 7, 79, 264
  cost, 36–37, 251
  inspectorate, *see* Hospital Advisory Service
  loyalty to colleagues, 6–7, 110, 117–118, 128
  responsibility for services for older people, 37–39, 46, 99
  Something for Nothing, 208, 213
  See also Complaints
National Old People's Welfare Committee, *see* Age UK
Nazi regime, 128–129
  Belsen, 128, 129, 163, 189
  concentration camps, 128
  nurses, 128
  public response to inhumanities, 129
News of the World, 144, 145, 147–148, 161–162, 190, 214, 217, 218
  See also Roxan, David
New Statesman, 99, 108, 127, 189, 211, 236
  See also Rolph, CH
Newstead, Keith, 123, 126
NHS, *see* National Health Service
Nightingale, Florence, 1, 256, 266
North West Metropolitan Regional Hospital Board, 145, 157
  alters *Sans Everything* inquiry report, 180
  meetings, 106, 111, 145
  See also Blofeld; Friern; Hackett; Harperbury
Norton, Doreen, 101, 232
Nurses, 25, 36
  attitudes towards older people, 22, 23, 32, 33, 70, 108, 178, 205, 227
  auxiliary nurses, 116, 118
  hierarchy, 24, 25, 122, 145, 146, 182, 194, 222
  matron, 20, 30, 106, 118, 120, 121, 123, 148, 152, 163, 178, 179
  protests 1968, 214

punishment/reprisals against/
victimisation of nurses who
criticize, 23, 25, 26, 117, 121,
122, 123, 146, 151, 152, 153,
156, 163, 216–217, 218–219,
226, 228, 230
recruitment, 41, 42, 43, 207,
212, 237
students, 25–26, 41, 146, 161–162,
222, 225, 263
See also Complainants; Complaints;
named nurses; Nursing Mirror;
Nursing practice
Nursing Homes Act 1963, 99
Nursing Mirror, 145, 146, 153, 158,
165, 263
See also Cross, Yvonne
Nursing practice
bathing, 23–24, 41, 111, 117, 118,
124, 184, 185
harsh, 33, 160, 178, 181–182, 185,
188, 194, 205, 216, 252, 263,
264, 265
physical care, 23, 72, 104, 205, 215
psychiatric care, 23, 24, 25–26, 85,
107, 184–185, 187–188, 225
See also named inquiries
NWMRHB, see North West
Metropolitan Regional Hospital
Board

O

Older people
admitted to the wrong sort of
ward, 38
ageism, 11–12
attitudes towards, 2, 11–12, 13, 22,
29, 32–39
domiciliary support, 28, 34–35, 39
economic cost, 20, 36–37, 126,
229, 251
epidemiology, 34
Local Authority provision, 29, 84,
99, 179, 191, 213
poverty, 8
rehabilitation, 2, 23, 26, 33–34,
85, 98
residential homes, 28, 34, 37,
72–76, 84
See also Dumping; Mental health
services for older people
Ombudsman, 108, 230, 263
direct access by NHS staff, 223, 230
opposition to, 230
proposals for, 112, 193, 206,
213, 226
Osbaldeston, Michael, see Moodie,
Dennis

P

PA, see Patients Association
Pantelides, Michael, 161, 162,
215–216, 217
Panting, Margaret, 4
Patients Association (PA), 10, 20–21,
82, 83, 98, 101, 103, 107, 108,
112, 113, 130, 154, 176, 209, 221
See also Hodgson, Helen
Pitt, Brice, 26, 32, 214, 229
Polson, George, 180–185, 218
See also St Lawrence's
Porter, Eileen, 116, 121, 190, 211
Post-Ely Working Party, 221
Post, Felix, 31, 34, 36, 85, 86
Powell, Enoch, 38, 46
Powell, Muriel, 180
Powick Hospital, 201, 205–206,
219, 227
Spencer, Arthur, 205–206, 219
Ward F13, 205–206
Worcester Development
Project, 206

Press Council, 144–145, 165, 207
Pressure group, 1, 8–11, 98, 99, 112, 159
  See also named pressure groups
Prestwich Asylum, 5, 122
Project, 70, 126–127, 225, 228
Psychiatric-geriatric assessment unit, 38
Psychiatric hospital
  bed occupancy, 78, 83, 85, 162
  buildings, 20, 21, 39, 40, 43, 79, 202, 221, 224, 228
  closure, 127, 202, 228
  improving, 36, 43, 202, 214, 220, 232, 237
  inspections, 21, 40–42, 146, 162, 226
  medical superintendents, 20, 43, 45, 85, 104, 106, 120, 204, 205, 258
  overcrowding, *see* Wards
  shift to general hospitals and community, 38, 120, 202, 233
  'total institution', 22, 87, 117
  two-tier provision, 26, 27, 163–164
  See also named hospitals;Project 70; Wards
Psychiatrist, 11, 20, 22, 26–27, 29–32, 33, 69, 71, 76, 79, 85, 87, 103, 123–124, 154, 158, 173, 184, 203, 207, 213–214, 226, 232, 238
Psychogeriatrician, 214, 228–229, 230, 253
Psychogeriatric services, *see* Mental health services for older people
Psychotherapy/psychotherapist, 58, 63–64, 69, 86, 254

R
RCN, *see* Royal College of Nursing
RCPsych, *see* Royal College of Psychiatrists
Regional Hospital Boards (RHBs), 20–21, 80, 107, 109, 110, 111, 112, 113, 159, 211, 228, 252
  and complaints, 109, 147, 150, 154, 160–161, 163
  excluding public from meetings, 145
  See also Complaints; named RHBs
RHB, *see* Regional Hospital Boards
Robb, Barbara
  ancestry and psudonyms, 115
  appearance, 65, 129, 257
  award, 256
  campaign style, 66, 256, 258
  childhood, 59–61, 259
  death, 254, 256, 258
  dreams, 64–65
  education, 58, 61–62, 63, 66
  family, 58–61
  marriage, 62
  personality, 63, 65, 66, 233, 236, 258
  religion, 58, 59, 254, 258
  Sans Varier, 114, 267
  sense of humour, 236
  See also AEGIS; *Sans Everything*
Robb, Brian, 58, 62, 63, 64, 65, 67, 69, 73, 80, 98, 211, 232, 233, 254, 255, 256, 258
  Last of the Centaurs, The, 259
  My Grandmother's Djinn, 259, 260, 262
Robb, Douglas, 88
Robinson, Anne, 14n6, 100, 143, 254, 257
Robinson, Elizabeth, 232–233

Robinson, Kenneth, 7, 78, 79–80,
    82–84, 106, 108, 148, 150, 203,
    204, 208, 231–234
  achievements, 78, 231–232
  attitude to Barbara Robb, 191,
    232–233, 234, 254
  Council on Tribunals
    reprimand, 192
  criticisms by press and public, 193,
    209–210, 213
  and Hackett, 101–102, 131, 156,
    157, 165, 231, 234, 235, 253
  interest in mental health, 78, 87
  Man Alive, 211–213
  in parliament, 79, 82–83, 113, 145,
    147, 150–151, 155, 201,
    208–209, 210
  Press Council, 144
  and Project 70, 127, 228
  and stripping, 82, 108, 147
  and Tooth, 82, 150
  24 Hours, 152–153, 159, 165
Robinson, Ronald 'Sam', 33, 34, 41,
    86
Rolph, CH., 99–100, 106, 107, 108,
    127, 129, 144, 164, 209, 210,
    211, 232, 256, 257, 258
  objectives for *Sans Everything*, 114
  See also New Statesman
Roth, Martin, 31, 34, 36, 85, 184,
    232
Rough handling of patients, *see*
    Nursing practice, harsh
Rowe, Phyllis, 123, 157, 192
Roxan, David, 147–148, 161–162,
    192, 214
Royal College of Nursing (RCN), 13,
    123, 148, 153, 157, 224, 238
Royal College of Psychiatrists
    (RCPsych), 3, 113, 214, 224,
    229, 253

Royal Medico-Psychological
    Association, 113
Royal Commissions on
  lunacy 1926, 5
  mental illness 1957, 36, 113, 221
  population 1949, 35
  tribunals 1966, 149, 175, 192
Royal Medico-Psychological
    Association, *see* Royal College of
    Psychiatrists

S
St James's, Leeds
  allegations, 120, 154
  Inquiry, 190
  See also Biss, Jean
St Lawrence's Inquiry, 174, 180–186
  bathing, 184–185
  committee's clinical
    understanding, 183–184, 185
  recommendations, 186
  response to Daniel, 185, 186
  RHB edits report, 186
  Sister W, 180–182, 184, 185
  standards used to make
    judgements, 186
  See also Daniel, Joyce; Polson,
    George
St Peter's Residence, 72–76
Sans Everything: A Case to Answer
  affidavits, 130, 183, 185
  author-witnesses, 115–122,
    155–156, 186, 252, 254
  choice of title, 114
  contributors, 115–127
  day of publication (30 June
    1967), 143, 151–153
  Ministry's response to, 143, 150–151
  Nelson (publisher), 130
  planning, 98, 113–114, 143–148

Sans Everything: A Case to Answer (*cont.*)
  public response to, 157–160
  See also named authors
Sans Everything inquiry
  committees, 180, 189, 193–195
  committees, composition, 156, 157, 173–174
  terms of reference, 173, 215
  See also Ministry of Health; named inquiries
Sans Everything white paper
  announcement of, 208–210
  plan to publish, 155, 175, 190–191
  press release, 209
Scandals of care (since 1960s), 3–4, 6–7, 261, 263–266
  similarities to *Sans Everything*, 261–262
  size and modernity of buildings, 264
Second World War, 24, 40, 58, 62–63, 128–129
Serota, Beatrice, 219, 221, 226, 233
Severalls Hospital, 20, 202, 211
  conference 1966, 123–124
  psychogeriatric services, 33, 76, 85, 214
  See also Barton, Russell; Whitehead, J Anthony
Shaftsbury, Lord, 256, 266
Shearer, Ann, 47n6, 236
  Davies Committee, 230
  Guardian, 144, 206–207, 257
  and Harperbury, 201, 206–207, 225
  opinion of Hackett, 235
  Press Council, 207
Shelter (charity), 9
Shelton Hospital, 30, 124, 201, 203–204, 223, 237
  See also Enoch, M David
Sister W, *see* St Lawrence's Inquiry

Skrine, Susan, 116, 121–122, 190, 211
Slapping patients, 70, 75, 160, 178, 182, 252, 265
Social work, 61, 80, 179
Social workers, 70–71, 79, 103, 116, 221
South Ockendon Hospital, 219, 222–224, 257, 264
South West Metropolitan Regional Hospital Board (SWMRHB), 109, 111, 112, 160
Spastics Society, 193, 209
Spencer, Arthur, *see* Powick Hospital
Springfield Inquiry, 118–119, 189–190, 216
  committee's response to Davie, 189
  Report, 190–191
  See also Davie, James
Stigma, 13, 29, 79, 87, 113, 132, 235
Storthes Hall Hospital, 118–120
  See also Storthes Hall Inquiry
Storthes Hall Inquiry, 187–189
  allegations, 118
  bathing, 118
  committee's response to Davie, 187, 189
  missing documents, 187, 191
  Report, 189
  See also Davie, James
Strabolgi, Lord, 58, 62, 69, 75, 79–80, 81–82, 83, 84, 85, 87, 98, 100–104, 106, 123, 219, 230, 256, 258
Stripping, 22, 69, 80, 81, 82, 100–101, 107–108, 114, 123–124, 128, 131–132, 147, 151, 160, 221, 238
  See also Lubbock, Eric; Robinson, Kenneth

INDEX   283

Sunday Times, 58, 143, 145, 146, 160
  See also Young, Hugo
Sutton, Isaac, 43, 180
Swinburne, Emily, *see* Porter, Eileen

T
Tasburg, Elizabeth, *see* Crofts, Dorothy
Taylor, Lord, 30, 84, 85
Teasing patients, 2, 177, 193, 215, 252
Thomson, Peter, 126, 127
Tooth, Geoffrey, 38, 58, 85, 147, 150, 151
  meeting with Barbara Robb, 80–82, 120, 126
Townsend, Peter, 8, 27–28, 30, 39, 69, 84, 102, 192, 198, 210, 221, 232
  See also Last Refuge
Typhoid, 41

U
UNISON, 264

V
Violence in hospitals
  guidance, 224, 253
  towards patients, 44, 118, 119, 120, 147, 161, 181, 188, 189

W
Ward E3, *see* Friern
Ward F13, *see* Powick
Wards
  back ward, 1, 2, 21, 22, 25, 27, 28, 37, 39, 42, 87, 97, 104, 106, 129, 163, 261, 264
  custodial care, 20, 22, 24, 40, 46, 87, 120, 125, 177, 187, 205

inspection, 21, 41–42, 76, 84, 162, 179, 188, 195
locked, 26, 104, 120, 177, 182–183, 203, 214
lockers, 41, 80, 83, 104, 177, 204
overcrowding, 21, 22–23, 34, 40, 41, 42, 44, 70, 75, 83, 104, 128, 145, 162, 179, 201, 204, 205, 216, 221, 251, 252, 264
privacy, 2, 23, 40, 41, 43, 83, 122, 124, 205, 252
staff level, 23, 39, 41, 42, 79, 104, 120, 121, 122, 179, 216, 217, 252, 264
unstaffed at night, 104, 179, 182–183, 203
  See also Dumping
Welsh Hospital Board, 161, 215, 217
WHB, *see* Welsh Hospital Board
Whistle-blower (since c.2000), 115, 164, 237, 263
Whitehead, J Anthony 'Tony', 31, 33–34, 85, 123–124, 191, 214, 229, 230, 238, 253
  See also Severalls
White, Victor, 63–65, 86, 254, 257
Whittingham Hospital, 162–164, 165, 222, 230
Wilberforce, William, 131, 266
Wilcox, Desmond, 211–213
Wills, Miss, *see* Gibbs, Amy
Wilson, Harold, 114, 201, 209
Women's movement, 194, 256
World in Action, *see* Powick
World Psychiatric Association, conference 1965, 85

Y
Young, Hugo, 145, 146
  praise for nurses, 145
  See also Sunday Times

The manufacturer's authorised representative in the EU is Springer Nature Customer Service Centre GmbH, Europaplatz 3, 69115 Heidelberg, Germany. If you have any concerns regarding our products, please contact ProductSafety@springernature.com

Printed and bound by CPI Group (UK) Ltd, Croydon, CR0 4YY
23/03/2026
02076667-0004